New Paradigms in Emergency Surgery

Edited by Amy Walker

hayle
medical

New York

Hayle Medical,
750 Third Avenue, 9th Floor,
New York, NY 10017, USA

Visit us on the World Wide Web at:
www.haylemedical.com

This book contains information obtained from authentic and highly regarded sources. Copyright for all individual chapters remain with the respective authors as indicated. All chapters are published with permission under the Creative Commons Attribution License or equivalent. A wide variety of references are listed. Permission and sources are indicated; for detailed attributions, please refer to the permissions page and list of contributors. Reasonable efforts have been made to publish reliable data and information, but the authors, editors and publisher cannot assume any responsibility for the validity of all materials or the consequences of their use.

ISBN: 978-1-63241-769-5

Trademark Notice: Registered trademark of products or corporate names are used only for explanation and identification without intent to infringe.

Cataloging-in-Publication Data

New paradigms in emergency surgery / edited by Amy Walker.
    p. cm.
Includes bibliographical references and index.
ISBN 978-1-63241-769-5
1. Surgical emergencies. 2. Medical emergencies. 3. Surgery, Operative.
I. Walker, Amy.
RD93 .N48 2019
617.026--dc23

Table of Contents

Permissions

List of Contributors

Index

Preface

The surgery which is performed immediately, in order to save life, limb or functional capacity is known as emergency surgery. It is done in the cases where immediate surgical intervention is the only possible way to solve the problem successfully. Some of the common cases in which the doctor often performs an emergency surgery include gastrointestinal perforation, cardiac tamponade, pneumothorax, acute appendicitis, peritonitis, bowel obstruction, urinary retention, limb ischemia, etc. The emergency department is the medical treatment facility that is concerned with the acute care of patients with a broad spectrum of life-threatening illnesses and injuries. The chances of survival for a patient are greatly improved if definitive treatment or surgery is provided as soon as possible. This book elucidates new techniques and their applications in a multidisciplinary manner. The topics included herein on emergency surgery are of utmost significance and bound to provide incredible insights to readers. This book includes contributions of experts and doctors which will provide innovative insights into this field.

This book is a comprehensive compilation of works of different researchers from varied parts of the world. It includes valuable experiences of the researchers with the sole objective of providing the readers (learners) with a proper knowledge of the concerned field. This book will be beneficial in evoking inspiration and enhancing the knowledge of the interested readers.

In the end, I would like to extend my heartiest thanks to the authors who worked with great determination on their chapters. I also appreciate the publisher's support in the course of the book. I would also like to deeply acknowledge my family who stood by me as a source of inspiration during the project.

Editor

Multi-organ protection of ulinastatin in traumatic cardiac arrest model

Shaoyun Liu[1,2], Jiefeng Xu[1,2,3], Yuzhi Gao[1,2], Peng Shen[1,2,4], Senlin Xia[1,2,5], Zilong Li[3] and Mao Zhang[1,2*]

Abstract

Background: Post-cardiac arrest syndrome, which has no specific curative treatment, contributes to the high mortality rate of victims who suffer traumatic cardiac arrest (TCA) and initially can be resuscitated. In the present study, we investigated the potential of ulinastatin to mitigate multiple organ injury after resuscitation in a swine TCA model.

Methods: Twenty-one male pigs were subjected to hemodynamic shock (40% estimated blood loss in 20 min) followed by cardiac arrest (electrically induced ventricular fibrillation) and respiratory suspension for 5 min, and finally manual resuscitation. At 5 min after resuscitation, pigs were randomized to receive 80,000 U/kg ulinastatin ($n = 7$) or the same volume of saline ($n = 9$) in the TCA group. Pigs in the sham group ($n = 5$) were not exposed to bleeding or cardiac arrest. At baseline and at 1, 3, and 6 h after the return of spontaneous circulation, blood samples were collected and assayed for tumor necrosis factor-alpha, interleukin 6, and other indicators of organ injury. At 24 h after resuscitation, pigs were sacrificed and apoptosis levels were assessed in samples of heart, brain, kidney, and intestine.

Results: One pig died in the ulinastatin group and one pig died in the TCA group; the remaining animals were included in the final analysis. TCA and resuscitation caused significant increases in multiple organ function biomarkers in serum, increases in tumor necrosis factor-alpha, and interleukin 6 in serum and increases in the extent of apoptosis in key organs. All these increases were lower in the ulinastatin group.

Conclusion: Ulinastatin may attenuate multiple organ injury after TCA, which should be explored in clinical studies.

Keywords: Ulinastatin, Traumatic cardiac arrest, Organ protection, Cardiopulmonary resuscitation, Post-resuscitation, Ischemia-reperfusion injury

Background

Traumatic cardiac arrest (TCA) is associated with poor outcome; traditionally, only 0–3.7% of TCA patients could be resuscitated [1], though advances in damage control resuscitation and understanding of TCA pathophysiology have increased the success rate to 5.6% (0–17%) [2], making it comparable to the rate with patients who suffer medical cardiac arrest [3]. Guidelines of the National Association of EMS Physicians and the Committee on Trauma of the American College of Surgeons do not recommend resuscitation for patients who suffer blunt trauma and out-of-hospital cardiac arrest and found pulseless, without organized ECG activity, or for patients who have suffered penetrating trauma and have no detectable pulse and signs of life [4]. TCA is associated with greater loss of productive life years than medical cardiac arrest because TCA usually affects young men [3]. More than 90% of TCA cases are caused by severe head injury or hypovolemia [4]. Even among TCA patients who achieve a return of spontaneous circulation (ROSC), mortality rates are high because of the prolonged whole-body ischemia during trauma and cardiac arrest and because of reperfusion injury after resuscitation.

It may be possible to reduce TCA-induced damage using the urinary trypsin inhibitor (UTI) ulinastatin,

* Correspondence: z2jzk@zju.edu.cn
[1]Department of Emergency Medicine, Second Affiliated Hospital, Zhejiang University School of Medicine, No. 88 Jiefang road, Hangzhou 310009, China
[2]Institute of Emergency Medicine, Zhejiang University, No. 88 Jiefang road, Hangzhou 310009, China
Full list of author information is available at the end of the article

which was first identified in human blood and urine in the 1980s. Ulinastatin, which inhibits the release of neutrophil elastase and inhibits the activation of various pro-inflammatory cytokines [3, 5], is used mainly to treat pancreatitis, sepsis, toxic shock, and hemorrhagic shock [5, 6]. In animal models of brain ischemia-reperfusion, ulinastatin decreased infarct volume and water content of brain tissue, and it inhibited cerebral apoptosis, thereby mitigating ischemia-reperfusion injury [7, 8]. A meta-analysis of randomized controlled trials concluded that ulinastatin can protect pulmonary tissue for patients undergoing cardiac surgery and reduce postoperative increases in the inflammatory agent's tumor necrosis factor (TNF)-alpha, polymorphonuclear neutrophil elastase, and interleukin (IL)-6 and IL-8 [9]. In addition, ulinastatin may be associated with a low incidence of acute kidney injury in patients undergoing robot-assisted laparoscopic partial nephrectomy or cardiac surgery [10, 11].

Few studies have examined the efficacy and safety of ulinastatin in patients who have suffered cardiac arrest, particularly TCA. In the present study, we examined whether ulinastatin can mitigate the effects of TCA and ischemia-reperfusion based on serum indicators and extent of apoptosis in major organs in a porcine TCA model.

Methods

The experimental procedures used in this study adhered to the US National Institutes of Health Guide for the Care and Use of Laboratory Animals.

TCA

Twenty-one male Chinese pigs (29–36 kg) were used for this study. Anesthesia was induced using an intramuscular injection of ketamine (500 mg) and midazolam (5 mg) and maintained with propofol (3 mg/kg/h) and fentanyl (1 µg/kg/h) during surgical procedures. Respiration was maintained using artificial ventilation (Syno-Vent E5; Mindray Biomedical Electronics, Shenzhen, China) with the following settings: respiratory rate, 12–15 bpm; inspired oxygen, 21% and PEEP, 3 mmHg. A catheter was inserted into the aortic artery through the left femoral artery and another catheter was inserted into the right atrium through the left jugular vein. Both catheters were connected to pressure transducers. Heart rate (HR), mean aortic blood pressure (MAP), and right atrial pressure (RAP) were monitored (Beneview T6; Mindray Biomedical Electronics, Shenzhen, China). The cannula in the right femoral artery was used for controlled blood-letting 40% of estimated blood volume at a constant rate during 20 min with a blood pump (JHBP-2000B; JIHUA Medical Apparatus & Instruments, Guangzhou, China). Then, ventricular fibrillation was induced using a modified voltmeter (85 L1-A; Yongsheng

Electric Instrument Co., Guangzhou, China). Respiration was suspended by separating the tracheal cannula from the ventilator. Artificial ventilation was resumed 5 min later, and pigs were defibrillated (Zoll Medical Corporation, USA) and manually resuscitated. Pigs that achieved ROSC were used in further interventions.

Experimental procedures

At 5 min after ROSC, pigs were infused with ulinastatin (80,000 U/kg; $n = 6$) or the same volume of normal saline (TCA group; $n = 8$) into the right femoral vein during 2 min. Half the blood withdrawn from the right femoral artery was reinfused through the right femoral vein during the first hour after ROSC. During the next 1-h period, pigs received a volume of normal saline equal to three times the volume of blood lost. As an additional control, sham pigs ($n = 5$) underwent surgery but were not subjected to bleeding, cardiac arrest or resuscitation.

Outcome measures

HR, MAP, RAP, and end-tidal carbon dioxide ($ETCO_2$) were recorded at baseline and at 1, 3, and 6 h after ROSC. Blood gases and coagulation function were also analyzed at these time points. Plasma samples stored at -80 °C were assayed for creatine kinase MB (CK-MB), cardiac troponin I (cTNI), neuron-specific enolase (NSE), S100 calcium-binding protein B (S100B), serum creatinine (sCr), blood urea nitrogen (BUN), intestinal fatty acid-binding protein (iFABP), diamine oxidase (DAO), IL-6, and TNF-α.

Animals were sacrificed at 24 h after ROSC. Samples of the apical myocardium, frontal cortex of the brain, infrarenal pole cortex, and terminal ileum were removed and stored at -80 °C. Then, the samples were assessed for the extent of apoptosis using terminal deoxynucleotidyl transferase-mediated dUTP nick end labeling (TUNEL), and they were analyzed for caspase-3 expression using immunohistochemistry.

Statistical analysis

Continuous data are presented as mean ± standard deviation (SD) and inter-group pairwise differences were analyzed using repeated measures one-way analysis of variance, followed by parametric Student's t test. All statistical analyses were performed using SPSS for Windows 20.0 (IBM, Chicago, IL, USA), and statistical significance was defined as $p < 0.05$.

Results

Baseline characteristics

The three groups were similar at baseline in terms of body weight, HR, MAP, and, $ETCO_2$ (all $p > 0.05$; Table 1). One pig died in the ulinastatin group and one

Table 1 Baseline characteristics[a]

Characteristic	Sham ($n = 5$)	TCA ($n = 9$)	Ulinastatin ($n = 7$)	p^{b}
Body weight (kg)	35.00 ± 1.41	31.75 ± 3.99	31.67 ± 1.51	0.119
Heart rate (bpm)	86 ± 8	85 ± 15	85 ± 13	0.978
ETCO$_2$/mmHg	40 ± 2	39 ± 2	39 ± 2	0.623
MAP (mmHg)	117 ± 5	104 ± 16	106 ± 13	0.221
Death/survival	0/5	1/8	1/6	0.725

[a]mean ± SD. *ETCO$_2$* end-tidal carbon dioxide, *MAP* mean aortic blood pressure, *TCA* traumatic cardiac arrest

[b]There were no significant differences among the groups (one-way analysis of variance)

in the TCA group. Additionally, all resuscitated animals survived to the end of the experiment.

Hemodynamics

After ROSC, HR was significantly higher in the TCA group than in the sham group ($p < 0.05$; Fig. 1a). HR was significantly lower in the ulinastatin group than

in the TCA group ($p < 0.05$). MAP after ROSC did not differ significantly among the three groups ($p > 0.05$; Fig. 1b).

Serum biomarkers of myocardial injury

Prior to surgery, neither serum CKMB nor cTNI differed significantly among the three groups (all $p > 0.05$; Fig. 1c, d). CKMB increased from the pre-operative baseline and peaked at 1 h after ROSC in the ulinastatin group or at 3 h after ROSC in the TCA group. Similarly, cTNI increased from baseline and peaked at 3 h after ROSC in the ulinastatin group or at 6 h in the TCA group. Serum CK-MB and cTNI in the TCA group were significantly higher after ROSC than in the sham group ($p < 0.01$). CKMB after ROSC did not differ significantly between the TCA and ulinastatin groups ($p > 0.05$). The level of cTNI after ROSC was lower in the ulinastatin group than in the TCA group ($p < 0.01$).

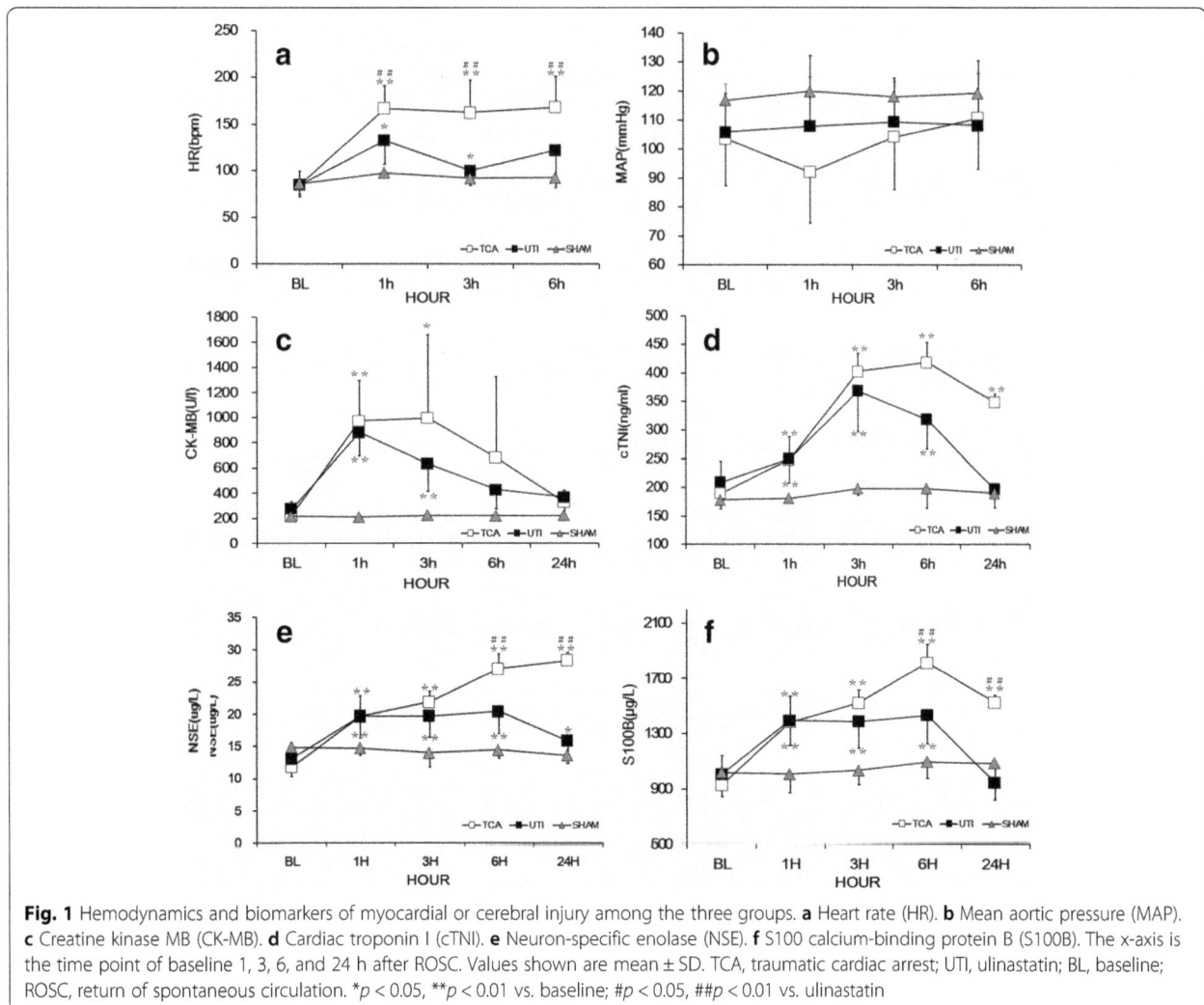

Fig. 1 Hemodynamics and biomarkers of myocardial or cerebral injury among the three groups. **a** Heart rate (HR). **b** Mean aortic pressure (MAP). **c** Creatine kinase MB (CK-MB). **d** Cardiac troponin I (cTNI). **e** Neuron-specific enolase (NSE). **f** S100 calcium-binding protein B (S100B). The x-axis is the time point of baseline 1, 3, 6, and 24 h after ROSC. Values shown are mean ± SD. TCA, traumatic cardiac arrest; UTI, ulinastatin; BL, baseline; ROSC, return of spontaneous circulation. *$p < 0.05$, **$p < 0.01$ vs. baseline; #$p < 0.05$, ##$p < 0.01$ vs. ulinastatin

Serum biomarkers of cerebral injury

Serum concentration of NSE and S100B did not differ among the three groups at baseline (all $p > 0.05$; Fig. 1e, f). Levels of both biomarkers were significantly higher after ROSC than at baseline in the TCA and ulinastatin groups (both $p < 0.01$). Levels of both biomarkers after ROSC were higher in the TCA group than in the sham control (both $p < 0.01$). The levels of both biomarkers after ROSC in the ulinastatin group were significantly lower than those in the TCA group (both $p < 0.01$).

Serum biomarkers of renal injury

At baseline, sCr and BUN did not differ among the three groups (both $p > 0.05$; Fig. 2a, b). The level of sCr after ROSC was similar among the three groups (all $p > 0.05$). BUN after ROSC was significantly higher in the ulinastatin group than at baseline ($p < 0.01$), whereas BUN was similar between the ulinastatin and sham groups ($p > 0.05$). BUN after ROSC was lower in the ulinastatin group than in the TCA group ($p < 0.01$).

Serum biomarkers of intestinal injury

At baseline, serum concentrations of NSE and S100B did not differ among the three groups (all $p > 0.05$; Fig. 2c, d). After ROSC, the levels of iFABP and DAO were significantly higher in the TCA group than in the sham group (both $p < 0.01$) and significantly lower in the ulinastatin group than in the TCA group (both $p < 0.05$).

Arterial blood gas analysis

Baseline PaO_2, SaO_2, pH, and lactate concentration were not significantly different among the three groups (all $p > 0.05$; Additional file 1: Table S1). PaO_2 and SaO_2 of arterial blood after ROSC were higher in the ulinastatin group than in the TCA group (both $p < 0.05$). The pH after ROSC was lower in the TCA group than in the sham group ($p < 0.05$), and it tended to be higher in the ulinastatin group than in the TCA group, although the difference did not achieve statistical significance ($p > 0.05$). Lactate after ROSC was significantly higher in the TCA group than in the sham group ($p < 0.01$), while lactate was significantly lower in the ulinastatin group than in the TCA group ($p < 0.05$).

Coagulation functions

Baseline PT, INR, APTT, and serum level of fibrinogen did not differ significantly among the three groups (all $p > 0.05$; Additional file 1: Table S2). PT, INR, and FIB after ROSC did not differ significantly among the three groups (all $p > 0.05$). APTT was significantly higher in the ulinastatin group than in the TCA group ($p < 0.05$), whereas it was similar between the TCA and sham groups ($p > 0.05$).

Serum TNF-α and IL-6

Preoperative TNF-α and IL-6 did not differ significantly among the three groups (all $p > 0.05$; Fig. 3a, b). Serum TNF-α and IL-6 in the TCA group were significantly higher after ROSC than in the sham group (both $p < 0.01$). Serum TNF-α and IL-6 were significantly lower

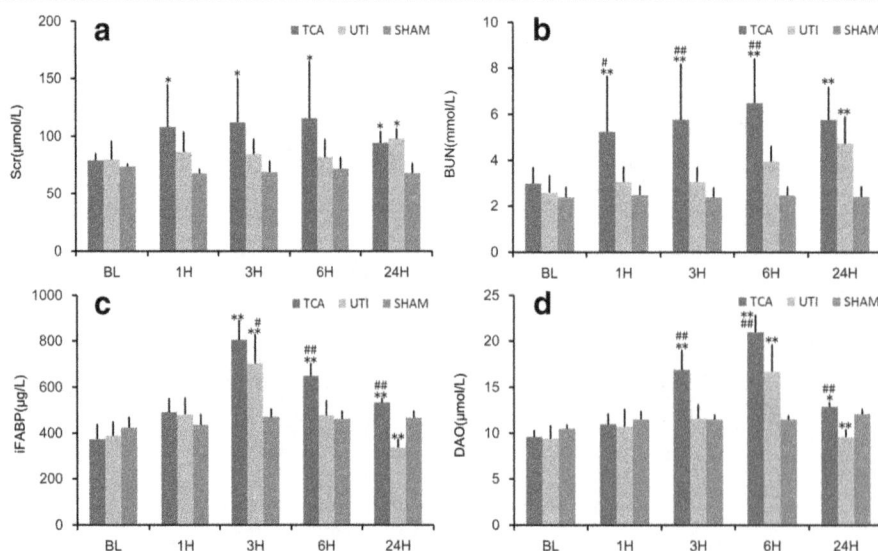

Fig. 2 Biomarkers of intestinal or renal injury in the three groups. a Serum creatinine (sCr). b Blood urea nitrogen (BUN). c Intestinal fatty acid-binding protein (iFABP). d Diamine oxidase (DAO). The x-axis is the time point of baseline 1, 3, 6, and 24 h after ROSC. Values shown are mean ± SD. TCA, traumatic cardiac arrest; UTI, ulinastatin; BL, baseline; ROSC, return of spontaneous circulation. *$p < 0.05$, **$p < 0.01$ vs. baseline; #$p < 0.05$, ##$p < 0.01$ vs. ulinastatin

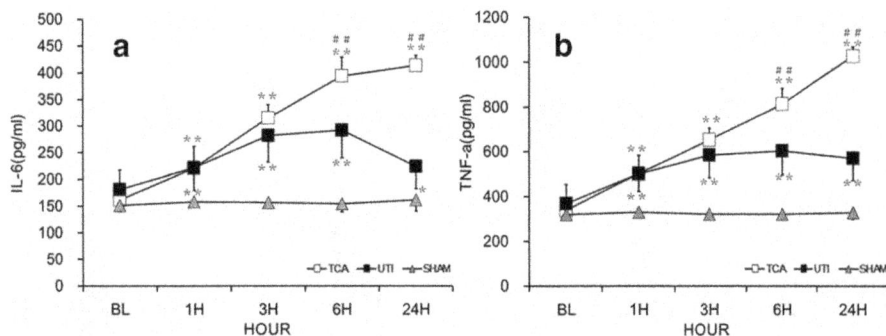

Fig. 3 IL-6 and TNF-α among the three groups. **a** Interleukin (IL)-6. **b** Tumor necrosis factor (TNF)-α. The x-axis is the time point of baseline 1, 3, 6, and 24 h after ROSC. Values shown are mean ± SD. TCA, traumatic cardiac arrest; UTI, ulinastatin; BL, baseline; ROSC, return of spontaneous circulation. $*p < 0.05$, $**p < 0.01$ vs. baseline; $\#p < 0.05$, $\#\#p < 0.01$ vs. ulinastatin

after ROSC in ulinastatin group than in the TCA group (both $p < 0.01$).

Histopathology of major organs

The optical density of immunostaining against caspase-3 as well as the number of TUNEL-positive cells in the apical myocardium were significantly higher in the TCA group than in the sham group (both $p < 0.01$; Fig. 4a, b), while both of these parameters were lower in the ulinastatin group than in the TCA control (both $p < 0.05$).

The optical density of caspase-3 immunostaining in cerebral frontal tissue was significantly higher in the TCA group than in the sham group ($p < 0.01$; Fig. 5a, b), while it was significantly lower in the ulinastatin group than in the TCA group ($p < 0.01$). The same results were observed for the number of TUNEL-positive cells ($p < 0.05$ and $p < 0.01$, respectively).

The optical density of caspase-3 immunostaining and the number of TUNEL-positive cells in the renal cortex

were significantly higher in the TCA group than in the sham group (both $p < 0.01$; Additional file 1: Table S3). Ulinastatin attenuated both measures of apoptosis (both $p < 0.01$ vs. TCA group).

The optical density of caspase-3 immunochemistry in terminal ileum was significantly higher in the TCA group than in the sham group ($p < 0.05$; Additional file 1: Table S3), whereas it was similar between the TCA and ulinastatin groups ($p > 0.05$). The number of TUNEL-positive cells was significantly higher in the TCA group than in the sham group ($p < 0.01$) and significantly lower in the ulinastatin group than in the TCA group ($p < 0.01$).

Discussion

The present study suggests that ulinastatin can improve hemodynamics and attenuate multiple organ injury following TCA in a porcine model. After ROSC, administration of ulinastatin suppressed the increase in HR and biomarkers of major organ injury. Ulinastatin was

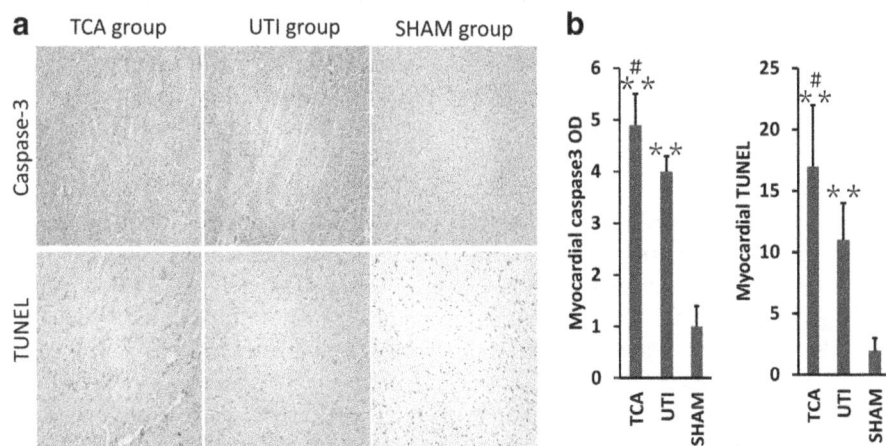

Fig. 4 Ulinastatin-mediated inhibition of apoptosis in the heart. **a** Anti-caspase-3 immunostaining and TUNEL assay results in the three groups. **b** Optical density of caspase-3 immunostaining and numbers of TUNEL-positive cells in the three groups. TCA, traumatic cardiac arrest; UTI, ulinastatin; BL, baseline; TUNEL, terminal deoxynucleotidyl transferase-mediated dUTP nick end labeling. $*p < 0.05$, $**p < 0.01$ vs. sham; $\#p < 0.05$, $\#\#p < 0.01$ vs. ulinastatin

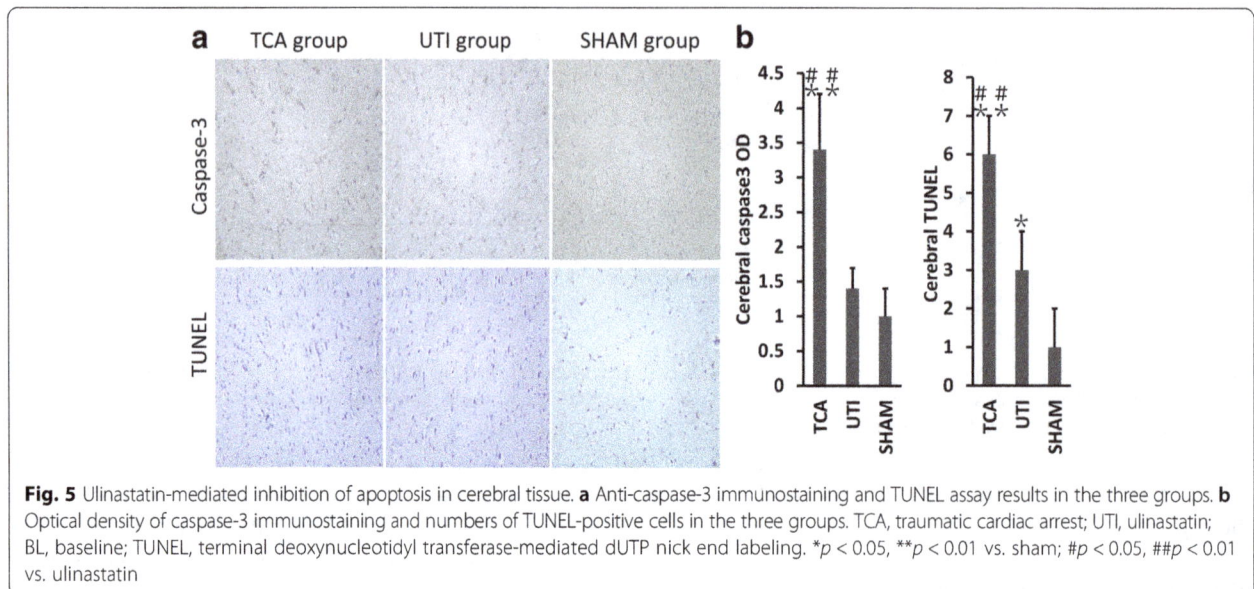

Fig. 5 Ulinastatin-mediated inhibition of apoptosis in cerebral tissue. **a** Anti-caspase-3 immunostaining and TUNEL assay results in the three groups. **b** Optical density of caspase-3 immunostaining and numbers of TUNEL-positive cells in the three groups. TCA, traumatic cardiac arrest; UTI, ulinastatin; BL, baseline; TUNEL, terminal deoxynucleotidyl transferase-mediated dUTP nick end labeling. $*p < 0.05$, $**p < 0.01$ vs. sham; $\#p < 0.05$, $\#\#p < 0.01$ vs. ulinastatin

associated with significantly higher PaO_2 and SaO_2 in arterial blood, as well as lower lactic acid, than in the TCA group. TCA in the present study was induced by controlled bleeding of 40% of total blood volume, followed by ventricular fibrillation. This model faithfully simulates the pathological causes of TCA in humans.

The main pathophysiological feature of TCA is ischemia-reperfusion injury [12], which is the main driver of morbidity and mortality in TCA patients. Ischemic damage occurs immediately during hemorrhage and cardiac arrest, whereas reperfusion injury occurs after ROSC. Such injury is associated with increases in oxygen free radicals and inflammatory factors, for example, superoxide anion free radical, hydrogen peroxide, hydroxyl radical, and TNF-α [7, 13–15]. In both animal studies and randomized clinical trials in humans, ulinastatin has shown protective effects against ischemia-reperfusion injury, leading to lower incidence of organ injury and higher survival rates [6, 9, 16–18]. How ulinastatin can mitigate ischemia-reperfusion injury remains unclear.

The present study showed that ulinastatin suppressed the increase in serum inflammatory factors after ROSC, consistent with previous studies of sepsis and septic shock [5, 6]. Inflammation plays an important role in ischemia-reperfusion injury and in apoptosis induction in multiple organs. Ulinastatin downregulates Toll-like receptors (TLRs) and NF-κB expression and protects the brain against ischemia-reperfusion injury [19]. TLRs form a complex with MyD88 to activate inflammatory cytokines and NF-κB, which regulates the expression of a wide array of genes involved in immune responses [19]. In the present study, we found that ulinastatin reduced TNF-α expression and IL-6 upregulation, consistent with previous studies [12, 20]. TNF-α can stimulate autophagy, and

IL-13 suppresses autophagy by stimulating the phosphoinositide 3-kinase/mTOR signal transduction pathway [20]. In cell culture, ulinastatin may downregulates the autophagy marker LC3-II by improving cell viability in the face of hypoxia/deoxygenation [20]. Ulinastatin also reverses the upregulation of water transporter aquaporin 4 induced in heart and brain tissue in response to cerebral hemorrhage, cerebral trauma or cardiopulmonary resuscitation, and ulinastatin mitigating damage to cardiac arrest function by decreasing the expression of aquaporin 4 [21]. These various studies suggest that ulinastatin may help protect against ischemia injury by inhibiting proteases, inflammatory responses, and cytokine-dependent signaling pathways.

In the present study, the extent of myocardial injury was assessed based on CK-MB and C-TNI; the extent of intestinal injury, based on iFABP and DAO; and the extent of brain injury, NSE and S-100B, which are the most commonly used blood markers of such injury. Elevated NSE and S-100B are associated with poor outcome [22].

In the present study, ulinastatin attenuated tissue injury and cell apoptosis in the brain, heart, kidneys, and intestine. Ulinastatin appears to attenuate ischemia-reperfusion injury in multiple organs by suppressing inflammation and oxidative stress [7, 11, 23], which reduces the generation of oxygen free radicals that accompanies many pathological states such as inflammation, ischemia, and reperfusion [12]. Ischemia-reperfusion injury can cause endothelial barrier dysfunction, resulting in high vascular permeability and tissue edema, and ulinastatin has been shown to inhibit vascular hyperpermeability [24, 25]. Tissue edema reduces the supply of oxygen and nutrients, as well as the removal of waste products from tissues. The ischemia-reperfusion injury also triggers endothelial cell inflammation that results in vascular dysfunction [8, 12]. Crystalloids have several disadvantages with respect to blood infusion: they improve circulation but cannot carry oxygen, they require the infusion of a greater volume of fluid, and they are associated with worse interstitial edema [4]. Ischemia-reperfusion injury induces endothelial production of vasoactive substances that cause vasoconstriction [12].

Factors that contribute to ischemia-reperfusion injury include energy metabolism, changes in the mitochondria and cellular membranes, initiation of different forms of cell death-like apoptosis, and necrosis [12, 26]. Energy metabolism depends on the delivery of blood and oxygen to the tissue, and it depends on the overall metabolic activity in the tissue. After ROSC, HR rises to increase stroke volume and maintain arterial blood pressure in order to compensate for hypovolemia. This increases ATP consumption and energy demand in the myocardium. In the present study, ulinastatin suppressed the increase in HR while maintaining aortic blood pressure. Ischemia-reperfusion initiates different forms of cell death-like apoptosis and necrosis, which recruits inflammatory cells to the necrotic areas and stimulates the release of cytokines [12]. Here, we showed that ulinastatin decreased apoptosis in major organs.

There are some limitations in the present study. First, cardiac arrest was induced by an electrode to produce ventricular fibrillation. However, ventricular arrhythmia occurs in < 3% of TCA patients, and 30–60% of patients present with pulseless electrical activity [4]. Second, ulinastatin in the present study was given at 80000 U/kg at 5 min after ROSC, but this regime may not be optimal for patients with TCA. Third, the observation period was only 24 h after ROSC, which is too short to capture the entire spectrum of post-cardiac arrest syndrome.

Conclusions
Ulinastatin can improve hemodynamics and attenuate multiple organ injury after TCA in a large animal model. Further clinical studies are needed.

Additional file

Additional file 1: Table S1. Blood gas analysis over time after ROSC in the TCA group (n = 8), ulinastatin group (n = 6) and sham group (n = 5). Table S2. Coagulation function over time after ROSC in the TCA group (n = 8), ulinastatin group (n = 6) and sham group (n = 5). Table S3. Caspase-3 levels and numbers of TUNEL-positive cells in the heart, cerebral, lung, renal, and intestinal tissues of the three groups. (DOCX 57 kh)

Abbreviations
BUN: Blood urea nitrogen; CK-MB: Creatine kinase MB; cTNI: Cardiac troponin I; DAO: Diamine oxidase; ETCO2: End-tidal carbon dioxide; HR: Heart rate; iFABP: Intestinal fatty acid-binding protein; IL: Interleukin; MAP: Mean aortic blood pressure; NSE: Neuron-specific enolase; RAP: Right atrial pressure; ROSC: Return of spontaneous circulation; S100B: S100 calcium-binding protein B; sCr: Serum creatinine; SD: Standard deviation; TCA: Traumatic cardiac arrest; TNF: Tumor necrosis factor; TUNEL: Terminal deoxynucleotidyl transferase-mediated dUTP nick end labeling; UTI: Urinary trypsin inhibitor

Acknowledgements
We thank Moli Li for assistance with animal preparation.

Funding
Mao Zhang is funded by the Welfare Scientific Research Project from the Chinese Ministry of Health (2015SQ00050), the Key Program Co-sponsored by Zhejiang Province and National Health and Family Planning Commission of China (2018271879), and the Welfare Scientific Research Project of Zhejiang Province (LGF18H150003). These agencies provided financial support but were not involved in any other aspect of the research.

Authors' contributions
ZM (corresponding author) was in charge of the study design and data analysis. LS (first author) was responsible for the data analysis and manuscript writing and cooperated with XJ, GY, SP, and SX in animal research work. All authors participated in the critical revision of the manuscript, and all authors approved the final version to be submitted.

Competing interests
The authors declare that they have no competing interests.

Author details
[1]Department of Emergency Medicine, Second Affiliated Hospital, Zhejiang University School of Medicine, No. 88 Jiefang road, Hangzhou 310009, China. [2]Institute of Emergency Medicine, Zhejiang University, No. 88 Jiefang road, Hangzhou 310009, China. [3]Department of Emergency Medicine, Yuyao People's Hospital, Medical School of Ningbo University, Yuyao 315400, China. [4]Department of Emergency Medicine, The First Hospital of Jiaxing/The First Affiliated Hospital of Jiaxing University, Jiaxing 314000, China. [5]Department of Emergency Medicine, Huzhou Central Hospital, Huzhou 313000, China.

References
1. Lockey D, Crewdson K, Davies G. Traumatic cardiac arrest: who are the survivors? Ann Emerg Med. 2006;48:240–4.
2. Harris T, Masud S, Lamond A, Abu-Habsa M. Traumatic cardiac arrest: a unique approach. Eur J Emerg Med. 2015;22:72–8.
3. Smith JE, Rickard A, Wise D. Traumtic cardiac arrest. J R Soc Med. 2015; 108:11–6.
4. Hopson LR, Hirsh E, Delgado J, Domeier RM, McSwain NE, Krohmer J, et al. Guidelines for withholding or termination of resuscitation in prehospital traumatic cardiopulmonary arrest: joint position statement of the National Association of EMS Physicians and the American College of Surgeons Committee on Trauma. J Am Coll Surg. 2003;196:106–12.
5. Feng Z, Shi Q, Fan Y, Wang Q, Yin W. Ulinastatin and/or thymosin α1 for severe sepsis: a systematic review and meta-analysis. J Trauma Acute Care Surg. 2016;80:335–40.

6.   Karnad DR, Bhadade R, Verma PK, Moulick ND, Daga MK, Chafekar ND, et al. Intravenous administration of ulinastatin (human urinary trypsin inhibitor) in severe sepsis: a multicenter randomized controlled study. Intensive Care Med. 2014;40:830–8.

7.   Chen HM, Huang HS, Ruan L, He YB, Li XJ. Ulinastatin attenuates cerebral ischemia-reperfusion injury in rats. Int J Clin Exp Med. 2014;7:1483–9.

8.   Liu M, Shen J, Zou F, Zhao Y, Li B, Fan M. Effect of ulinastatin on the permeability of the blood-brain barrier on rats with global cerebral ischemia/reperfusion injury as assessed by MRI. Biomed Pharmacother. 2017; 85:412–7.

9.   He QL, Zhong F, Ye F, Wei M, Liu WF, Li MN, et al. Does intraoperative ulinastatin improve postoperative clinical outcomes in patients undergoing cardiac surgery: a meta-analysis of randomized controlled trials. Biomed Res Int. 2014;2014:630835.

10. Lee B, Lee SY, Kim NY, Rha KH, Choi YD, Park S, et al. Effect of ulinastatin on postoperative renal function in patients undergoing robot-assisted laparoscopic partial nephrectomy: a randomized trial. Surg Endosc. 2017;31: 3728–36.

11. Wan X, Xie X, Gendoo Y, Chen C, Ji X, Cao C. Ulinastatin administration is associated with a lower incidence of acute kidney injury after cardiac surgery: a propensity score matched study. Crit Care. 2016;20:42.

12. Salvadori M, Rosso G, Bertoni E. Update on ischemia-reperfusion injury in kidney transplantation: pathogenesis and treatment. World J Transplant. 2015;5:52–67.

13. Korthuis RJ, Granger DN, Townsley MI, Taylor AE. The role of oxygen-derived free radicals in ischemia-induced increases in canine skeletal muscle vascular permeability. Circ Res. 1985;57:599–609.

14. Werns SW, Shea MJ, Driscoll EM, Cohen C, Abrams GD, Pitt B, et al. The independent effects of oxygen radical scavengers on canine infarct size. Reduction by superoxide dismutase but not catalase. Circ Res. 1985;56:895–8.

15. Baker GL, Corry RJ, Autor AP. Oxygen free radical induced damage in kidneys subjected to warm ischemia and reperfusion. Protective effect of superoxide dismutase Ann Surg. 1985;202:628–41.

16. Lili X, Zhiyong H, Jianjun S. A preliminary study of the effects of ulinastatin on early postoperative cognition function in patients undergoing abdominal surgery. Neurosci Lett. 2013;541:15–9.

17. Lv ZT, Huang JM, Zhang JM, Zhang JM, Guo JF, Chen AM. Effect of ulinastatin in the treatment of postperative cognitive dysfunction: review of current literature. Biomed Res Int. 2016;2016:2571080.

18. Inoue K, Takano H. Urinary trypsin inhibitor as a therapeutic option for endotoxin-related inflammatory disorders. Expert Opin Investig Drugs. 2010; 19:513–20.

19. Li X, Su L, Zhang X, Zhang C, Wang L, Li Y, et al. Ulinastatin downregulates TLR4 and NF-κB expression and protects mouse brains against ischemia re/ perfusion injury. Neurol Res. 2017;39:367–73.

20. Xiao J, Zhu X, Ji G, Yang Q, Kang B, Zhao J, et al. Ulinastatin protects cardiomyocytes against ischemia-reperfusion injury by regulating autophagy through mTOR activation. Mol Med Rep. 2014;10:1949–53.

21. He W, Liu Y, Geng H, Li Y. The regulation effect of ulinastatin on the expression of SSAT2 and AQP4 in myocardial tissue of rats after cardiopulmonary resuscitation. Int J Clin Exp Pathol. 2015;8:10792–9.

22. Callaway CW, Donnino MW, Fink EL, Geocadin RG, Golan E, Kern KB, et al. Part 8: post–cardiac arrest care: 2015 American Heart Association Guidelines Update for Cardiopulmonary Resuscitation and Emergency Cardiovascular Care. Circulation. 2015;132:S465–S82.

23. Guan L, Liu H, Fu P, Li Z, Li P, Xie L, et al. The protective effects of trypsin inhibitor on hepatic ischemia-reperfusion injury and liver graft survival. Oxidative Med Cell Longev. 2016;2016:1429835.

24. Ma L, Zhang H, Liu YZ, Yin YL, Ma YQ, Zhang SS. Ulinastatin decreases permeability of blood--brain barrier by inhibiting expression of MMP-9 and t-PA in postoperative aged rats. Int J Neurosci. 2016;126:463–8.

25. Lin B, Liu Y, Li T, Zeng K, Cai S, Zeng Z, et al. Ulinastatin mediates protection against vascular hyperpermeability following hemorrhagic shock. Int J Clin Exp Pathol. 2015;8:7685–93.

26. Cho YS, Shin MS, Ko IG, Kim SE, Kim CJ, Sung YH, et al. Ulinastatin inhibits cerebral ischemia-induced apoptosis in the hippocampus of gerbils. Mol Med Rep. 2015;12:1796–802.

2

Plasma calprotectin level: usage in distinction of uncomplicated from complicated acute appendicitis

Murat Cikot[1], Kivanc Derya Peker[1]* , Mehmet Abdussamet Bozkurt[1], Ali Kocatas[1], Osman Kones[1], Sinan Binboga[1], Asuman Gedikbasi[2] and Halil Alis[1]

Abstract

Background: The aim of this study was to identify the diagnostic role of plasma calprotectin value for a distinction of presence acute appendicitis and the indifference of uncomplicated from complicated acute appendicitis.

Methods: Plasma calprotectin, white blood cell and C-reactive protein values of 89 patients, who have undergone laparoscopic appendectomy between January 2013 and May 2013 were evaluated.

Results: Calprotectin was 91 ng/mL (range 45–538) for acute appendicitis and 47 ng/ml (range 28–205) for the control group. There was a positive, statistically significant relation between calprotectin and C-reactive protein values ($r = 0.292$ $p = 0.001$, respectively). There was no statistically significant difference was determined between calprotectin and white blood cell values ($r = 0.142$ $p = 0.187$, respectively). CRP and Cal values were significantly higher in patients with a complicated AA group than in those with uncomplicated AA ($p = 0.014$, $p = 0.0001$, respectively) whereas white blood cell counts did not differ significantly between two groups ($p = 0.164$).

Conclusion: Plasma calprotectin levels were increased in patients with acute appendicitis and should use in a distinction of uncomplicated from complicated acute appendicitis patients.

Keywords: Acute appendicitis, Plasma Calprotectin, Uncomplicated acute appendicitis, Complicated acute appendicitis

Background

The lifetime occurrence of acute appendicitis (AA) is approximately 7–8 % and it is the most common disease, which find in emergency surgery [1, 2]. Although the most severe of all adverse events, mortality in developed health systems is low (between 0.09 % and 0.24 %) and does not have a sensitivity to detect differences in care processes that lead to variation in other outcomes [3, 4]. No inflammatory marker alone, such as white blood cell (WBC) count, C-reactive protein (CRP) or other novel tests, including procalcitonin, can identify AA with high specificity and sensitivity [5]. However, WBC count is obtained in virtually all patients who are assessed for AA, when available. A range of novel biomarkers has been suggested during the past decade, including bilirubin, but these do not have external validity and suffer repeatedly from low sensitivity, which means they are unlikely to come into clinical practice [6]. Initial reliance on ultrasound (USG) has become more guarded recently because of moderate sensitivity (86 %, CI 83–88) and specificity (81 %, CI 78–84) as shown through pooled diagnostic accuracy of 14 studies [7], limiting its diagnostic ability. In adolescent and adult patients, computed tomography (CT) has become the most widely accepted imaging strategy. It is used in 86 % of patients, with a sensitivity of $92 \cdot 3$ % [8]. The rate of negative appendectomy decreased significantly over time, from $12 \cdot 7$ % in 1995 to $2 \cdot 8$ % in 2006 [9–11].

Calprotectin (Cal) S-100 is a 36-kDa heterodimer that belongs to the family of calcium-binding proteins, which involve both lights (MRP8) and heavy (MRP14) chains

---
* Correspondence: pekerkivancderya@gmail.com
[1]Department of General Surgery, Istanbul Bakirkoy Dr. Sadi Konuk Training and Research Hospital, Zuhuratbaba Mh, Tevfik Saglam Cad. No: 11, 34147 Bakirkoy/Istanbul, Turkey
Full list of author information is available at the end of the article

and were identified as an antimicrobial protein in granules of neutrophils and to a lesser extent in monocytes and reactive macrophages [12]. Cal was counting 60 % of the total cytosolic protein in neutrophils [13], which provide to separate these from monocytes during cell death and cell rupture [12]. In the presence of an ongoing cycle of inflammation, Cal levels are increased in plasma, synovial fluid, urine and tool [14–16]. Thus, Cal levels in plasma and various body fluids have been proposed as a marker of inflammation [12].

In this prospective study, the authors have aimed to compare of inflammatory markers, which use in routine practice and plasma Cal values and to identify the role of plasma Cal values in the diagnosis of complicated and uncomplicated AA. Therefore, in this study, we measured plasma Cal and CRP levels in patients with AA to investigate the diagnostic accuracy of the combined use of these markers.

Methods

The Strengthening the Reporting of Observational Studies in Epidemiology (STROBE) statement was used in the design and implementation of the study and to prepare the manuscript [17]. The study was approved by the Local Ethics Committee of our hospital (01-2013) and judged that informed consent from patients was not necessary because of the observational study design with no additional burden for the patient.

Eighty-nine patients with AA, with an ASA (American Society of Anesthesiologists) score of I–III, who underwent laparoscopic appendectomy in our general surgery clinic between January 2013 and May 2013 included the study. The control group consisted of 30 patients, which were selected from a group of 67 patients, who admitted to the emergency clinic with the complaint of abdominal pain in the right or right and left lower quadrants, after laboratory tests and abdominal imaging, necessary consultations were performed and follow-up for 48 h, during which time neither antibiotics nor non-steroidal anti-inflammatory drugs were administered, diagnostic laparoscopy was performed in these patients. In 18 of 67 patients were determined a pelvic inflammatory disease, 16 patients had hemorrhagic ovarian cyst or cyst rupture, and 3 patients had diverticulitis at laparoscopic exploration. Since Cal values of plasma have been increased with inflammatory process in these pathological cases and if patients in the control group have these pathologic findings, excluded the study. The control group was created from 30 patients without intra-abdominal pathology and thus diagnosed as non-specific abdominal pain.

A pilot study, which were conducted with 20 patients in each group. As a result of the study, the effect size for Cal values was determined to be 0.609. Three patients

for each control group member were taken. With 0.05 Type I error rate, %80 power and allocation size of 3, the minimum needed numbers were determined as 29 and 87 for control group respectively.

At our hospital, the normal laboratory values for CRP and WBC are 0.01–0.5 mg/dL and $4–11 \times 103$/mm, respectively. The detection limit for Cal, according to Hycult Biotech is 46.8 ng/ml [18]. The Cal values of the AA group were compared with the control group, which were in normal range. Blood samples were centrifuged for 15 min at $2000 \times g$. Aliquots of plasma were stored at–80 °C until used in the assays. Serum Cal was determined using a human Cal ELISA kit (East Biopharm, China) according to the manufacturer's instructions. Cal level was expressed ng/ml. The limit of detection of the ELISA is 20 ng/mL. The intra-assay and inter-assay coefficients of variation were < 8.1 % and <7.6 %, respectively.

Cal was measured in blood samples obtained from both the AA and control groups. To patients, who presented with abdominal pain, a physical examination, laboratory tests and abdominal USG and CT were performed. In the AA group, blood samples for Cal, WBC and CRP measurements were obtained after diagnosis and before medical and surgical treatment. The abdominal cavities of these patients were explored during the laparoscopic appendectomy. Only those without any additional intra-abdominal inflammatory pathologies were included the study. Complicated AA was defined as AA in which perforation, gangrenous or an intra-abdominal abscess [19].

Statistical analysis

Statistical analysis was performed using the Statistical Software Package Program (Utah, USA), NCSS (Number Cruncher Statistical System) 2007. When evaluating data, besides routine statistical analysis, such as mean, standard deviation, median, frequency and rate, in the intergroup comparison of variables with normal distribution, Independent Sample test and in the intergroup comparison of variables in the normal distribution Mann-Whitney U test were used. Yates' continuity correction test (Yates corrected chi-square) was used in the comparison of qualitative data. Cut-off values for Call were assessed using ROC curves. The results were assessed within a confidence interval of 95 % and significance was assessed at $p < 0.05$ level.

Results

The male-to-female ratio was 54/35 in the study of patients and 20/10 in the control patients. The mean age was 28 (range 19–45) and 31 (range 21–56), respectively. AA was histopathologically confirmed in 89 patients and determination of acute mucosal inflammation was in 22 patients (24.7 %), AA with phlegmon formation in 48 patients (53.9 %), and AA with gangrene in 19 patients (21.3 %). A ruptured appendix was detected in 18 of 89 cases with AA. Findings of peritonitis and evaluation of appendix microscope with histopathological results have shown, 23 (26 %) of patients had complicated and 66 (74 %) of patients had uncomplicated AA.

WBC levels were significantly higher in the AA group than in the control group ($p = 0. 0001$), as high as in CRP ($p = 0. 0001$) and Cal ($p = 0. 0001$) levels. The relationship between Cal and CRP values was statistically significant ($p = 0.001$, $r = 0.292$), whereas this was not the case for Cal and WBC values ($p = 0.187$, $r = 0.141$) (Table 1). Average plasma Cal values were 59 ng/ml (range 46–107) in the group of patients with acute mucosal inflammation, 68 ng/ml (45–109) in those with phlegmonous AA, and 185 ng/ml (range 85–538) in those with gangrenous or ruptured AA. CRP and Cal values were significantly higher in patients with a complicated AA group than in those with uncomplicated AA ($p = 0. 014$ and $p = 0. 0001$, respectively) whereas WBC counts did not differ significantly between two groups ($p = 0. 164$) (Table 2). However, WBC, CRP and Cal values were significantly higher in patients with positive USG findings [USG (+)], than in those AA patients with negative USG findings [USG (–)] with AA ($p = 0. 0001$) (Table 3).

In terms of the presence of AA, statistically significant differences ($p = 0. 001$; $p < 0.01$) was observed between the values of Cal, and the results clearly had showed that Cal level is high if AA is the presence. Following these results, it has been decided to study the cut-off point for Cal. In terms of the presence of AA, ROC analyzes and the full-screen test were used to determine cut-off point. In terms of the presence of AA, it has been observed that the cut-off point for Cal is 46 and higher. For the 46 ng/mL cutoff value of Cal; sensitivity is %98. 88, specificity is %83. 33, positive cutoff value 94.62 and

Table 1 WBC, CRP and Cal values in the AA and control group

		AA	Control	p
WBC	Mid ± SS	14,11 ± 5,62	7,21 ± 3,79	0,0001
	Median (IQR)	13,9 (10,9–17,3)	6,75 (5,9–7,9)	
CRP	Mid ± SS	5,92 ± 5,48	0,50 ± 0,42	0,0001
	Median (IQR)	4,2 (2,14–7,7)	0,40 (0,26–0,66)	
Cal	Mid ± SS	91,56 ± 77,40	47,18 ± 32,55	0,0001
	Median (IQR)	67,12 (53,87–67,12)	39,50 (34,81–42,71)	
		Cal		
CRP	r	0,292		
	p	0,001		
WBC	r	0,141		
	p	0,187		

Table 2 WBC, CRP and Cal values in the uncomplicated and complicated AA groups

		Uncomplicated AA	Complicated AA	p
WBC	Mid ± SS	5,78 ± 5,6	6,43 ± 5,15	0,164
	Median (IQR)	3,78 (1,75–8,28)	6,43 ± 5,15	
CRP	Mid ± SS	13,54 ± 4,74	16,21 ± 3,52	0,014
	Median (IQR)	13,35 (10,4–16,93)	16,21 ± 3,52	
Cal	Mid ± SS	65,44 ± 17,12	187,78 ± 125,45	0,0001
	Median (IQR)	59,58 (52,29–72,75)	187,78 ± 125,45	

negative cutoff value is 96.15. On the ROC curve, the standard error for the below part %91. 2 is %4. 3 (Fig. 1).

Statistically significant relation between the presence of AA and 46 cut-off value of Cal was observed ($p = 0.001$; $p < 0.01$). When Cal level is 46 and higher, the risk to see AA is 7.33 times more. While the below part of the ROC curve is 0.912 for Cal, it is 0.952 for WBC and 0.824 for CRP. Significant differences in the below ROC curve was observed ($p = 0. 942$; $p = 0. 952$; $p = 0. 824$; $p > 0.05$, respectively). (Table 4) If leukocyte, CRP and Cal values below the ROC curve were evaluated, value for Cal was 0.935 below ROC curve, 0.640 for WBC and 0.597 for CRP and values below the ROC curve was statistically significant ($p < 0.01$) (Fig. 2). These findings helped us to find the value of Cal in complicated AA was more effective than WBC and CRP values ($p = 0.001$; $p = 0.001$; $p < 0.01$, respectively). Any significant difference wasn't determined between WBC and CRP in pre-diagnosis of complicated AA ($p = 0. 603$; $p > 0.05$) (Table 5).

Discussion

There is currently no evidence for suggesting, that serum Cal is superior to standard inflammatory markers for the exclusion or confirmation of suspected AA [20]. However, uncomplicated and complicated AA is considered to be two entities. The curability of uncomplicated disease without surgery is proven in studies comparing to antibiotic therapy, whereas complicated AA with necrosis or perforation of the appendix cannot be treated successfully without invasive modality. The preferred surgical approach in complicated AA is more unclear, therefore of lack of evidence in this group [21]. In this

Table 3 WBC, CRP and Cal values in the USG (+/−)

		USG (−)	USG (+)	p
WBC	Mid ± SS	13,85 ± 4,54	14,31 ± 4,71	0,0001
	Median (IQR)	14,75 (10,75–17,3)	13,60 (10,8–18,2)	
CRP	Mid ± SS	7,38 ± 6,31	4,83 ± 4,54	0,0001
	Median (IQR)	5,5 (2,7–9,77)	3,75 (1,76–5,93)	
Cal	Mid ± SS	90,46 ± 87,9	92,37 ± 69,45	0,0001
	Median (IQR)	63,62 (52,3–98,42)	68,5 (55,57–97,1)	

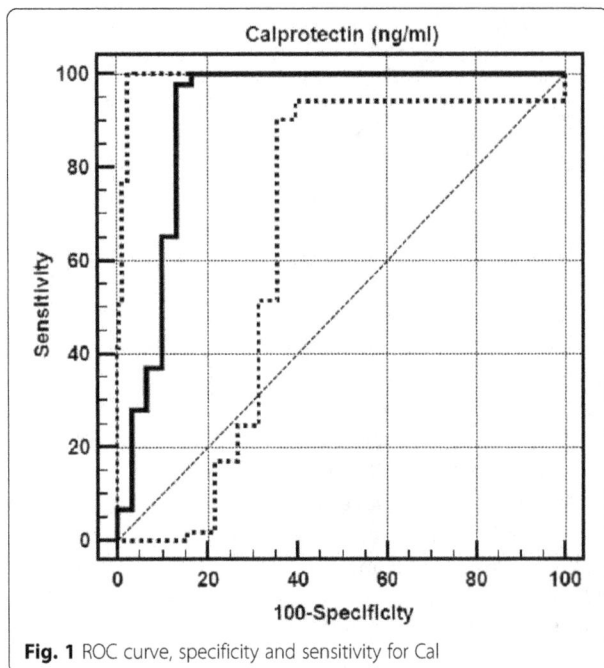

Fig. 1 ROC curve, specificity and sensitivity for Cal

Table 4 The area under the ROC curve (AUC) for Cal, WBC and CRP in the AA

	AUC	SE	%95 CI
Cal	0,912	0,044	0,846–0,956
WBC	0,909	0,027	0,842–0,954
CRP	0,914	0,026	0,849–0,958
Cal- WBC	p= 0,942		
Cal-WBC	p = 0,952		
WBC -CRP	p = 0,824		

study has supported, that plasma CRP level increase was nonspecific, as in literature. Another fact that, we wanted to emphasize the identification of Cal was a useful inflammatory parameter. In distinction of complicated and uncomplicated AA, Cal was statistically more effective than the other inflammatory parameters according to imaging and laboratory methods [21]. When inflammatory process progresses and peritonitis findings have occurred, Cal level has also increased. Due to thickening of appendix wall, inflammation around fat plans or the liquid amount around the appendix, plasma Cal level has increased, and, therefore, Cal levels were

determined USG (+) patients higher than USG (–) patients [21].

In this study, the average plasma Cal value of the control group was 47.18 ng/ml, which was close to the value, which was reported by Hycult Biotechnology (46.8 ng/ml). Cal levels in AA group were significantly higher than the control group. Although this increase was non-specific for AA, it was specifically for the acute inflammatory process, as well as CRP value, which has a plasma half-life of 19 h and is produced by the liver [22–25]. The relationship between plasma Cal and CRP levels was statistically meaningful.

Cal was an acute-phase reactant, which increases in local and systemic inflammatory diseases [23]. According to Yui et al. This increase was caused by the migration of leukocytes in the region of inflammation and tissue disruption [26, 27]. Thus, in colorectal cancer, inflammatory bowel disease, necrotizing enterocolitis and celiac diseases fecal Cal levels have increased. According to this, fecal Cal has been proposed as a non-invasive, nonspecific marker for the diagnosis of these diseases and for detection of disease activation and remission in patients with ulcerative colitis and Crohn's Disease

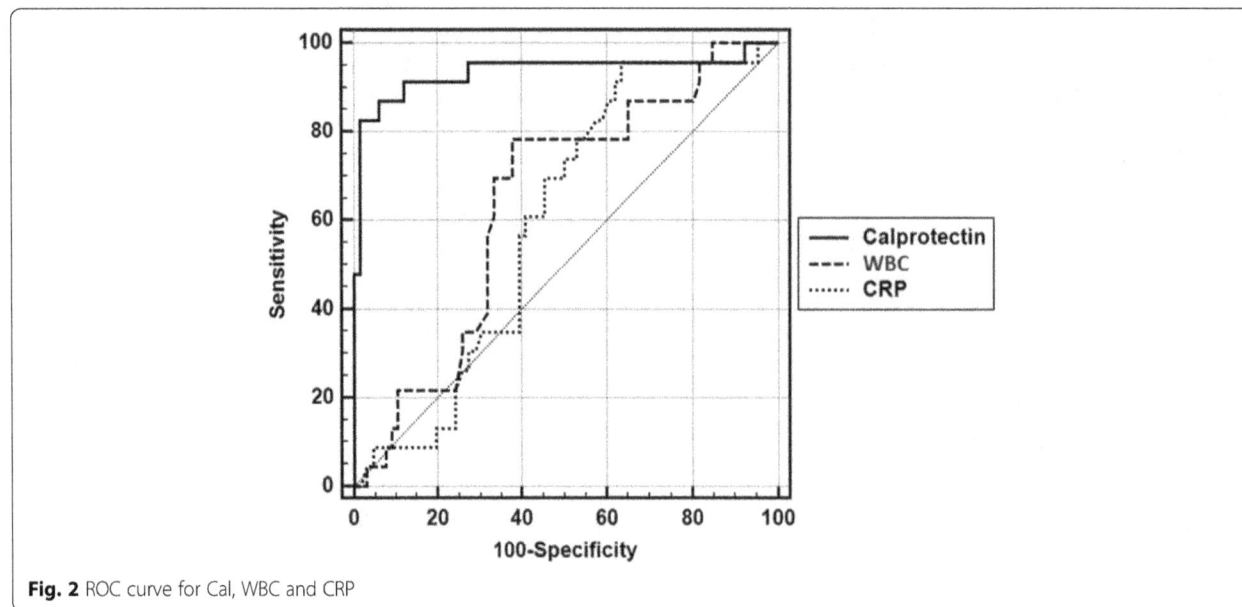

Fig. 2 ROC curve for Cal, WBC and CRP

Table 5 The area under the ROC curve (AUC) for Cal, WBC and CRP in the uncomplicated and complicated AA groups

	AUC	SE	%95 CI
Calprotectin	0,935	0,042	0,862–0,976
WBC	0,640	0,064	0,532–0,739
CRP	0,597	0,062	0,488–0,700
Calprotectin- WBC	p = 0,001		
Calprotectin-CRP	p = 0,001		
WBC -CRP	p = 0,603		

[27–32]. In AA, increased plasma Cal levels, when were used together with WBC and CRP levels might allow a more accurate diagnosis of AA [33, 34]. While plasma Cal levels also increase in acute pancreatitis, whether similar increases could be measured in the pancreatic inflammation included further study [35].

Despite the use of laboratory tests, imaging techniques and clinical examinations in patients with suspected AA, both the number of negative laparotomy/laparoscopy and surgery-related morbidity and mortality were remaining high [36, 37]. On the other hand, routine diagnostic laparoscopy has been proposed as an alternative to in-hospital observation in patients with suspicion of AA [10]. Two recent reviews of randomized trials, comparing early laparoscopy to observation did not perform, however, determine not any clear advantage [38, 39]. Investigations to help distinguish those patients in the mid-Alvarado Score group includes CRP, USG and CT. CRP as a blood test for AA has a relatively high specificity: according to this, a patient with normal CRP level is unlikely to have AA [5]. Compared to WBC and procalcitonin, a meta-analysis determined, CRP was more accurate [5]. One study recommends that Cal, CRP or WBC count did not have high sensitivity and specificity to be clinically useful in the evaluation of subjects with suspected AA. Likewise, procalcitonin had little effect in diagnosing AA, with lower diagnostic accuracy than CRP and WBC [40].

The diagnosis of AA depends on the patient's history, a detailed physical examination, completed with laboratory tests and imaging methods. In patients with suspected AA, together elevated CRP levels and increased plasma Cal levels could provide further support for the diagnosis. Whether the use of CRP and Cal levels in the diagnosis of AA, decreased the rate of unnecessary and delayed laparotomies/laparoscopies remains to be determined in larger groups of patients.

Our study has several limitations, such as a low number of patients and was a single-center design. This study was prospective, but the study design and data analysis were performed retrospectively. Once the diagnosis was confirmed and the study group was selected retrospectively. There is a lack of validation cohort in this study.

Conclusion

Plasma Cal levels could be used indistinctness of uncomplicated from complicated acute appendicitis as a diagnostic marker of acute appendicitis.

Competing interests
The authors declare that they have no competing interests. The funders had no role in the study design, data collection and analysis, decision to publish, or preparation of the manuscript.

Authors' contributions
MC carried out conception and design, acquisition of data, analysis, interpretation and writing manuscript; KDP carried out conception and design, data analysis, interpretation and writing manuscript; OK carried out data extraction, interpretation and drafting manuscript, AK carried out data extraction, interpretation and drafting manuscript; AG and HA carried out data extraction interpretation and drafting manuscript; MAB and SB carried out data extraction, interpretation and drafting manuscript. All authors read and approved the final manuscript.

Acknowledgments
We would like to thank Mr. David F. Chapman for his assistance with the language in the manuscript.

Author details
[1]Department of General Surgery, Istanbul Bakirkoy Dr. Sadi Konuk Training and Research Hospital, Zuhuratbaba Mh, Tevfik Saglam Cad. No: 11, 34147 Bakirkoy/Istanbul, Turkey. [2]Department of Biochemistry, Istanbul Bakirkoy Dr. Sadi Konuk Training and Research Hospital, Bakirkoy/Istanbul, Turkey.

References
1. Jacobs JE. CT and sonography for suspected acute appendicitis: a commentary. AJR Am J Roentgenol. 2006;186(4):1094–6.
2. Bhangu A, Søreide K, Di Saverio S, Assarsson JH, Drake FT. Acute appendicitis:modern understanding of pathogenesis, diagnosis, and management. Lancet. 2015;386(10000):1278–87.
3. Bliss LA, Yang CJ, Kent TS, Ng SC, Critchlow JF, Tseng JF. Appendicitis in the modern era: universal problem and variable treatment. Surg Endosc. 2014;146:1057.
4. Faiz O, Clark J, Brown T, et al. Traditional and laparoscopic appendectomy in adults: outcomes in English NHS hospitals between 1996 and 2006. Ann Surg. 2008;248:800–6.
5. Yu CW, Juan LI, Wu MH, Shen CJ, Wu JY, Lee CC. Systematic review and meta-analysis of the diagnostic accuracy of procalcitonin, C-reactive protein and White blood cell count for suspected acute appendicitis. Br J Surg. 2013;100:322–9.
6. Andersson M, Ruber M, Ekerfelt C, Hallgren HB, Olaison G, Andersson RE. Can new inflammatory markers improve the diagnosis of acute appendicitis? World J Surg. 2014;38:2777–83.
7. Terasawa T, Blackmore CC, Bent S, Kohlwes RJ. Systematic review: computed tomography and ultrasonography to detect acute appendicitis in adults and adolescents. Ann Intern Med. 2004;141:537–46.
8. Cuschieri J, Florence M, Flum DR, et al. Negative appendectomy and imaging accuracy in the Washington State Surgical Care and Outcomes Assessment Program. Ann Surg. 2008;248:557–63.
9. Van Rossem CC, Bolmers MD, Schreinemacher MH, van Geloven AA, Bemelman WA, Snapshot Appendicitis Collaborative Study Group. Prospective nationwide outcome audit of surgery for suspected acute appendicitis. Br J Surg. 2015;103(1):144–51.
10. Andersson RE. Short-term complications and long-term morbidity of laparoscopicand open appendectomy in a national cohort. Br J Surg. 2014;101(9):1135–42.
11. Güller U, Rosella L, McCall J, Brügger LE, Candinas D. Negative appendectomyand perforation rates in patients undergoing laparoscopic surgery for suspected appendicitis. Br J Surg. 2011;98(4):589–95.

12. Dale I, Fagerhol MK, Naesgaard I. Purification and partial characterization of highly immunogenetic human leukocyte protein, the L1 antigen. Eur J Biochem. 1983;134:1–6.

13. Stockley RA, Dale I, Hill SI, Fagerhol MK. Relationship of neutrophil cytoplasmic protein (L1) to acute and chronic lung disease. Scand J Clin Lab Invest. 1984;44:629–39.

14. Ton H, Brandsnes, Dale S, Holtlund J, Skuibina E, Schjønsby H, et al. Improved assay for fecal Cal. Clin Chim Acta. 2000;292:41–54.

15. Konikoff MR, Denson LA. Role of fecal Call as a biomarker of intestinal inflammation in inflammatory bowel disease. Inflamm Bowel Dis. 2006;12:524–34.

16. Roseth AG, Aadland E, Jhansen J, Raknerud N. Assessment of disease activity in ulcerative colitis by fecal Cal, a novel granulocyte marker protein. Digestion. 1997;58:176–80.

17. von Elm E, Altman DG, Egger M, Pocock SJ, Gotzsche PC, Vandenbroucke JP. The Strengthening the Reporting of Observational Studies in Epidemiology (STROBE) statement: guidelines for reporting observational studies. Lancet. 2007;370:1453–7.

18. Hanssen SJ, Derikx JP, VermeulenWindsant IC, Heijmans JH, Koeppel TA, Schurink GW, et al. Visceral injury and systemic inflammation in patients undergoing extracorporeal circulation during aortic surgery. Ann Surg. 2008;248:117–25.

19. Al-Omran M, Mamdani MM, McLeod RS. Epidemiologic features of acute appendicitis in Ontario, Canada. Can J Surg. 2003;46:263–8.

20. Horner D, Long AM. Towards evidence-based emergency medicine: best BETs fromthe Manchester Royal Infirmary. BET 3: Super calprotectin will not expedite yourdischarge. Emerg Med J. 2013;30(8):691–3.

21. Atema JJ, van Rossem CC, Leeuwenburgh MM, Stoker J, Boermeester MA. Scoring system to distinguish uncomplicated from complicated acute appendicitis. Br J Surg. 2015;102(8):979–90.

22. Matthiessen P, Henriksson M, Hallböök O, Grunditz E, Norén B, Arbman G. Increase of serum C-reactive protein is an early indicator of subsequent symptomatic anastomotic leakage after anterior resection. Colorectal Dis. 2008;10:75–80.

23. Mustard RA, Bohnen JM, Haseeb S, Kasina R. C-reactive protein levels predict postoperative septic complications. Arch Surg. 1987;122:69–73.

24. Welsch T, Müller SA, Ulrich A, Kischlat A, Hinz U, Kienle P, et al. C-Reactive protein as early predictor for infectious postoperative complications in rectal surgery. Int J Colorectal Dis. 2007;22:1499–507.

25. Golden BE, Clohessy PA, Russell G, Fagerhol MK. Calprotectin as a marker of inflammation in cystic fibrosis. Arch Dis Child. 1996;74:136–9.

26. Yui S, Mikami M, Yamazaki M. Induction of apoptotic cell death in Mouse lymphoma and human leukemia cell lines by a calcium-binding protein complicated, calprotectin, derived from inflammatory peritoneal exudate cells. J Leuk Biol. 1995;58:650.

27. Stritz I, Trebichavsky I. Calprotectin - a pleiotropic molecule in acute and chronic inflammation. Physiol Res. 2004;53:245–53.

28. Zhao L, Wang H, Sun X, Ding Y. Comparative proteomic analysis identifies proteins associated with the development and progression of colorectal carcinoma. FEBS J. 2010;277:4195–204.

29. Burri E, Beglinger C. Faecal calprotectin - a useful tool in the management of in flammatory bowel disease. Swiss Med Wkly. 2012;142:135.

30. Aomatsu T, Yoden A, Matsumoto K, Kimura E, Inoue K, Andoh A, et al. Fecalcalprotectin is a useful marker for disease activity in pediatric patients with in flammatory bowel disease. Dig Dis Sci. 2011;56:2372–7.

31. Ho GT, Lee HM, Brydon G, Ting T, Hare N, Drummond H, et al. Fecal calprotectin predicts the clinical course of acute severe ulcerative colitis. Am J Gastroenterol. 2009;104:673–8.

32. Jensen MD, Kjeldsen J, Nathan T. Fecal calprotectin is equally sensitive in Crohn's disease affecting the small bowel and colon. Scand J Gastroenterol. 2011;46:694–700.

33. Thuijls G, Derikx JP, Prakken FJ, Huisman B, van BijnenIng AA, van HeurnEL BWA, et al. A pilot study on potential new plasma markers for diagnosis of acute appendicitis. Am J Emerg Med. 2011;29:256–60.

34. Bealer JF, Colgin M. S100A8/A9: a potential new diagnostic aid for acute appendicitis. Acad Emerg Med. 2010;17:333–6.

35. Carroccio A, Rocco P, Rabitti PG, Di Prima L, Forte GB, Cefalù AB, et al. Plasma calprotectin levels in patients suffering from acute pancreatitis. Dig Dis Sci. 2006;51:1749–53.

36. Sugi K, Saitoh O, Hirata I, Katsu K. Fecal lactoferrin as a marker for disease activity in inflammatory bowel disease: comparison with other neutrophil-derived proteins. Am J Gastroenterol. 1996;91:927–34.

37. Lee SL, Walsh AJ, Ho HS. Computed tomography and ultrasonography do not improve and may delay the diagnosis and treatment of acute appendicitis. Arch Surg. 2001;136:556–62.

38. Domínguez LC, Sanabria A, Vega V, Osorio C. Early laparoscopy for the evaluation of nonspecific abdominal pain: a critical appraisal of the evidence. Surg Endosc. 2011;25:10–8.

39. Maggio AQ, Reece-Smith AM, Tang TY, Sadat U, Walsh SR. Early laparoscopy versus active observation in acute abdominal pain: systematic review and meta-analysis. Int J Surg. 2008;6:400–3.

40. Schellekens DH, Hulsewé KW, van Acker BA, van Bijnen AA, de Jaegere TM, Sastrowijoto SH, et al. Evaluation of the diagnostic accuracy of plasma markers for early diagnosis in patients suspected for acute appendicitis. Acad Emerg Med. 2013;20(7):703–10.

3

Benefits of WSES guidelines application for the management of intra-abdominal infections

Belinda De Simone[1*], Federico Coccolini[2], Fausto Catena[1], Massimo Sartelli[3], Salomone Di Saverio[4], Rodolfo Catena[5], Antonio Tarasconi[6] and Luca Ansaloni[2]

Abstract

Introduction: The use of antibiotics is very high in the departments of Emergency and Trauma Surgery above all in the treatment of the intra-abdominal infections, to decrease morbidity and mortality rates; often the antimicrobial drugs are prescribed without a rationale and they are second-line antibiotics; this clinical practice increases costs without decreasing mortality.

Aim of our study is to report the results in the application to the clinical practice of the World Society Emergency Surgeons (WSES) guidelines for the management of intra-abdominal infections, at the department of Emergency and Trauma Surgery of the University Hospital of Parma (Italy) in 2012.

Methods: A retrospective observational analysis was carried out about patients admitted in the department of Emergency and Trauma Surgery of Parma (Italy), between January 2011 and December 2012. The data are expressed as percentages (%) and means (± SD). The results of the compared groups were analyzed using the Pearson's Chi-Square and Fisher's tests. For means involving continuous numerical data, the independent sample T test and the Mann–Whitney U-test were used for normally and abnormally distributed data, respectively (the data had been previously tested for normality using the Kolmogorov-Smirnov test). A p-value < 0.05 was considered statistically significant.

Results: Between January 2011 and December 2012, 2121 (968 in 2011 and 1153 in 2012) patients were admitted in the department of Emergency and Trauma Surgery (Italy) of Parma University Hospital with a diagnosis of acute IAI. Morbidity in 2012 was 10,2% compared to 22.7% in 2011 and mortality in 2012 was 1,1% compared to 3,2% in 2011 ($p < 0,05$). Costs for antibiotics in 2012 was 51392 euro, with a reduction of 31% compared to 2011.

Conclusions: This study demonstrates that an inexpensive and easily application of guidelines based on medicine evidence in the use of antibiotics can lead to a significative reduction of hospital costs with outcomes improvement.

Keywords: Intra-abdominal infections, Antibiotics, WSES guidelines, Cost-effectiveness

Introduction

Antibiotics are the essential drugs that we have to fight and prevent bacterial infectious diseases. Improper and excessive use of antibiotics is the major worldwide problem because it has an important economic impact on increasing healthcare costs, caused by the selection of multi-drug resistant bacteria, resulting in a longer hospital stay and an higher mortality [1]. For the World Health Organization (WHO), the rational use of drugs requires that patients receive medications appropriate to their clinical needs, in doses that meet their own individual requirements, for an adequate period of time and at the lowest cost, to them and their community [2]; because each antibiotic has different unit dose of daily administration, a specific standardized method to evaluate the in-hospital antibiotic use was suggested and periodically update by WHO, the ATC/DDD index (Anatomical Therapeutic Chemical/Defined Daily Dose): it is considered the universal parameter to calculate the antibiotic use intensity [3]. Furthermore, the use of

* Correspondence: desimoneB@hotmail.it
[1]Department of Emergency and Trauma Surgery, University Hospital of Parma, Via Gramsci 11, 43100 Parma, Italy
Full list of author information is available at the end of the article

antibiotic prophylaxis, according to standardized protocols, has been shown to prevent post-surgical wound infections, which are the primary cause of morbidity and mortality in patients undergoing surgery.

The use of antibiotics is very high in the departments of Emergency and Trauma Surgery, above all in the treatment of the intra-abdominal infections (IAIs) to decrease morbidity and mortality rates. Often the antimicrobial drugs are prescribed without a rationale and they are second-line antibiotics; this clinical practice increases costs without decreasing mortality [4]. Sartelli et al., during the 1st Congress of the World Society of Emergency Surgeons (WSES), discussed in a multidisciplinary approach these problems, approving evidence based recommendations for the management of IAIs [1]. According to the WSES guidelines, the initial antibiotic therapy for IAIs is always empiric because the patient is often critically ill and microbiological data (culture and susceptibility results) usually take at least 48 hours to become fully available [1]. IAIs are classified as uncomplicated and complicated. The uncomplicated infections involve a single organ and do not spread to the peritoneum (antimicrobial therapy is indicated as first line approach); the complicated IAIs proceed beyond a single organ, causing localized or diffuse peritonitis and need for surgical and antimicrobial therapy.

IAIs are divided in 3 sub-groups: 1. community acquired extrabiliary infections: gastroduodenal perforations, small bowel perforations, acute appendicitis, acute diverticulitis, large bowel perforations; 2. community acquired biliary infections:acute cholecystitis, cholangitis; 3. hospital acquired infections: postoperative and non-postoperative peritonitis. Once the diagnosis of intra-abdominal infection is suspected, it is necessary to begin, as soon as possible, the empiric antimicrobial therapy, even if routine use of antimicrobial therapy is not appropriate for all patients with intra-abdominal infections. Source control should be obtained as early as possible after the diagnosis of postoperative intra-abdominal peritonitis has been confirmed [1].

The principles of empiric antibiotic treatment should be defined according to the most frequently isolated germs, always taking into consideration the local trend of antibiotic resistance. The choice of the antimicrobial regimen depends on the source of intra-abdominal infection, the risk factors for specific microorganisms, the resistance patterns and the clinical patient's condition. In uncomplicated IAIs, when the focus of infection is treated effectively by surgical excision of the involved tissue, the administration of antibiotics is unnecessary beyond prophylaxis. In complicated IAIs, antimicrobial therapy is mandatory. Hospital acquired infections are commonly caused by larger and more resistant flora, and for these infections, complex multi-drug regimens are always recommended [1].

We report the results in the application to the clinical practice of the WSES guidelines for the management of intra-abdominal infections at the Department of Emergency and Trauma Surgery of Parma University Hospital (Italy) in 2012.

Materials and methods

A retrospective observational analysis was carried out about patients with IAIs admitted to the Department of Emergency and Trauma Surgery of Parma University Hospital, between January 2011 and December 2012 The following parameters were collected: patients demographics, diagnosis, surgical procedures performed, antibiotic treatment, length of hospital stay (day) and outcomes. In 2011 and 2012, the same antibiotic drugs were available in our hospital, at the same price.

In 2011, no guidelines were used, whereas in 2012 WSES IAIs guidelines were utilized. (Figure 1) Community acquired extra-biliary IAIs (gastro-duodenal perforations, small bowel perforations, acute appendicitis, acute diverticulitis, large bowel perforations) were treated with Ampicillin/Sulbactam or Ciprofloxacin (in patients with allergic reaction to Penicillin) +/− Metronidazole.

Community acquired biliary IAIs (cholecystitis, cholangitis) were treated with Ampicillin/Sulbactam or Ciprofloxacin, if allergic reaction to Penicillin, +/− Metronidazole, as first line therapy, if an ESBL or MDR pathogens were suspected.

Hospital acquired IAIs needed for a large spectrum therapy (high risk of ESBL or MDR pathogens involved) with Piperacillin/Tazobactam or Meropenem +/−Fluconazole +/− Tigecycline. Critically ill patients were often hospitalized in ICU.

All antibiotic treatments started with an i.v. administration followed by oral switch when appropriate (normal infection signs, normal infection laboratory parameters and resumption of oral feeding).

The data are expressed as percentages (%) and means (± SD). The results of the compared groups were analyzed using the Pearson's Chi-Square and Fisher's Exact tests, as appropriate, for proportions involving discrete data. The Fisher's Exact test was used when the data were unequally distributed among the cells of the table, when the expected frequency of any cell was less than 5, or when the total number (N) was less than 50.

For means involving continuous numerical data, the independent sample T test and the Mann–Whitney U-test were used for normally and abnormally distributed data, respectively (the data had been previously tested

Type of patient	Hospital acquired IAIs	Hospital extra-biliary acquired IAIs
Non critical pts; risk factors for MDR	Piperacillin + Tigecycline + Fluconazole	
Critically ill pts; risk factors for MDR		Piperacillin + Tigecycline + Echinocandin (Caspofungin,Anidulafungin, Micofungin) or Meropenem Imipenem Doripenem + Teicoplanin + Echinocandin

Type of patient	Community acquired extra-biliary IAIs	Community acquired biliary IAIs
Stable pts; no risk factors for ESBL	Amoxicillin/Clavulanate or, if pt allergic to beta-lactams, Ciprofloxacin+ Metronidazole	Amoxicillin/Clavulanate or, if pt allergic to beta-lactams, Ciprofloxacin+ Metronidazole
Stable pts; risk factors for ESBL	Ertapenem or Tigecycline	Tigecycline
Critically ill pts; no risk factors for ESBL	Pipericillin/Tazobactam	Pipericillin/Tazobactam
Critically ill pts; risk factors for ESBL	Meropenem or Imipenem +/- Fluconazole	Piperacillin + Tigecycline +/- Fluconazole

Figure 1 WSES IAIs guidelines.

for normality using the Kolmogorov-Smirnov test). A p-value < 0.05 was considered statistically significant.

Results

Between January 2011 and December 2012, 2121 (968 in 2011 and 1153 in 2012) patients were admitted in the Department of Emergency and Trauma Surgery of Parma University Hospital with a diagnosis of acute IAI. The mean age was 58,8 years (SD ⊥ 9,1) in 2011 and 59,1 in 2012 (SD ± 8.9); (p = n.s.). Male/ female ratio was 1,04 in 2012 and 1,02 in 2011 (p = n.s.). Complicated IAIs were 41,1% in 2012 and 38,7% in 2011. (p = n.s.).

Empirical treatment was performed in 91,8% of patients in 2012 and in 95,3% of patients in 2011 (p = n.s.).

In the Figure 2 patients were divided according to admission diagnosis: the majority of patients were affected by acute cholecystitis, followed by acute appendicitis and complicated abdominal hernias, including incisional hernias, without any statistical difference in distribution between 2011 and 2012. (p = n.s.). Surgical procedures, performed as source control on these patients, are shown in Figure 3: again there was not any statistical difference in distribution between 2011 and 2012. (p = n.s.).

All patients with IAIs were treated with antibiotics according to WSES guidelines.

The administrated antibiotic treatments is shown in Figure 4. Between 2011 and 2012 there was a statistical significant difference for 5 antibiotic regimens: Ampicillin/ Sulbactam, Ciprofloxacin plus Metronidazole, Meropenem,

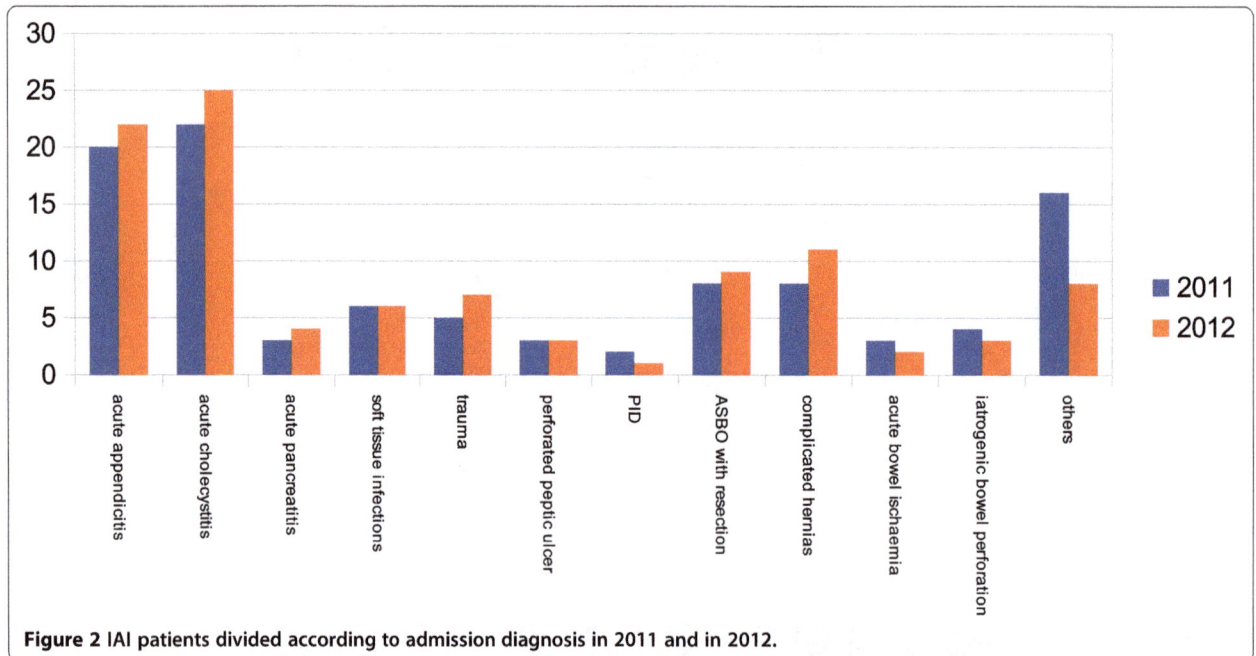

Figure 2 IAI patients divided according to admission diagnosis in 2011 and in 2012.

Ampicillin/Sulbactam plus Metronidazole, and Piperacillin/Tazobactam. The oral switch was performed in 540/ 968 (55,7%) patients in 2011 and in 691/1153 (59,9%) in 2012. (p = n.s.).

The mean length of intravenous therapy was 4.9 days (range 21–1) (DS 3,67) and the mean lenght of oral therapy was 3.23 days (range 13–3) (DS 3,18) in 2012, whereas the mean length of intravenous therapy was 5.4 days (range 33–2) (DS 4,22) and the mean lenght of oral therapy was

4,59 days (range 18–4) (DS 2,25); (p = n.s.) in 2011. Mean lenght of hospital stay was 7.5 days (range 43–1) (DS 6,08) in 2012 and 8,9 days (range 49–1) (DS 5,36) in 2011 (p = n.s.).

In-hospital mortality rate was 1.10% in 2012 vs 3.2% in 2011 (p < 0.05.) and morbidity was 10,2% in 2012 vs 22,7% in 2011 (p < 0.05). Costs for antibiotics in 2012 was 51392 euro compared to 75327 euro in 2011 (31,7% reduction). More common bacteria isolates were comparable between 2011 and 2012.

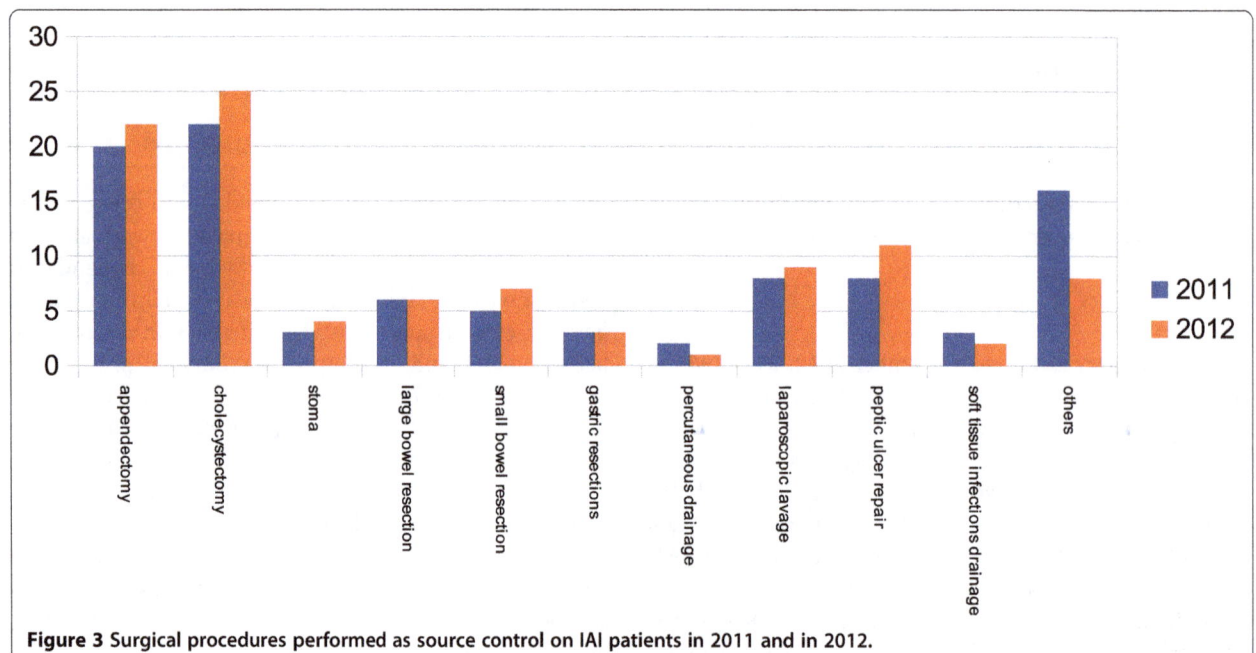

Figure 3 Surgical procedures performed as source control on IAI patients in 2011 and in 2012.

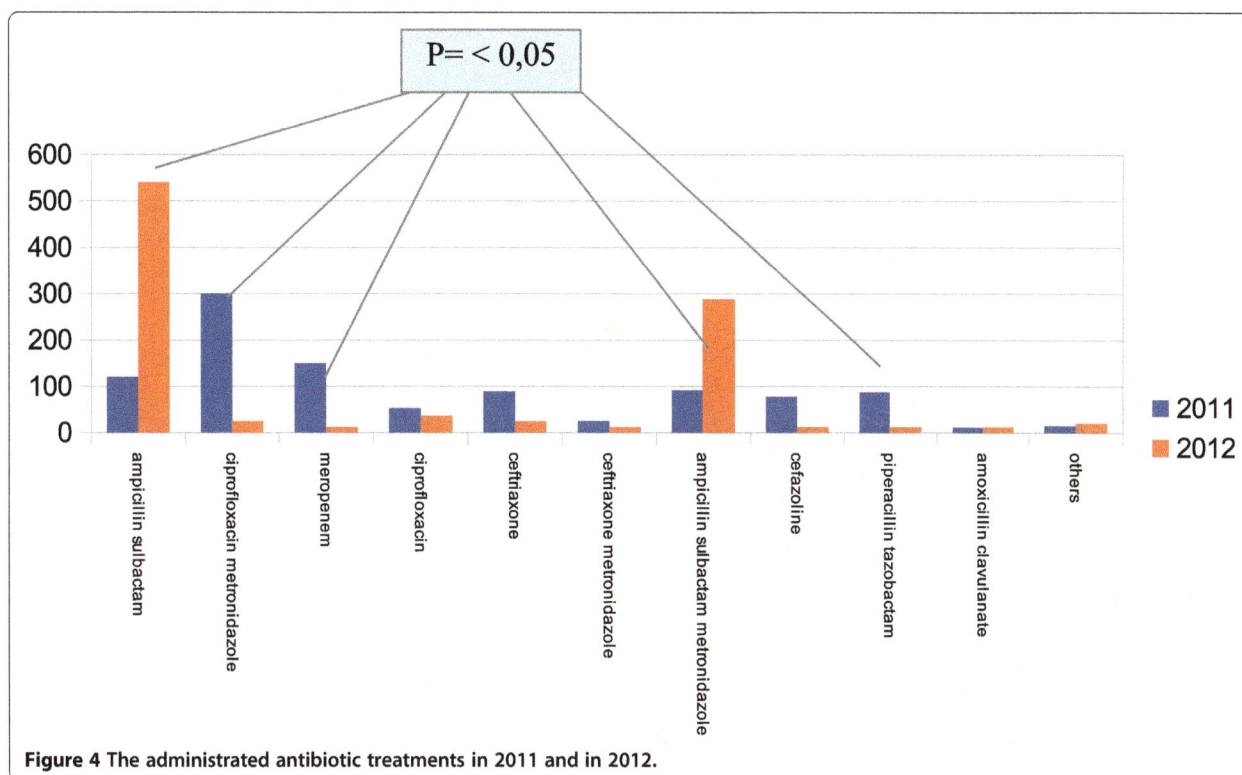

Figure 4 The administrated antibiotic treatments in 2011 and in 2012.

Discussion

It's worldwide accepted that a remarkable amount of antibiotics used in hospitalized patients is excessive or inappropriate; this irrational use of antibiotics leads to the emergence of drug resistant bacteria, associated with an higher rates of death, illness and prolonged hospital stay, with a considerable increasing of the healthcare costs. Besides the research involved with the development of new antibiotics has no progressed in parallel with the increasing rates of resistance, leaving clinicians with fewer options, often more expensive, for the treatment of some resistant infections.

In the recent literature, several studies argue on the necessity of the diffusion of valid guidelines, based on clinical evidence and on the bacterial resistance epidemiology, to rationalize the use of antibiotics [2-6]. Many authors highlight on the importance of the application of validated guidelines in clinical practice and of the surgical prophylaxis protocols, associated with adequate education programs for physicians and surgeons on the "diligent" prescription and administration of antibiotics, in reducing healthcare costs with considerable benefits in terms of cost-effectiveness [7-11].

In the present study, the application of WSES guidelines for the management of intra-abdominal infections was highly effective in reducing the number of unnecessary second-line antibiotics prescriptions and costs; it led to a 31% reduction of costs for antimicrobial drugs,

keeping low morbidity and low mortality rates. The source control associated with an adequate antimicrobial therapy are efficacy to decrease morbidity and mortality rates.

This study demonstrates that an inexpensive and easily application of guidelines based on medicine evidence in the use of antibiotics can lead to a significant reduction of hospital costs. There is an urgent need to develop education programs, to spread valid guidelines in the use of antimicrobial agents, to limit the emergence of bacterial resistance, responsible of the increasing in the incidence of "difficult" infectious diseases and deaths, and to reduce costs resulting from this global problem [10-12].

Competing interests
The authors declare that they have no competing interests.

Authors' contributions
BDS collected data and wrote the manuscript. FCt did the statistical analysis and reviewed the manuscript. All authors read and approved the final manuscript.

Author details
[1]Department of Emergency and Trauma Surgery, University Hospital of Parma, Via Gramsci 11, 43100 Parma, Italy. [2]Department of General and Emergency Surgery, Papa Giovanni XIII Hospital, Bergamo, Italy. [3]Department of Surgery, Macerata Hospital, Macerata, Italy. [4]Department of Surgery, Maggiore Hospital of Bologna, Bologna, Italy. [5]Oxford University, Oxford, Great Britain. [6]Ospedali Civili di Brescia, Brescia, Italy.

References

1. Sartelli M, Viale P, Catena F, Ansaloni L, Moore E, Malangoni M, et al. 2013 WSES guidelines for management of intra-abdominal infections. World J Emerg Surg. 2013;8(1):3.
2. Antimicrobial resistence:global report on surveillance 2014,WHO Library Cataloguing-in-Publication Data ISBN 978 92 4 156474 8 (NLM classification: QV 250)
3. Fanning M, McKean M, Seymour K, Pillans P, Scott I. Adherence to guideline based antibiotic treatment for acute exacerbations of COPD in an Australian tertiary hospital. Intern Med J. 2014;44(9):903–10.
4. Avorn J, Solomon DH. Cultural and economic factors that (mis)shape antibiotic use: the nonpharmacologic basis of therapeutics. Ann Intern Med. 2000;133(2):128–35.
5. Bantar C, Sartori B, Vesco E, Heft C, Saúl M, Salamone F, et al. A hospital wide intervention program to optimize the quality of antibiotics, use: impact on prescribing practice, antibiotic consumption, cost savings and bacterial resistance. Clin Infect Dis. 2003;37(2):180–6.
6. Rodrigues RM, Fontes AM, Mantese OC, Martins RS, Jorge MT. Impact of an intervention in the use of sequential antibiotic therapy in a Brazilian University Hospital. Rev Soc Bras Med Trop. 2013;46(1):50–4.
7. Nausheen S, Hammad R, Khan A. Rational use of antibiotics–a quality improvement initiative in hospital setting. J Pak Med Assoc. 2013;63(1):60–4.
8. Fonseca LG, de Oliveira CL. Audit of antibiotic use in a Brazilian University Hospital. Braz J Infect Dis. 2004;8(4):272–80. Epub 2004 Nov 19.
9. Rüttimann S, Keck B, Hartmeier C, Maetzel A, Bucher HC. Long term antibiotic cost savings from a comprehensive intervention program in a medical department of a University affiliated teaching Hospital. Clin Infect Dis. 2004;38(3):348–56.
10. Mylotte JM, Neff M. Trends in antibiotic use and cost and influence of case mix and infection rate on antibiotic-prescribing in a long term care facility. Am J Infect Control. 2003;31(1):18–25.
11. Natsch S, Hekster YA, de Jong R, Heerdink ER, Herings RM, van der Meer JW. Application of the ATC/DDD methodology to monitor antibiotic drug use. Eur J Clin Microbiol Infect Dis. 1998;17(1):20–4.
12. Sartelli M, Catena F, Ansaloni L, Leppaniemi A, Taviloglu K, van Goor H, et al. Complicated Intra-Abdominal Infections Observational European study (CIAO Study). World J Emerg Surg. 2012;7(1):36. Doi: 10.1186/1749-7922-7-36.

4

Trauma resuscitation requiring massive transfusion: a descriptive analysis of the role of ratio and time

Ruben Peralta[1], Adarsh Vijay[1], Ayman El-Menyar[2,3]*, Rafael Consunji[1], Husham Abdelrahman[1], Ashok Parchani[1], Ibrahim Afifi[1], Ahmad Zarour[1,3], Hassan Al-Thani[1] and Rifat Latifi[1,4]

Abstract

Objective: We aimed to evaluate whether early administration of high plasma to red blood cells ratios influences outcomes in injured patients who received massive transfusion protocol (MTP).

Methods: A retrospective analysis was conducted at the only level 1 national trauma center in Qatar for all adult patients(≥18 years old) who received MTP (≥10 units) of packed red blood cell (PRBC) during the initial 24 h post traumatic injury. Data were analyzed with respect to FFB:PRBC ratio [(high ≥ 1:1.5) (HMTP) vs. (low < 1:1.5) (LMTP)] given at the first 4 h post-injury and also between (>4 and 24 h). Mortality, multiorgan failure (MOF) and infectious complications were studied as well.

Results: During the study period, a total of 4864 trauma patients were admitted to the hospital, 1.6 % (n = 77) of them met the inclusion criteria. Both groups were comparable with respect to initial pH, international normalized ratio, injury severity score, revised trauma score and development of infectious complications. However, HMTP was associated with lower crude mortality (41.9 vs. 78.3 %, p = 0.001) and lower rate of MOF (48.4 vs. 87.0 %, p = 0.001). The number of deaths was 3 times higher in LMTP in comparison to HMTP within the first 30 days (36 vs. 13 cases). The majority of deaths occurred within the first 24 h (80.5 % in LMTP and 69 % in HMTP) and particularly within the first 6 h (55 vs. 46 %).

Conclusions: Aggressive attainment of high FFP/PRBC ratios as early as 4 h post-injury can substantially improve outcomes in trauma patients.

Keywords: Trauma, Transfusion ratio, Massive transfusion protocol, Outcome

Background

In severe trauma patients, exsanguinating hemorrhage is the most common cause of early death, which occurs within the first few hours of hospital admission [1, 2]. Up to 30 % of severely injured patients are coagulopathic upon arrival to the emergency department [3]. Moreover, the coagulopathy status developed early post traumatic injury invariably complicates the massive blood transfusion and damage control resuscitation pattern and outcome. Prior reports of the military and civilian experience that advocated the use of higher ratios of fresh frozen plasma (FFP) to packed red blood cells (PRBCs) showed an improvement in survival of trauma patients [4, 5]. These studies have addressed the implications of early aggressive hemostatic resuscitation to control coagulopathy, which potentially reduces the mortality rate. However, some investigators suggested that transfusion of inappropriate volumes of plasma might result in a higher incidence of infection or transfusion-associated acute lung injury [6–8]. According to the current guidelines of hemostatic resuscitation, severe trauma patients should be supplemented with a considerable amount of blood products (PRBC, FFP and platelet) in an early and continuous manner [9]. However, there is no consensus on the optimal ratio of FFP to PRBC for trauma patients requiring massive transfusion protocol

* Correspondence: traumaresearch@hamad.qa
[2]Clinical Research, Trauma Surgery Section, Hamad General Hospital, HMC, PO Box 3050, Doha, Qatar
[3]Clinical Medicine, Weill Cornell Medical College, Doha, Qatar
Full list of author information is available at the end of the article

(MTP). Borgman et al. [4] proposed a predictive model of MTP in severe trauma patients. The authors suggested that a high ratio (FFP: RBC) (≥15 TASH score) was an independent predictor of survival; whereas, the low ratio (<15 TASH score) was correlated well with higher complication rates.

There is still ongoing debate to define the most appropriate time and ratio of MTP that should be given to patients undergoing hemostatic resuscitation. Specifically, the appropriate timing and resuscitation ratio during the early hours of severe trauma remain unclear. Herein, we aimed to evaluate whether early administration of high plasma ratios to RBC influences outcomes in trauma patients receiving massive blood transfusion.

Methods

We conducted a retrospective analysis of the prospectively collected data of all adult trauma (≥18 years old) patients who received MTP. The study was conducted at the Hamad Trauma Center which is the only level 1 national trauma referral center in Qatar from January 2010 to December 2012. Blood bank records were used to identify patients who received more than 6 units PRBC. The records were then screened for subset of patients who received more than 10 units PRBC in the first 24 h. The medical records of patients were obtained to evaluate the ratio based on actual blood products transfused, the actual time of transfusion along with the details of other comorbid conditions, complications and outcome. All patients who died on arrival were excluded. We defined MTP as the infusion of ≥10 units of PRBC over the initial 24 h post-injury [10]. Injury Severity Scores (ISS) and Revised Trauma Scores (RTS) were collected from the hospital trauma database for all cases. Based on FFP: PRBC ratio at 4 h post-injury; patients were categorized into two groups i.e. high MTP (HMTP) who received FFP: PRBC ratio ≥ 1:1.5 and low MTP (LMTP) who received a FFP: PRBC ratio of < 1:1.5. The ratio of FFP: PRBC administered was calculated for each patient at 4 h and the ratios were also calculated based on the blood products given from 4 to 24 h post injury in the same cohort to look for the effect of timing and transfusion ratios. Our analysis is based on the actual transfusion of blood products and MTP of our institution including 6 units of RBC, 6 units of FFP, and 6 units of platelets. Two units of uncross-matched blood were available to each patient without delay. All patients were followed-up until hospital discharge or death. The outcomes measures included mortality, 1st MTP International Normalized Ratio (INR), multiorgan failure (MOF) and infectious complications.

We intended to analyze the outcomes in relation to the transfusion ratios calculated initially at 4 h and at 4–24 h.

In particular, we looked at the effect of early (<4 h) MTP ratios on the final outcome.

Definitions

The diagnosis of MOF was based on a maximum Marshall Multiple Organ Dysfunction score > 5. Ventilator associated pneumonia (VAP) diagnosis was based on the quantitative culture threshold of ≥10^4 CFU/mL for broncho-alveolar lavage [11]. Blood stream infection (BSI) is a positive blood culture that not necessarily related to an indwelling central venous catheter. Whereas, line related infection was defined as catheter-related blood stream infections (CRBSI) which required positive peripheral cultures with the identical organism obtained from either a positive semi-quantitative culture (≥15 CFU/segment), or positive quantitative culture (≥10^3 CFU/segment) from a catheter segment specimen. Urinary tract infection (UTI) was confirmed if the urine specimen revealed ≥10^5 organisms/ml. This study was approved by the medical research center at Hamad Medical Corporation, Qatar (IRB # 11153/11).

Statistical analysis

Data were presented as proportions, mean ± standard deviation (SD) or median as appropriate. Baseline demographic characteristics, clinical presentation, and outcomes were compared according to FFP: PRBC ratio at 4 h (HMTP vs. LMTP). Pearson chi-square (X^2) test was used for categorical variables and student-t test for continuous variables. The Fisher's exact test was used, if the expected cell frequencies were below 5. A significant difference was considered when the 2-tailed p value was less than 0.05. Data analysis was carried out using the Statistical Package for Social Sciences version 18 (SPSS Inc. USA).

Results

During the 3- year study period, there were 4864 trauma admissions, of which 100 patients received massive blood transfusion. Finally, the study included 77 (1.6 %) cases in which ratios were attainable and the remaining 23 cases were excluded as they did not receive FFP within the first 4 h post-injury and so no ratio could be calculated. The mean age of patients was 33.7 ± 14 years and the majority of them were males (91 %). Blunt trauma accounted for most of cases (88.3 %). The median ISS, GCS and RTS were 29 (8–75), 4.4 ± 3.8, and 4 (1.2-7.8), respectively (Table 1). Lung contusion (62.3 %), head injury (50 %), pelvic (46.7 %) and rib fracture (35.5 %) were the most commonly associated injuries. The most frequent used operative interventions included exploratory laparatomy (66.2 %), Thoracotomy (24.7 %), repair of major vessels (22 %) and angioembolization (13 %). Among patients who underwent emergency operative interventions, 39 %

Table 1 Demographics and presentation of study cohort (n = 77)

Variable		Variable	
Age (mean ± SD; years)	33.7 ± 14	**Injured body region**	
Males	69 (90.8 %)	Head	32 (50 %)
Blunt trauma	68 (88.3 %)	Lung contusion	48 (62.3)
Mechanism of injury		Rib fracture	27 (35.5 %)
Traffic Pedestrian	22 (28.6 %)	Pelvic fracture	35 (46.7 %)
Traffic Driver	20 (26 %)	Long bone fracture	24 (32.0 %)
Traffic Passenger	12 (15.6 %)	Spleen	21 (27.3 %)
Fall From Height	10 (13 %)	Liver	25 (32.5 %)
fall of heavy object	5 (6.5 %)	Bowel	15 (19.5 %)
crush injury	1 (1.3 %)	Pancreas	9 (11.7 %)
Gunshot	1 (1.3 %)	Cardiac	4 (5.2 %)
Stab	5 (6.5 %)	**Operative interventions**	
SBP (mmHg)	85.2 ± 35.5	Exploratory Laparotomy	51 (66.2 %)
Heart rate (b/min)	119.3 ± 27.6	Thoracotomy	19 (24.7 %)
Temperature in ED (°C)	36.1 ± 0.66	Repair of major vessels	17 (22.1 %)
FAST positive	41 (53.2 %)	Chest tube insertion	7 (9.1 %)
Laboratory Findings		Craniotomy	1 (1.3 %)
Initial Hemoglobin (g/dL)	10.3 ± 2.6	External fixation	6 (7.8 %)
Initial Platelets (×10^9/L)	187.7 ± 69.8	ORIF	1 (1.3 %)
Initial INR	1.6 ± 1.2	Mangled extremity amputation	3 (3.9 %)
Initial APTT (median)	30.3 (22–149)	Successful Angioembolization	10 (13 %)
Initial Fibrinogen (g/L)	0.96 ± 0.58	**Intra-operative status**	
Initial pH	7.1 ± 0.2	Stable + damage control	30 (39 %)
Initial HCO3 (mmol/L)	15.6 ± 3.8	Unstable + damage control	24 (31.2 %)
Saline	3739 ± 1411	Stable + procedure completed	8 (10.4 %)
Ringer Lactate (mmol/L)	1300 ± 958	unstable + procedure completed	1 (1.3 %)
Blood products transfused <4 h		**Intra-operative mortality**	13 (20.6 %)
PRBC	10.9 ± 4.9 [10 (2–23)]	**ICU LOS**	3 (1–45)
FFP	6.5 ± 3.8 [6(1–21)]	**Overall Hospital LOS (days)**	1.5 (1–112)
Platelet	6.4 ± 3.4 [6(1–22)]	**Hospital LOS**	28 (8–112)
Severity Scores		**Multi Organ Failure**	49 (63.6 %)
Injury Severity Score	29 (8–75)	**Overall mortality**	55 (71.4 %)
Revised Trauma Score	4 (1.2–7.8)		
Glasgow Coma Score	3 (3–15)		

FFP Fresh frozen plasma, *PRBC* packed red-blood-cells, *ICU* Intensive Care Unit, *LOS* length of stay, *FAST* Focused Assisted Sonography for Trauma, *INR* international normalized ratio, *APTT* Activated Partial Thromboplastin Time, *SBP* Systolic Blood Pressure, *ORIF* Open reduction internal fixation
bold means heading variable non-bold means subheadings of the main variable

had damage control surgery. The intra-operative mortality was 17 %. Focused assessment with sonography for trauma (FAST) was positive in more than half of the cases (53 %). The median intensive care unit (ICU) stay was 3 (1–45) days, the overall hospital length of stay was 2 (1–112) days and the hospital length of stay for patients who survived was 28 (8–112). Transport time to the trauma center was 64 ± 32.3 min. According to our institutional policy, blood transfusion begins only

after arrival to the hospital, whereas prehospital crystalloid (normal saline) administration is initiated by EMS.

Table 2 shows the clinical presentation and outcome of patients based on FFP: PRBC ratio (HMTP and LMTP) within the first 4 h. The mean age of the LMTP group was higher (37.6 ± 16.5 vs. 29.7 ± 9.5; P = 0.03) in comparison to HMTP group. However, both the HMTP (n = 31) and LMTP (n = 46) groups were comparable with respect to gender, mechanism of injury, prehospital intubation,

Table 2 Clinical presentation and complications based on high and low transfusion ratios within the first 4 h post-injury

	HMTP (n = 31)	LMTP (n = 46)	P value
Age (mean ± SD)	29.7 ± 9.5	37.6 ± 16.5	0.03
Blunt injury (%)	87.1	89.1	0.53
Penetrating injury (%)	12.9	10.9	
Saline (Prehospital)	1193 ± 666	1197 ± 737	0.97
Transport Time (min.)	64.4 ± 29.8	63.7 ± 34.3	0.93
Prehospital interventions			
Intubation	36 %	41 %	0.60
Thoracostomy	3 %	9 %	0.32
Laboratory findings			
Initial Hemoglobin (mean ± SD)	10.6 ± 3	10 ± 2.3	0.37
Initial INR	1.3 (1–10)	1.3 (1–3)	0.09
Initial pH	7.2 ± 0.14	7.1 ± 0.2	0.09
*1ST MTP INR	1.35 (1–2)	1.7 (1–12)	0.09
1st MTP pH	7.2 ± 0.16	7.1 ± 0.23	0.04
2nd MTP INR	1.1 (1–3)	1.5 (1–3)	0.03
2nd MTP pH	7.3 ± 0.1	7.2 ± 0.2	0.04
3rd MTP INR	1.1 (1–2)	1.2 (1–10)	0.17
3rd MTP pH	7.2 ± 0.18	7.2 ± 0.2	0.55
Saline	3456 ± 1591	3929 ± 1258	0.15
Ringer Lactate	883 ± 431	1550 ± 1099	0.01
Saline + Ringer lactate	3883 ± 1580	4771 ± 1466	0.01
Cryoprecipitate	9.5 ± 0.7	8.4 ± 3.5	0.70
Calcium Gluconate/Chloride	1933 ± 1334	2250 ± 1674	0.54
Sodium Bicardonate	92.9 ± 73	152.3 ± 96	0.05
Fibrinogen	2800 ± 1095	3000 ± 1341	0.77
Factor VII	5.2 ± 2.4	3.8 ± 1.3	0.19
Injuries			
Head injury	52	48.6	0.80
Lung contusion	68	59	0.42
Rib fracture	47	28	0.10
Pelvic fracture	52	43	0.47
Long bone fracture	45	23	0.04
Spleen	19	33	0.2
Liver	26	37	0.3
Cardiac	0	9	0.09
Injury Severity Score	29.4 ± 11.6	32.5 ± 10.7	0.24
Revised Trauma Score	5.2 ± 2.3	5.2 ± 2.02	0.97
Glasgow Coma Score	8.5 ± 5	8 ± 5.1	0.72
Hyperkalemia (%)	17.2	29.3	0.19
Hypomagnesemia (%)	68.2	61	0.42
Hypocalcemia (%)	93	82	0.17

Table 2 Clinical presentation and complications based on high and low transfusion ratios within the first 4 h post-injury (Continued)

Complications			
Ventilator-associated Pneumonia (%)	32.3	14	0.05
Wound infection (%)	32.3	18.6	0.14
Bloodstream Infection (%)	6.5	11.6	0.37
CRBSI (%)	3.2	7	0.44
Urinary tract infections (%)	3.2	4.7	0.62
ACS (%)	6.5	2.2	0.35

HMTP high transfusion ratios, *LMTP* low transfusion ratios, *INR*, international normalized ratio, *ACS* abdominal compartment syndrome, *CRBSI* Catheter related Blood Stream Infection, *MTP* massive transfusion protocol

thoracotomy, volume of normal saline administration, initial hemoglobin reading, INR, arterial pH and severity of injury (ISS & RTS). The incidence of hyperkalemia, hypomagnesemia and hypocalcemia were also comparable in the two groups. The mean arterial pH was higher among HMTP group post 1st MTP (7.2 ± 0.16 *vs.* 7.1 ± 0.23; P = 0.04) and 2nd MTP (7.3 ± 0.1 *vs.* 7.2 ± 0.2; P = 0.04) as compared to LMTP group. HMTP patients had better mean INR values after the 2nd MTP shipment (1.1 (1–3) *vs.* 1.5(1–3); p = 0.03) than LMTP. Significantly greater amount of Ringer lactate (1550 ± 1099 *vs.* 883 ± 431; p = 0.01) and combination of saline and Ringer lactate (4771 ± 1466 *vs.* 3883 ± 1580; P = 0.01) were transfused to patients with LMTP.

Though, the frequency of VAP, wound infection and abdominal compartment syndrome were higher in the HMTP group, these trends did not reach statistical significance. However, BSI and UTI were non-significantly higher in LMTP group (Fig. 1).

The overall mortality was 63.6 % (Table 3). Patients who died mainly had lung contusion (42.9 %), head injury (29.9 %), pelvic fracture (28.6 %), liver injury (24.7 %) and rib fractures (23.4 %). Moreover, significant number of patients in HMTP group who died had

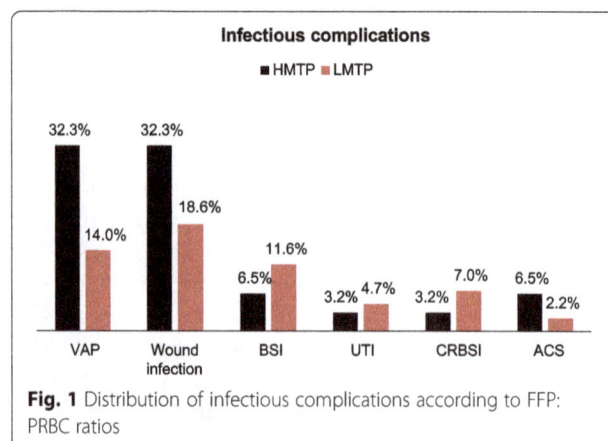

Fig. 1 Distribution of infectious complications according to FFP: PRBC ratios

Table 3 Outcome based on transfusion ratios

	HMTP (n = 31)	LMTP (n = 46)	P value
Mortality by associated injuries (ratios at <4 h)			
Head injury	88.9	55.6	0.07
Lung contusion	69.2	66.7	0.86
Rib fracture	66.7	27.8	0.01
Pelvic fracture	53.8	44	0.55
Long bone fracture	30.8	23.5	0.61
Spleen	15.4	27.8	0.37
Liver	30.8	41.7	0.48
Cardiac	0.0	8.3	0.28
Outcomes* based on MTP ratios calculated at <4 h			
Multi Organ Failure (%)	48.4	87	0.001
Mortality (%)	41.9	78.3	0.001
Outcomes* based on MTP ratios calculated at 4–24 h			
Multiorgan failure (%)	58.3	72.7	0.29
Mortality (%)	46.7	63.6	0.24

*It represents the overall outcome (MOF and mortality) and its correlation with the transfusion ratios calculated initially at 4 h and at 4-24 h

Fig. 2 Outcome according to time post-injury (hours) and transfusion ratio (HMTP vs. LMTP) (**a**) multiorgan failure (MOF) (**b**) overall mortality

more rib fractures (66.7 % vs. 27.8 %; P = 0.01) than LMTP group. A non-significantly higher proportion of patients in LMTP group died within 6 h post-injury in comparison to HMTP. During the early period of resuscitation (<4 h), the incidence of MOF (48.4 % vs. 87.0 %, p = 0.001) and crude mortality (41.9 % vs.78.3 %, p = 0.001) were significantly lower in HMTP compared to LMTP group. However, in the later period (4–24 h) MOF and mortality were comparable among the two groups (Fig. 2).

Figure 3 demonstrates the time to all-cause mortality in those who received LMTP vs. HMPT (<4 h). The number of deaths was 3 times higher in LMTP in comparison to HMTP within the first 30 days (36 vs. 13 cases). The vast majority of deaths occurred within the first 24 h (80.5 % in LMTP and 69 % in HMTP) and particularly within the first 6 h (55 % vs. 46 %).

Discussion

The present study evaluates the implication of FFP to PRBC ratio and its appropriate timing in trauma patients who required MTP. Our findings support the survival advantage of attaining high FFP to PRBC ratio for trauma patients who are identified early (within the first 4 h post-injury). Historically, Kashuk et al. [12] suggested a 'bloody vicious cycle' in which hemorrhage, cellular shock and tissue injury contributed to the formation of the lethal triad of coagulopathy, hypothermia, and acidosis. About 24 % of severely injured patients had acute traumatic coagulopathy on the hospital arrival [3]. Recent evidence suggests that co-agulopathy should be thought of as a primary event, which

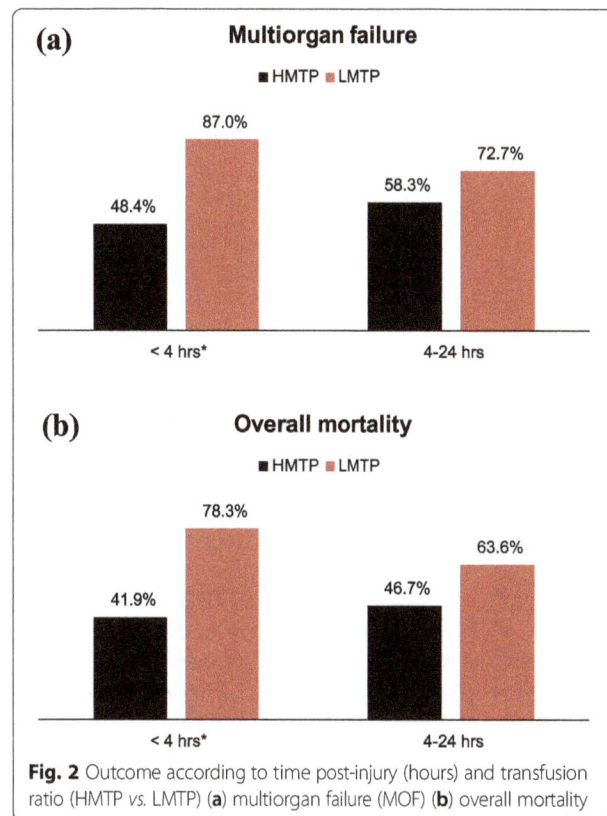

is independently associated with detrimental outcomes. Therefore, more attention has been given to control the worse outcomes of acute traumatic coagulopathy through hemostatic resuscitation which improves patient outcomes [13]. Particularly, the role of FFP in managing traumatic co-agulopathy is well documented. Despite the fact that use of high transfusion ratios is still a debatable issue, the majority of studies supported early and aggressive plasma use to attain FFP: PRBC transfusion ratios as high as 1:1 [4, 14, 15]. However, in the current practice there is no consensus on the optimal cut-off between adequately high and low plasma to PRBC ratios. Table 4 presents a comparison of several studies with respect to different FFP: PRBC cut-off ratios, timing and outcomes [4, 5, 14–24].

Our study revealed a significant improvement in the crude mortality and MOF rate when a FFP: PRBC transfusion ratio ≥1:1.5 was attainable within the initial 4 h of admission. As it have been shown in Fig. 3; the number of deaths within the first 30 days was 3 times higher in LMTP group and most deaths occurred within the first 24 h and particularly within the first 6 h in the 2 study groups.

Comparable survival benefit was documented in other studies that have used similar high transfusion ratios at different time durations [14–16]. However, achievement of such ratio as early as in the first 4 h and its impact

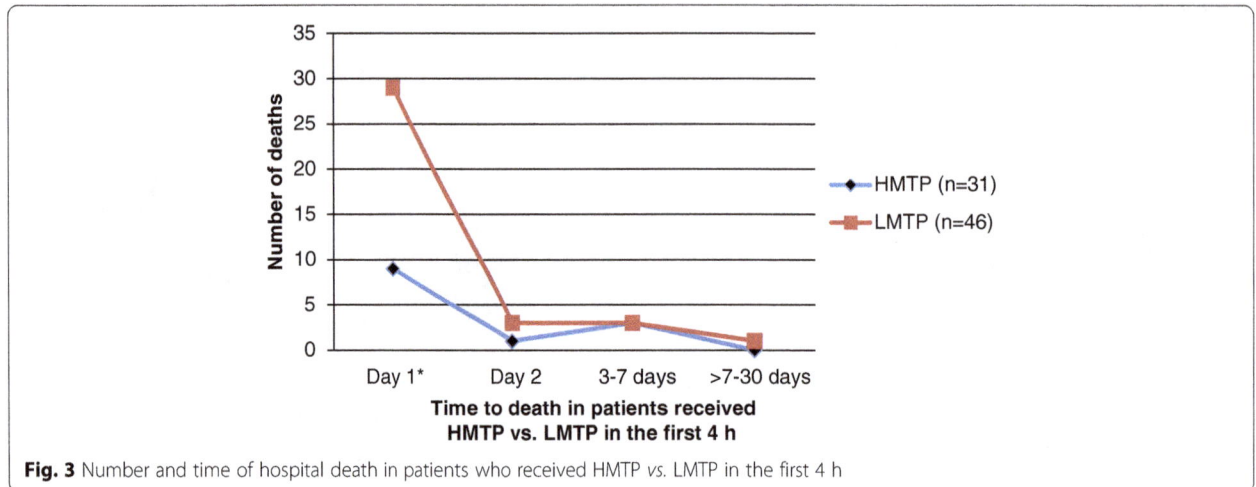

Fig. 3 Number and time of hospital death in patients who received HMTP vs. LMTP in the first 4 h

on patient outcome has been described recently by Mitra et al. [19]. Consistent with our findings, the authors reported survival benefit for higher FFP: PRBC ratios during the first 4 h of resuscitation in severely injured blunt trauma patients. Moreover, the low FFP: PRBC ratio during the early phase was independently associated with the risk of mortality.

Of note, the improvement in mortality and MOF rates with high transfusion ratios were observed only during the early period of hemostatic resuscitation and were not seen later on (>4 – 24 h) in our study. Hence, we believe that the survival benefit observed in other studies when the ratios were calculated at 24 h is possibly a dilution effect.

Snyder et al. [17] introduced the question of survival bias for transfusion ratio in massively transfused trauma patients. The authors observed a significant association between improved survival and high transfusion ratios during the first 24 h. But this relationship did not sustain after adjustment for survival bias in the study cohort.

Similarly, Teixeira et al. [18] conducted a 6-year retrospective study to analyze the effect of plasma transfusion (≥10 PRBC) among massively transfused patients and observed a survival benefit for higher FFP: PRBC ratio during initial 24 h. De Baisi et al. [25] reported that mortality was significantly correlated with worse plasma deficit during the initial 2 h of resuscitation but no association with plasma ratio was reported. A similar association was observed among the massive transfusion group at 24 h.

Several studies have shown a correlation between FFP transfusion and the development of hospital complications. Khan et al. [26] suggested that FFP transfusion is independently associated with the risk of acute lung injury and acute respiratory distress syndrome (ARDS). In addition, Sperry et al. [5] observed 2 times higher risk of ARDS in patients resuscitated with a high FFP: PRBC ratio. In contrast, our study reported a lower MOF rate

among the high ratio group within the early as well as late phase. Both groups were comparable in terms of the initial coagulopathy, injury severity and demographic status except for age. We also noted progressive improvement in the coagulopathy status in the high ratio group. These results substantiate our current understandings of the utility of aggressive plasma use to prevent and treat early onset coagulopathy after injury. Furthermore, the rate of nosocomial infections did not reach statistical significance in either group. However, high ratio group patients had higher rates of wound infection and pneumonia which might explain the potential complications and risks attributable to this type of resuscitative practice.

Our study has some limitations including its retrospective nature. Being a single institution study, we are limited with the small sample size and power in addition to the lack of detailed description of the coagulation management. We were also not able to account for the incidence of ARDS. Also, the possibility of survival bias and incompleteness of collected data cannot be ruled out. We were looking for the MTP and the death burden from exsanguination, not the over-all death burden. After all, an MTP's main objective is to reduce deaths from traumatic hemorrhage. All deaths due to the severity of injury were 'pre-ordained' already. To date most of the studies have calculated FFP: PRBC ratios at 24 h. Therefore, analysis of ratios at 4 h would help to counter survival bias to some extent [19]. The proper ratios and time for administrating MTP in trauma patients are not well defined yet in the literatures (Table 4). In our institute, the MTP protocol was fully implemented in 2011 and so the difference in transfusion practice can be attributed to practice variation as well as the 'learning curve' that attends the implementation of any new clinical protocol. Furthermore the data were collected retrospectively so we cannot assume the

Table 4 Review of massive transfusion studies

Reference	N of pts	Mechanism	Massive transfusion definition	Time ratio calculated	Plasma : PRBC ratio	Results
Borgman et al., 2007 [4]	246	94 % penetrating (military)	≥9 U RBC in 1st 24 h	24 h	Low: 1:8, Medium: 1:2.5 High:1:1.4	Overall Mortality in low −65%, medium-34%, high-19 %, (P < .001).
Sperry et al., 2008 [5]	415	100 % blunt	≥8 U RBC in 1st 8 h	12 h	Low: < 1 : 1.5 High: ≥ 1 : 1.5	24-h mortality in low-12.8%, high - 3.9% (P = 0.012). Benefit gone by 48 h
Holcomb et al., 2008 [14]	466	35 % penetrating	≥9 U RBC in 1st 24 h	24 h	Low: < 1 : 2 High: ≥ 1 : 2	Improved 30-day survival in high ratio (59.6 vs. 40.4 %; P < 0.01)
Gunter et al. 2008 (15)	259	55 % penetrating	≥10 U RBC in 1st 24 h	24 h	Low: < 1 : 1.5 High: ≥ 1 : 1.5	reduction in 30-day mortality: high (41 %) vs. low (62 %) ratio group p = 0.008
Maegele et al., 2008 [16]	713	92 % blunt	≥10 U RBC ED → ICU admission	NA	PRBC:FFP > 1.1, PRBC:FFP 0.9-1.1 PRBC:FFP < 0.9	6 h mortality 24.6, 9.6 & 3.5 % (P < 0.0001) 24 h mortality 32.6, 16.7 & 11.3 % (P < 0.0001) 30 day mortality 45.5, 35.1 & 24 % (P < 0.001)
Snyder et al., 2009 [17]	134	60 % penetrating	≥10 U RBC in 1st 24 h	24 h	Low: < 1 : 2 High: ≥ 1 : 2	24-h mortality in low-58%, High - 40 %; but effect disappears when analyzed as time-dependent variable
Teixeira et al., 2009 [18]	383	NA	≥10 U RBC in 1st 24 h	24 h	Low: ≤ 1:8, Medium: >1:8 & ≤1:3 High: >1:3 & ≤ 1:2	Mortality rate decreased significantly with increased FFP; but effect disappears after a 1:3 ratio.
Mitra et al., 2010 [19]	331	86 % blunt	≥5 U RBC in 1st 4 h	4 h	>1:1.5 >1:2.5 to 1:1.5 >1:3.5 to 1:2.5 ≤1:3.5	higher ratios were associated with significantly improved mortality rates
Magnotti et al., 2011 [20]	103	63 % blunt	≥10 U RBC in 1st 24 h	6 h	Low: < 1 : 2 High: ≥ 1 : 2	6-h mortality was less in the high-group (10% vs. 48 %, p < 0.002)
Lustenberger et al. 2011 [21]	229	100 % blunt	≥10 U RBC in 1st 24 h	12, 24 h	Low: < 1 : 1.5 High: ≥ 1 : 1.5	High ratio was associated with improved survival at 12 and 24 h
Brown et al., 2012 [22]	604	100 % blunt	≥10 U RBC in 1st 24 h	6, 12, 24 h	Low: < 1 : 1.5 High: ≥ 1 : 1.5	High 6-h ratios were associated with a reduction in mortality risk at 6, 12, and 24 h (p < 0.05).
Kudo et al., 2013 [23]	NA	NA	≥10 U RBC in 1st 24 h	6 h	High: >1:1.5, Medium: 1:1.5-1:2 Low: <1:2	Mortality rate: high (44.4 %); Middle (16.7 %); low (33.3 %)
Holcomb et al., 2015 [24]	680	Severely injured (55 % blunt)	≥10 U of RBCs within 24 h	6 h	1:1:1 transfusion ratio of plasma, platelets, and RBCs to a 1:1:2 ratio	early administration of plasma, platelets, and red blood cells in a 1:1:1 ratio compared with a 1:1:2 ratio did not result in significant differences in mortality at 24 h or at 30 days
Present study	77	88.3 % Blunt 11.7 % penetrating	≥10 U RBC in 1st 24 h	4 h	Low: < 1 : 1.5 High: ≥ 1 : 1.5	higher ratios were significantly associated with lower rate of mortality and MOF within initial 4 h of injury

exact reason behind this time and ratio variations except for physician discretion in the absence of hospital protocol at that time. Lastly, multi-year retrospective studies might suffer from the same 'potential bias' that could be encountered in our analysis.

Conclusions

The mortality risk associated with low FFP: PRBC ratios of <1:1.5 may occur very early, possibly secondary to ongoing coagulopathy and hemorrhage. Aggressive attainment of high FFP/PRBC ratios as early as 4 h post injury can substantially improve coagulopathy and reduce mortality and MOF rates. The present study is an audit of massive transfusion strategies used at our center which highlights the current experience of managing exsanguinating trauma patients. The analysis of appropriate transfusion ratios and timings provides useful information regarding the correct ratios of blood component and avoiding wastage of the blood products. This information can form the basis for developing research based uniform massive transfusion guidelines for the appropriate use of various blood components. Furthermore, it can be the basis for designing massive transfusion research focusing high transfusion ratios targeted within the first 4 h. Therefore, large prospective studies are needed to validate our findings for a balanced FFP: PRBC ratio that would decrease the overall PRBC utilization and the decision needed for massive transfusion.

Abbreviations
MTP: Massive transfusion protocol; MOF: multiorgan failure; FFP: fresh frozen plasma; PRBC: Packed red blood cells; ISS: Injury Severity Score; RTS: Revised Trauma Score; HMTP: high MTP; LMTP: low MTP; INR: International Normalized Ratio; VAP: Ventilator associated pneumonia; BSI: blood stream infection; CRBSI: Catheter-related blood stream infections; UTI: Urinary tract infection.

Competing interests
The author(s) declare that they have no competing interests.

Authors' contributions
RP: study design data interpretation, and manuscript drafting; AV: study design data interpretation, and manuscript drafting; AE: data analysis and interpretation, drafting and manuscript review; RC: study design data interpretation, and manuscript drafting; HA: data analysis, interpretation, and drafting; AP: was involved in study design, data collection and writing manuscript; IA: was involved in study design, data collection and writing manuscript; AZ: data analysis, interpretation, and drafting, HA: study design, data interpretation, and review manuscript, AP: study design data interpretation, and manuscript review; and RL: study design data interpretation, and manuscript review. All authors read and approved the final manuscript.

Authors' information
RP: Trauma Surgery Section, Hamad General Hospital, Qatar; AV: Trauma Surgery Section, Hamad General Hospital, Qatar; AE: Clinical Research, Trauma Surgery Section, Hamad General Hospital, Qatar and Weill Cornell Medical School, Doha, Qatar; RC: Trauma Surgery Section, Hamad General Hospital, Qatar; HA: Trauma Surgery Section, Hamad General Hospital, Qatar; AP: Trauma Surgery Section, Hamad General Hospital, Qatar; IA: Trauma Surgery Section, Hamad General Hospital, Qatar; AZ: Trauma Surgery Section, Hamad General Hospital, Qatar; HA: Trauma Surgery Section, Hamad General Hospital, Qatar; RL: Trauma Surgery Section, Hamad General Hospital, Qatar and Department of Surgery, Arizona University, Tucson, AZ, USA.

Acknowledgement
We thank the entire registry database team in the section of trauma surgery. All authors read the manuscript and approved it and had no financial issues to disclose. Medical Research Center (IRB# 11153/11) at Hamad Medical Corporation, Qatar has approved the study.
This study has been presented in part at the 43rd Annual Congress of the Society of Critical Care Medicine, San Francisco, California, USA.

Author details
[1]Trauma Surgery Section, Hamad Trauma Center, Hamad General Hospital, Doha, Qatar. [2]Clinical Research, Trauma Surgery Section, Hamad General Hospital, HMC, PO Box 3050, Doha, Qatar. [3]Clinical Medicine, Weill Cornell Medical College, Doha, Qatar. [4]Department of Surgery, University of Arizona, Tucson, AZ, USA.

References
1. Peng R, Chang C, Gilmore D, Bongard F. Epidemiology of immediate and early trauma deaths at an urban Level I trauma center. Am Surg. 1998;64:950–4.
2. Demetriades D, Murray J, Charalambides K, Alo K, Velmahos G, Rhee P, et al. Trauma fatalities: time and location of hospital deaths. J Am Coll Surg. 2004;198:20–6.
3. Brohi K, Singh J, Heron M, Coats T. Acute traumatic coagulopathy. J Trauma. 2003;54:1127–30.
4. Borgman MA, Spinella PC, Perkins JG, Grathwohl KW, Repine T, Beekley AC, et al. The ratio of blood products transfused affects mortality in patients receiving massive transfusions at a combat support hospital. J Trauma. 2007;63:805–13.
5. Sperry JL, Ochoa JB, Gunn SR, Alarcon LH, Minei JP, Cuschieri J, et al. Inflammation the Host Response to Injury Investigators: An FFP:PRBC transfusion ratio >/=1:1.5 is associated with a lower risk of mortality after massive transfusion. J Trauma. 2008;65:986–93.
6. Gajic O, Dzik WH, Toy P. Fresh frozen plasma and platelet transfusion for non-bleeding patients in the intensive care unit: benefit or harm? Crit Care Med. 2006;34 Suppl 5:170–3.
7. MacLennan S, Williamson LM. Risks of fresh frozen plasma and platelets. J Trauma. 2006;60 Suppl 6:46–50.
8. Silliman CC, Ambruso DR, Boshkov LK. Transfusion-related acute lung injury. Blood. 2005;105:2266–73.
9. Dutton RP. Resuscitative strategies to maintain homeostasis during damage control surgery. Br J Surg. 2012;99 Suppl 1:21–8.
10. Meißner A, Schlenke P. Massive Bleeding and Massive Transfusion. Transfus Med Hemother. 2012;39:73–84.
11. Minei JP, Nathens AB, West M, Harbrecht BG, Moore EE, Shapiro MB, et al. Inflammation and the Host Response to Injury Large Scale Collaborative Research Program Investigators. Inflammation and the Host Response to Injury, a Large-Scale Collaborative Project: patient-oriented research core–standard operating procedures for clinical care. II. Guidelines for prevention, diagnosis and treatment of ventilator-associated pneumonia (VAP) in the trauma patient. J Trauma. 2006;60:1106–13.
12. Kashuk JL, Moore EE, Millikan JS, Moore JB. Major abdominal vascular trauma – a unified approach. J Trauma. 1982;22:672–9.
13. Kautza BC, Cohen MJ, Cuschieri J, Minei JP, Brackenridge SC, Maier RV, et al. Inflammation and the Host Response to Injury Investigators: Changes in massive transfusion over time: an early shift in the right direction? J Trauma Acute Care Surg. 2012;72:106–11.
14. Holcomb JB, Wade CE, Michalek JE, Chisholm GB, Zarzabal LA, Schreiber MA, et al. Increased plasma and platelet to red blood cell ratios improves outcome in 466 massively transfused civilian trauma patients. Ann Surg. 2008;248:447–58.
15. Gunter Jr OL, Au BK, Isbell JM, Mowery NT, Young PP, Cotton BA. Optimizing outcomes in damage control resuscitation: identifying blood product ratios associated with improved survival. J Trauma. 2008;65:527–34.
16. Maegele M, Lefering R, Paffrath T, Tjardes T, Simanski C, Bouillon B. Working Group on Polytrauma of the German Society of Trauma Surgery (DGU). Red-blood-cell to plasma ratios transfused during massive transfusion are associated with mortality in severe multiple injury: a retrospective analysis from the Trauma Registry of the Deutsche Gesellschaft für Unfallchirurgie. Vox Sang. 2008;95:112–19.
17. Snyder CW, Weinberg JA, McGwin Jr G, Melton SM, George RL, Reiff DA, et al. The relationship of blood product ratio to mortality: Survival benefit or survival bias? J Trauma. 2009;66:358–62.
18. Teixeira PG, Inaba K, Shulman I, Salim A, Demetriades D, Brown C, et al. Impact of plasma transfusion in massively transfused trauma patients. J Trauma. 2009;66:693–7.
19. Mitra B, Mori A, Cameron PA, Fitzgerald M, Paul E, Street A. Fresh frozen plasma (FFP) use during massive blood transfusion in trauma resuscitation. Injury. 2010;41:35–9.
20. Magnotti LJ, Zarzaur BL, Fischer PE, Williams RF, Myers AL, Bradburn EH, et al. Improved survival after hemostatic resuscitation: does the emperor have no clothes? J Trauma. 2011;70:97–102.
21. Lustenberger T, Frischknecht A, Brüesch M, Keel MJ. Blood component ratios in massively transfused blunt trauma patients a time-dependent covariate analysis. J Trauma. 2011;71:1144–50.
22. Brown JB, Cohen MJ, Minei JP, Maier RV, West MA, Billiar TR, et al. Inflammation and Host Response to Injury Investigators: Debunking the survival bias myth: characterization of mortality during the initial 24 h for

patients requiring massive transfusion. J Trauma Acute Care Surg. 2012;73:358–64.

23. Kudo D, Sasaki J, Akaishi S, Yamanouchi S, Koakutsu T, Endo T, et al. Efficacy of a high FFP:PRBC transfusion ratio on the survival of severely injured patients: a retrospective study in a single tertiary emergency center in Japan. Surg Today. 2014;44:653–61.

24. Holcomb JB, Tilley BC, Baraniuk S, Fox EE, Wade CE, Podbielski JM, et al. Transfusion of plasma, platelets, and red blood cells in a 1:1:1 vs a 1:1:2 ratio and mortality in patients with severe trauma: the PROPPR randomized clinical trial. JAMA. 2015;313(5):471–82.

25. de Biasi AR, Stansbury LG, Dutton RP, Stein DM, Scalea TM, Hess JR. Blood product use in trauma resuscitation: plasma deficit versus plasma ratio as predictors of mortality in trauma (CME). Transfusion. 2011;51:1925–32.

26. Khan H, Belsher J, Yilmaz M, Afessa B, Winters JL, Moore SB, et al. Fresh-frozen plasma and platelet transfusions are associated with development of acute lung injury in critically ill medical patients. Chest. 2007;131:1308–14.

5

Epidemiology and socioeconomic features of appendicitis in Taiwan: a 12-year population-based study

Kai-Biao Lin[1,2†], K. Robert Lai[2,6*†], Nan-Ping Yang[3,4†], Chien-Lung Chan[5,6†], Yuan-Hung Liu[2,6,7], Ren-Hao Pan[6] and Chien-Hsun Huang[8]

Abstract

Introduction: This paper presents an epidemiologic study of appendicitis in Taiwan over a twelve-year period. An analysis of the incidence in the low-income population (LIP) is included to explore the effects of lower socioeconomic status on appendicitis.

Methods: We analyzed the epidemiological features of appendicitis in Taiwan using data from the National Health Insurance Research Database (NHIRD) from 2000 to 2011. All cases diagnosed as appendicitis were enrolled.

Results: The overall incidences of appendicitis, primary appendectomy, and perforated appendicitis were 107.76, 101.58, and 27.20 per 100,000 per year, respectively. The highest incidence of appendicitis was found in persons aged 15 to 29 years; males had higher rates of appendicitis than females at all ages except for 70 years and older. Appendicitis rates were 11.76 % higher in the summer than in the winter months. A multilevel analysis with hierarchical linear modeling (HLM) revealed that male patients, younger patients (aged ≤14 years), and elderly patients (aged ≥60 years) had a higher risk of perforated appendicitis; among adults, the incidence increased with age. Moreover, the risk of perforation was higher in patients with one or more comorbidities. LIP patients comprised 1.25 % of the total number of patients with appendicitis from 2000 to 2011. The overall incidence of appendicitis was 34.99 % higher in the LIP than in the normal population (NP), and the incidence of perforated appendicitis was 40.40 % higher in the LIP than in the NP. After multivariate adjustment, the adjusted hospital costs and length of hospital stay (LOS) for the LIP patients were higher than those for the NP patients.

Conclusions: Appendicitis and appendectomy in Taiwan had similar overall incidences, seasonality patterns, and declining trends compared to numerous previous studies. Compared to NP patients, LIP patients had a higher risk of appendicitis, longer LOS and higher hospital costs as a result of appendectomy.

Keywords: Appendicitis, Appendectomy, Epidemiology, Socioeconomic status

Introduction

Appendectomy is one of the most common operations worldwide [1]. Although numerous epidemiological studies on appendicitis have been conducted, most have focused on Western populations [2–7]; relatively few epidemiological studies have focused on appendicitis in Asian populations. Lee et al. [8] reported the epidemiological features and lifetime risk of appendicitis and appendectomy in South Korea using epidemiological data from 2005 to 2007. However, considering the relatively short observation period, determining long-term trends was challenging. In addition, several studies have been conducted in Taiwan regarding the epidemiological features of appendicitis [9–17]. These studies were chiefly concerned with the monthly variation in the incidence of acute appendicitis [11], the volume-outcome relationship of acute appendicitis [13], trend differentials in the incidence of ruptured appendicitis between rural and urban populations [15], and

* Correspondence: krlai@cs.yzu.edu.tw
†Equal contributors
[2]Department of Computer Science and Engineering, Yuan Ze University, Taoyuan 32003, Taiwan
[6]Innovation Center for Big Data and Digital Convergence, Yuan Ze University, Taoyuan 32003, Taiwan
Full list of author information is available at the end of the article

a comparison of the perforation rate of acute appendicitis between nationals and immigrants [16]. No comprehensive study has evaluated the epidemiology of appendicitis in Taiwan from 2000 to 2011. Furthermore, only a few studies have paid attention to the effect of socioeconomic status (SES) on appendicitis, particularly studies focusing on the low-income population (LIP) [18].

We performed a comprehensive study to investigate the epidemiological features of age, gender, comorbidities, readmission, length of hospital stay (LOS), hospital cost, incidences, seasonal variation and the effect of lower SES on appendicitis and appendectomy. We also compared the differences in adjusted costs and LOS for appendicitis between the LIP and normal population (NP). A multi-level analysis with hierarchical linear modeling (HLM) was performed using data from all appendicitis patients to assess the odds ratio of the occurrence of perforated appendicitis. The data were retrieved from the National Health Insurance Research Database (NHIRD) for all years from 2000 to 2011.

Methods

Data source

Taiwan launched the single-payer National Health Insurance (NHI) program in 1995; by 2000, the NHI coverage rate had expanded to 96.16 % of the Taiwanese population, and by 2011, coverage had reached 99.88 %. All eligible enrollees can access health care services from most clinics and hospitals by making a small copayment [19]. The National Health Insurance Bureau (NHIB) established a nationwide research database, which included nationwide population-based data with high quality control and representation. The NHIRD includes various data subsets, such as inpatient expenditures by admissions (DD), details of inpatient orders (DO), ambulatory care expenditures by visits (CD), and details of ambulatory care orders (OO). In this study, the DD dataset was used for further analysis.

To evaluate temporal trends, the estimated population of Taiwan from 2000 to 2011 was used to calculate the annual incidences of appendicitis and appendectomy. For all other analyses, the mean annual incidence for the aforementioned years was determined by combining the annual discharges and using the Taiwan census data as the denominator, which are created and maintained by the Taiwan Department of Household Registration of the Ministry of the Interior.

Data protection and permission

To protect patient privacy, all personal information was encrypted using a double scrambling protocol. Before using the NHIRD and its data subsets, all researchers signed a written agreement declaring that they had no intention of obtaining information that could violate the privacy of patients or care providers. This study was

approved by the Institutional Review Board (IRB) of Taoyuan General Hospital, which has been certified by the Ministry of Health and Welfare in Taiwan (IRB Approval Number: TYGH103015). The study protocol was also evaluated by the NHI Research Institutes, which consented to the planned analysis of the NHIRD data (Agreement Numbers: NHIRD-103-160 and NHIRD-104-081).

Study design

The NHIRD contains registration files and original claims data, including patient demographics, diagnoses, and treatment details related to inpatient and outpatient claims for reimbursement. Every claimant of the NHI program from 2000 to 2011 was included in the study population (22,276,672 persons in 2000, which increased to 23,224,912 persons by 2011). The registration and claims data of the study cohort were obtained from the NHIRD, and the various expenditure categories were established according to the DD. One exclusion criterion and two inclusion criteria were used to select cases that were admitted because of appendicitis or appendectomy. The exclusion criterion was patients who had undergone incidental appendectomy (ICD-9-CM procedure code of 47.1). The inclusion criteria were the following International Classification of Disease, Version 9 (ICD-9) code items: (1) diagnostic codes 540–543; and (2) procedure code 47.0.

The analysis included four steps: (1) identification of data sources and extracting data; (2) investigation of the epidemiological features of age, gender, comorbidities, readmission, LOS, hospital costs, incidences, seasonal variation and the effect of SES on appendicitis and appendectomy; (3) conversion of the extracted data to a comparable metric; and (4) application of statistical models to evaluate hazard ratios for the risk of perforation.

Data definition

To investigate the incidence of appendicitis in Taiwan, International Classification of Diseases, Ninth Revision, Clinical Modification (ICD-9-CM) diagnostic codes were used. The major diagnostic codes for appendicitis were 540 (acute appendicitis), 541 (appendicitis unqualified), 542 (other appendicitis), and 543 (other diseases of the appendix). Furthermore, code 540 was further classified as 540.0 (acute appendicitis with generalized peritonitis), 540.1 (acute appendicitis with peritoneal abscess), and 540.9 (acute appendicitis without mention of peritonitis). The procedure code was defined as 47.0 (appendectomy, excludes incidental). Perforated appendicitis was considered for appendectomies revealing evidence of perforation, peritonitis, rupture, or abscess (ICD-9-CM diagnostic codes 540.0 and 540.1). The perforation ratio was defined as the ratio of the number of perforated appendicitis diagnoses to the number of appendectomies. The case-fatality ratio was defined as the percentage of patients with an appendectomy who died during hospitalization.

Classification of LIP and NP

To evaluate the effect of socioeconomics, the enrolled subjects were divided into NP and LIP groups based on Taiwan's Social Assistance Act criteria and registration in Taiwan's NHI database [18]. Low-income households were defined as those with a monthly average per-member gross income of less than the monthly minimum living expense standard of that residence region. The minimum living expense standard was defined as 60 % of the average monthly disposable income for each region. The family property could not exceed the amount announced by the central or municipal authorities in the corresponding year [20]. This segment of the population was recorded as the fifth class insured in Taiwan's NHI database [19]. The NP was all individuals who were not in the LIP.

Statistical analysis

The descriptive statistics for comparing the baseline characteristics included the number of cases, percentages, annual incidences (per 100,000 individuals), and 95 % Confidence Interval (CI) for the estimated rates. The Analysis of Variance (ANOVA) was used to describe and compare the continuous variables among the various subgroups. Statistical significance was set at 0.05. To evaluate the risk factors for perforated appendicitis, a multiple logistic regression analysis was performed, and the Adjusted Odds Ratio (AOR) was calculated. Multilevel analysis (or the hierarchical linear modeling, HLM method) was used as an analytical strategy, which allowed the evaluation of group-level and individual-level factors [21]. The hypothesis and formulas of the HLM analysis used in the present study were as follows.

Level 1 HLM Model

$$
\begin{aligned}
Yij = {}& \beta 0 + \beta 1 \times (gender) + \beta 2 \times (age\ group\ 1) + \beta 3 \\
& \times (age\ group\ 2) + \beta 4 \times (age\ group\ 3) + \beta 5 \\
& \times (age\ group\ 4) + \beta 6 \times (comorbidities\ 1) + \beta 7 \\
& \times (comorbidities\ 2) + \beta 8 \times (regional\ hospital) \\
& + \beta 9 \times (medical\ center) + \beta 10 \times (suburban) \\
& + \beta 11 \times (readmission) + \gamma.
\end{aligned}
\tag{1}
$$

Level 2 HLM Model

$$
\beta 0 = \gamma 00 + \gamma 01 \times (SES) + \mu 0.
\tag{2}
$$

To estimate the incidence for the various populations in each age group, we constructed a life table in 5-year age intervals using combined incidence data from 2000 to 2011. To compare the incidence of appendicitis

during various months and seasons, months with fewer than 31 days were adjusted to fit a standard 31-day month. To reduce the effect of extreme data on the mean LOS and hospital cost values, 1 % maximum and 1 % minimum values were excluded from the raw data. All statistical analyses were performed using the Statistical Package for the Social Sciences (SPSS) for Windows (Version 18.0).

Results

From 2000 to 2011, 294,544 patients were diagnosed with appendicitis (24,545/year on average). Of these, 53.09 % were male, 45.54 % were female, and the remaining 1.37 % of the patients had missing gender information. The median ages of the patients with appendicitis and perforated appendicitis were 35 years (23, 51) and 44 years (27, 61), respectively. As shown in Table 1, 3.98 % of the patients with appendicitis exhibited one comorbidity, and 0.36 % exhibited two or more comorbidities; 19.54 % of the patients chose a laparoscopic appendectomy. The proportions of patients residing in urban, suburban and rural areas were 85.72 %, 13.07 % and 1.22 %, respectively. We observed a higher proportion of patients residing in urban areas compared to suburban and rural areas. The proportions of patients hospitalized in medical centers, regional hospitals and district hospitals were 46.93 %, 33.39 % and 19.68 %, respectively. This result indicated that a large proportion of patients were more likely to choose medical centers and regional hospitals for better medical care. All of these demographic characteristics were similar between male and female patients; however, the ratio of readmission for complications was higher in male patients than in female patients (3.89 % vs. 2.27 %), and the overall case-fatality ratio of appendectomies was higher for male patients than for female patients (0.14 % vs. 0.09 %, Table 1).

Appendicitis

The overall incidence of appendicitis was 107.76 per 100,000 per year (95 % CI: 101.33–114.19), including 114.38 per 100,000 per year (95 % CI: 107.76–121) for males and 100.96 per 100,000 per year (95 % CI: 94.74–107.18) for females. The age-specific incidence of appendicitis displayed a similar pattern for both genders; the lowest incidence was observed in the 0-to-4-year age group, with an incidence of 16.62 per 100,000 per year (95 % CI: 14.10–19.15) for males and 12.90 per 100,000 per year (95 % CI: 10.67–15.12) for females. As shown in Fig. 1, the incidence gradually increased in subsequent age groups and peaked at 15-to-19-years (152.92 per 100,000/year) for males and at 20-to-24-years (137.20 per 100,000/year) for females. Subsequently, the incidence decreased gradually

Table 1 Demographic characteristics of patients with appendicitis in Taiwan from 2000 to 2011

Variable	Total(n = 294,544)		Male(n = 156,371)		Female(n = 134,141)		P
	n	%	n	%	n	%	
Age Stratum							< 0.001
0–14 y/o	38,222	12.98 %	23,382	14.95 %	14,803	11.04 %	
15–29 y/o	91,965	31.22 %	48,056	30.73 %	41,589	31.00 %	
30–44 y/o	78,384	26.61 %	41,305	26.41 %	35,528	26.49 %	
45–59 y/o	48,590	16.50 %	25,001	15.99 %	23,478	17.50 %	
60 y/o or more	37,383	12.69 %	18,627	11.91 %	18,743	13.97 %	
Comorbidities [a]							< 0.001
0	281,756	95.66 %	149,510	95.61 %	128,227	95.59 %	
1	11,732	3.98 %	6,235	3.99 %	5,485	4.09 %	
≥ 2	1056	0.36 %	626	0.40 %	429	0.32 %	
Readmission for complication [b]							< 0.001
No	285,359	96.88 %	150,293	96.11 %	131,091	97.73 %	
Yes	9,185	3.12 %	6,078	3.89 %	3,050	2.27 %	
Hospital Mortality							< 0.001
No	294,197	99.88 %	156,147	99.86 %	134,019	99.91 %	
Yes	347	0.12 %	224	0.14 %	122	0.09 %	
Operation Type							< 0.001
OA	223,145	80.46 %	119,052	80.88 %	100,278	79.41 %	
LA	54,178	19.54 %	28,147	19.12 %	26,007	20.59 %	
Hospital Level [c]							< 0.001
District Hospital	58,303	19.68 %	30,513	19.40 %	26,160	19.38 %	
Regional Hospital	139,070	46.93 %	74,210	47.17 %	63,211	46.83 %	
Medical Center	98,946	33.39 %	52,585	33.43 %	45,597	33.78 %	
Area level							< 0.001
Urban	252994	85.72 %	133,743	85.34 %	115,859	86.20 %	
Suburban	38568	13.07 %	21,004	13.40 %	17,014	12.66 %	
Rural	3594	1.22 %	1,965	1.25 %	1,536	1.14 %	

OA Open Appendectomy LA Laparoscopic Appendectomy

A total of 4,032 records of appendicitis patients were missing information regarding gender

The denominator for "Operation Type" was the total number of patients who underwent a primary appendectomy (277,323)

[a] Comorbidities were identified by referring to the ICD-9-CM codes, as described in Appendix C in [17]

[b] Readmission for complication was defined as readmission with the diagnosis of a commonly encountered postoperative complication within 1 month after an appendectomy (Appendix B in [17])

[c] In Taiwan, there are four types of accreditation (medical center, regional hospital, district hospital, and unaccredited hospital). Unaccredited hospital refers to clinic, special pharmacy, and home care organizations; they cannot treat appendicitis patients. Therefore, in the present paper, we separate hospitals into three groups by accreditation status: medical center, regional hospital, and district hospital

and reached the low point for the 55-to-59 year age group in both genders. The incidence then gradually increased again until it reached another peak at the age of 75 years and older. Overall, the 15-to-29-year age group was the highest risk group for both genders, and males exhibited a higher incidence at all ages except for 70 years and older (Fig. 1).

Acute appendicitis

A total of 280,725 patients were diagnosed with acute appendicitis (23,394/year on average), which accounted for 95.31 % of the total number of patients diagnosed with

appendicitis. The overall incidence of acute appendicitis was 102.69 per 100,000 per year (95 % CI: 96.41–108.97). The age-specific incidence of acute appendicitis exhibited a similar trend as that of appendicitis. The only difference was that the incidences of acute appendicitis in each age group were slightly lower than those of appendicitis, as acute appendicitis is a subcategory of appendicitis.

Primary appendectomy

A primary appendectomy was defined as a non-incidental appendectomy. A total of 277,323 patients underwent an appendectomy from 2000 to 2011. Among these, 268,288

Incidence of Appendicitis

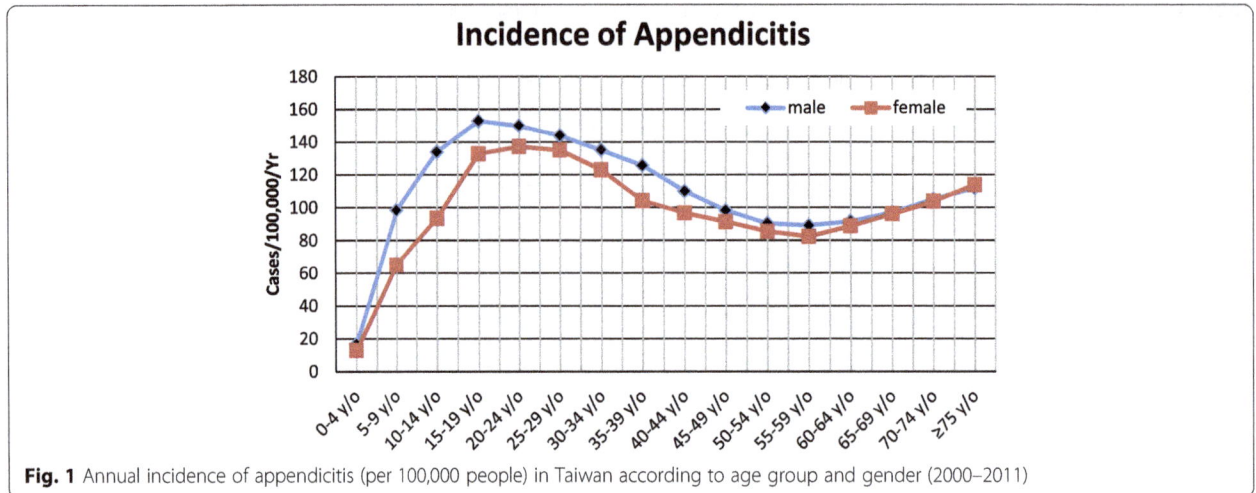

Fig. 1 Annual incidence of appendicitis (per 100,000 people) in Taiwan according to age group and gender (2000–2011)

patients were diagnosed with appendicitis at discharge, and the remaining 9,035 patients were not diagnosed with appendicitis at discharge, indicating that they may have been misdiagnosed. The overall incidence of primary appendectomy was 101.58 per 100,000 per year (95 % CI: 95.34–107.82). The incidence of primary appendectomy was higher in males than in females (male-to-female ratio of 1.13:1), with values of 107.83 per 100,000 per year (95 % CI: 101.40–114.27) and 95.15 per 100,000 per year (95 % CI: 89.11–101.20) for males and females, respectively. The age-specific incidences of primary appendectomy were similar for both genders, but males exhibited higher rates at almost all ages; in the 60-to-69-year age group, females exhibited a slightly higher incidence than males.

Perforated appendicitis

A total of 74,326 patients exhibited appendiceal perforation, rupture, abscess, or generalized peritonitis. Among these, 58.28 % were males, 40.75 % were females, and the remaining 0.97 % of patients had missing gender information. The overall incidence of perforated appendicitis was 27.20 per 100,000 per year (95 % CI: 23.97–30.44). Male patients had a higher risk of having perforated appendicitis than female patients at all ages. The incidence by gender was 31.59 per 100,000 per year (95 % CI: 28.11–35.08) for males and 22.69 per 100,000 per year (95 % CI: 19.74–25.65) for females, respectively, with an overall male-to-female ratio of 1.39:1. The overall perforation ratio was 25.23 % (27.70 % for male patients and 22.58 % for female patients). The age-specific perforation ratios were similar for both genders; these ratios were higher in the older and younger patients but lower at intermediate ages, thus exhibiting a V-shaped pattern (Fig. 2).

A multilevel analysis with HLM was used to evaluate the individual effects (i.e., gender, age, comorbidities, hospital level, area level, and readmission) and the group effect (i.e., SES) on the incidence of perforated appendicitis. Male patients had a higher risk of suffering from perforated appendicitis than female patients. Compared to the 15-to-29-year age group, the younger patients (aged ≤14 years) and adults (aged ≥30 years and older) exhibited a higher risk of perforated appendicitis; among adults, the incidence of ruptured appendicitis increased with age (Table 2). In addition, the risk of perforation was higher in patients with one or more comorbidities, and this risk increased further as the number of comorbidities increased. The risk of perforation was higher in patients admitted to regional hospitals and medical centers than in patients admitted to district hospitals. Furthermore, the risk of ruptured appendicitis increased significantly in patients who were readmitted to a hospital for complications (AOR = 4.930, $p < 0.001$). Compared to the NP, the LIP exhibited a higher risk of ruptured appendicitis (AOR = 1.098, $p = 0.016$). These patterns were consistent in both genders (Table 2).

Utilization of care: LOS and hospital cost

The period between admission and discharge was defined as the LOS (measured in days). For patients who were discharged on the day of admission, the LOS was recorded as 1 day [17]. From 2000 to 2011, the estimated LOS for appendicitis was 1,510,007 days (125,833/year) in total. As shown in Table 3, the mean LOS values for appendicitis, acute appendicitis, and primary appendectomy were similar, whereas the LOS for perforated appendicitis was longer. The male-to-female ratio for the mean LOS values ranged from 1.01 to 1.05:1, which indicated that the mean LOS values were slightly higher for male patients than for female patients. The overall age-specific trend of LOS was a U-shaped pattern. The incidence was higher in the older

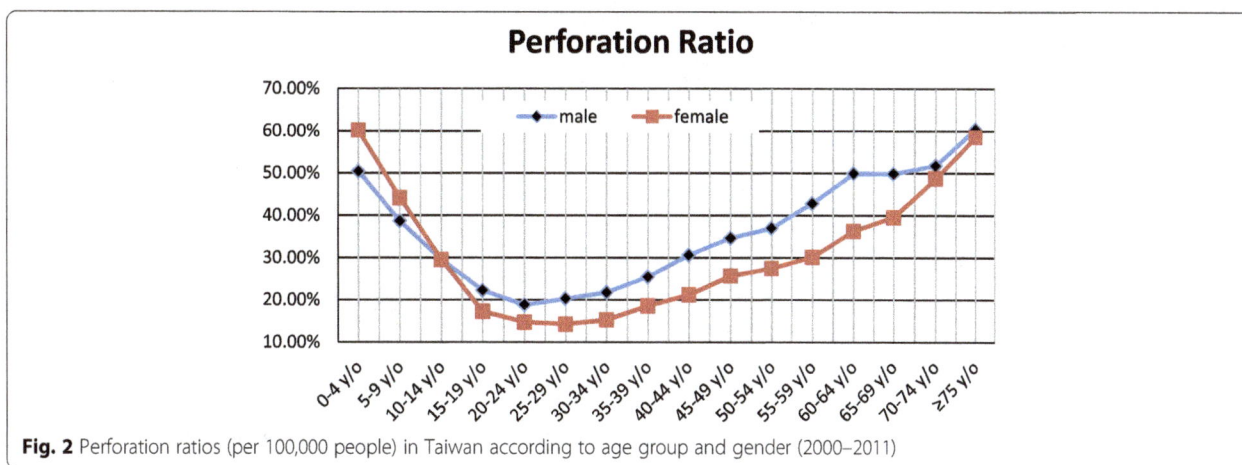

Fig. 2 Perforation ratios (per 100,000 people) in Taiwan according to age group and gender (2000–2011)

Table 2 Multilevel analysis (with HLM) of the risk factors for perforation among male and female patients with appendicitis in Taiwan (2000–2011)

Variable	Total			Male			Female		
	β value	AOR	P	β value	AOR	P	β value	AOR	P
Gender									
Female[c]		1.0							
Male	0.264	1.302 (1.279,1.324)	< 0.001						
Age(years)[a]									
0–14 y/o	0.779	2.179 (2.119,2.241)	< 0.001	0.620	1.858 (1.793,1.927)	< 0.001	1.048	2.851 (2.727,2.980)	< 0.001
15–29 y/o[c]		1.0			1.0			1.0	
30–44 y/o	0.283	1.327 (1.295,1.361)	< 0.001	0.302	1.353 (1.310,1.397)	< 0.001	0.268	1.307 (1.257,1.359)	< 0.001
45–59 y/o	0.758	2.134 (2.078,2.191)	< 0.001	0.774	2.167 (2.092,2.245)	< 0.001	0.758	2.134 (2.049,2.222)	< 0.001
≥60 y/o	1.290	3.633 (3.532,3.737)	< 0.001	1.234	3.433 (3.304,3.568)	< 0.001	1.336	3.805 (3.647,3.969)	< 0.001
Comorbidities[a]									
0[c]		1.0			1.0			1.0	
1	0.353	1.424 (1.367,1.483)	< 0.001	0.367	1.443 (1.365,1.525)	< 0.001	0.335	1.398 (1.316,1.484)	< 0.001
≥2	0.529	1.697 (1.495,1.926)	< 0.001	0.473	1.604 (1.361,1.892)	< 0.001	0.607	1.834 (1.508,2.231)	< 0.001
Hospital Level[a]									
District Hospital[c]		1.0			1.0			1.0	
Regional Hospital	0.223	1.250 (1.219,1.281)	< 0.001	0.233	1.262 (1.222,1.304)	< 0.001	0.229	1.258 (1.210,1.308)	< 0.001
Medical Center	0.394	1.483 (1.444,1.523)	< 0.001	0.381	1.464 (1.413,1.516)	< 0.001	0.428	1.534 (1.472,1.598)	< 0.001
Area level[a]									
Urban[c]		1.0			1.0			1.0	
Suburban	0.038	1.038 (1.011,1.067)	0.007	0.044	1.045 (1.009,1.083)	0.015	0.008	1.008 (0.966,1.051)	0.713
Rural	0.269	1.308 (1.210,1.415)	< 0.001	0.251	1.285 (1.160,1.423)	< 0.001	0.256	1.292 (1.140,1.463)	< 0.001
Readmission[a]									
No[c]		1.0			1.0			1.0	
Yes	1.595	4.930 (4.712,5.159)	< 0.001	1.528	4.608 (4.361,4.870)	< 0.001	1.706	5.506 (5.087,5.961)	< 0.001
Socioeconomic status[b]									
Normal population[c]		1.0			1.0			1.0	
Low-income population	0.093	1.098 (1.018,1.184)	0.016	0.139	1.149 (1.038,1.273)	0.008	0.048	1.049 (0.936,1.176)	0.410

[a]Individual level. [b]Cluster level. AOR: adjusted odds ratio.[c]: Reference group
A multivariate analysis was conducted after adjusting for age, gender, comorbidities, hospital level, area level, readmission, and socioeconomic status

Table 3 The mean LOS and hospital cost for patients with appendicitis, acute appendicitis, primary appendectomy, and perforated appendicitis in Taiwan (2000–2011)

Variable	Gender	Appendicitis	Acute appendicitis	Primary appendectomy	Perforated appendicitis
Mean hospital stay ± SE (days)	Male	4.85 ± 0.01	4.77 ± 0.01	4.82 ± 0.01	7.63 ± 0.03
	Female	4.65 ± 0.01	4.56 ± 0.01	4.77 ± 0.01	7.44 ± 0.03
	Total	4.76 ± 0.01	4.67 ± 0.01	4.80 ± 0.01	7.55 ± 0.19
	Male–female ratio	1.04	1.05	1.01	1.03
Mean hospital cost ± SE (US$)	Male	1,052 ± 1	1,039 ± 1	1,091 ± 2	1,462 ± 5
	Female	1,030 ± 2	1,016 ± 1	1,120 ± 2	1,449 ± 6
	Total	1,042 ± 1	1,029 ± 1	1,104 ± 1	1,457 ± 4
	Male–female ratio	1.02	1.02	0.97	1.01

SE standard error of the mean
To reduce the effect of extreme data on the mean LOS and hospital cost values, the 1 % maximum and 1 % minimum values were excluded from the raw data

and younger age groups but lower in the intermediate age group. The age-specific LOS for appendicitis displayed a similar pattern in both sexes, but males had higher rates at virtually all ages except the 0-14-year age group (Fig. 3). The mean LOS was 9.01 days for patients with one commodity and 12.25 days for patients with two or more commodities, which indicated that the mean LOS greatly increases for patients with one or more commodities compared to patients without commodity.

Hospital costs were calculated by adding all items in the hospital discharge summary together, including operation-associated costs and ward costs. Operation-associated costs included anesthesia and surgery fees and the costs of medical supplies used during the operation. Ward costs included surplus costs [17]. All costs were expressed in U.S. dollars (USD). In 2007, 1 USD was equivalent to approximately 32.64 New Taiwan dollars. As shown in Table 3, a positive association was observed between the hospital costs and the mean LOS: the longer the mean LOS, the higher the cost. The male-to-female ratio for the mean

hospital cost ranged from 0.97 to 1.17:1; the cost was similar in both genders (Table 3).

Seasonal variation
The incidence of appendicitis revealed clear seasonality in both males and females, peaking in the summer and reaching troughs in the winter. Among males, the average incidence of appendicitis was 10.25 per 100,000 per month (adjusted to 31 days per month) in the summer and 9.04 per 100,000 per month in the winter. Therefore, the incidence of appendicitis in males in the summer was 11.76 % higher than the incidence in the winter. Among females, the average incidence was 9.10 per 100,000 per month in the summer and 7.78 per 100,000 per month in the winter. Therefore, the incidence of appendicitis in females in the summer season was 14.56 % higher than the incidence in the winter season. Similar seasonal variation was observed in the incidence of acute appendicitis and appendectomy. Slight seasonal variation was observed in the incidence of perforated appendicitis (the incidence was higher in the

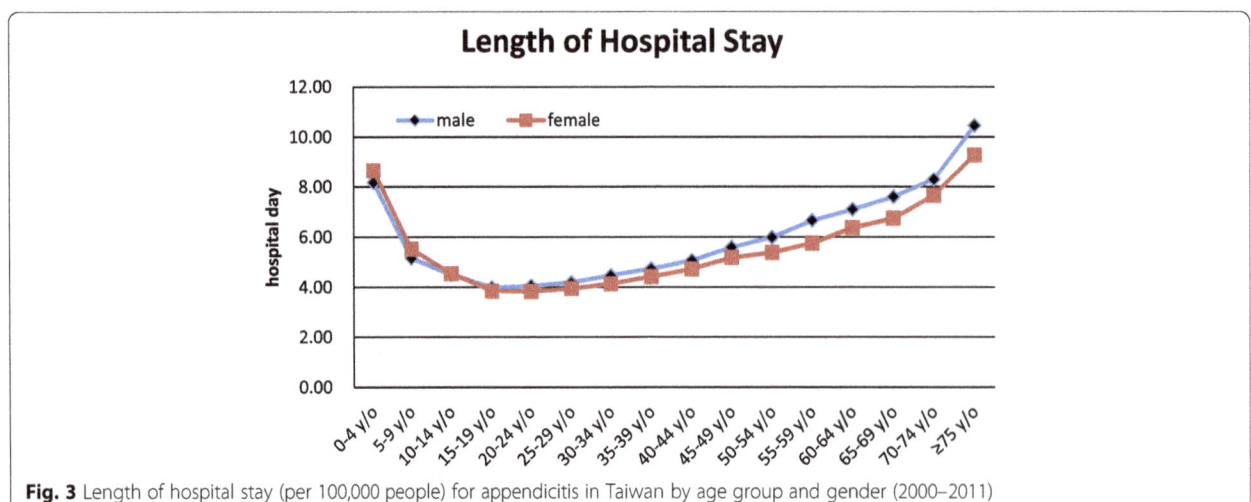

Fig. 3 Length of hospital stay (per 100,000 people) for appendicitis in Taiwan by age group and gender (2000–2011)

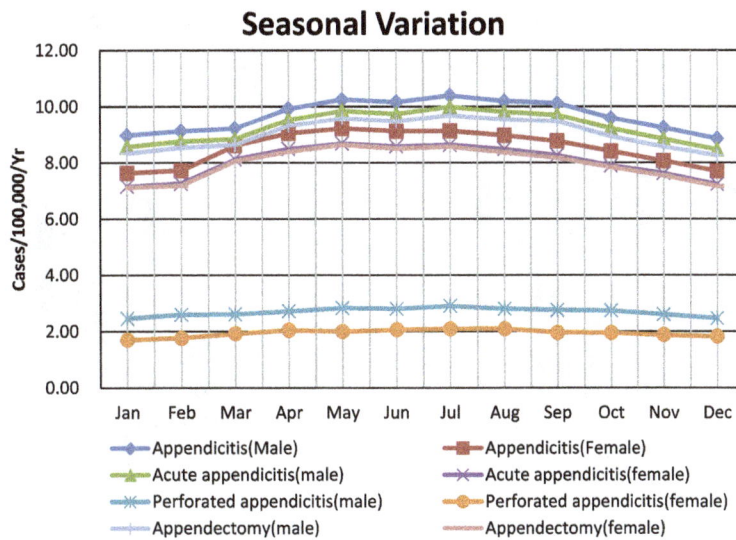

Fig. 4 Monthly incidences of appendicitis, acute appendicitis, primary appendectomy, and perforated appendicitis in Taiwan (2000–2011)

summer than in the winter), but the difference between the seasonal incidences was not as remarkable as those observed for appendicitis (Fig. 4).

Socioeconomic status: LIP versus NP

The descriptive statistics of the NP and LIP with appendicitis are presented in Table 4. LIP patients accounted for 1.25 % of the total number of patients with appendicitis. The proportion of LIP patients gradually increased from 2000 to 2011.

The overall incidence of appendicitis was 145.46 per 100,000 per year (95 % CI: 137.99–152.93) for the LIP, which was 34.99 % higher than the NP incidence of 107.76 per 100,000 per year (95 % CI: 101.33–114.19). The overall incidence of appendicitis for the LIP exhibited an annual wave-like trend but decreased in overall. Moreover, the annual incidence of appendicitis for the LIP was higher than the incidence for the NP (Fig. 5). The overall incidence of perforated appendicitis was 38.19 per 100,000 per year (95 % CI: 34.36–42.02) and 27.20 per 100,000 per year (95 % CI: 23.97–30.44) for the LIP and the NP, respectively, with an LIP-to-NP ratio of 1.40:1. Also displaying a wave-like trend, the annual incidence of perforated appendicitis was higher for the LIP than for the NP (Fig. 6).

The mean LOS for the LIP patients with appendicitis was 5.34 ± 0.09 days, which was 13.14 % higher than the LOS for the NP patients with appendicitis (4.72 ± 0.01 days). The mean hospital cost for the LIP patients with appendicitis was $1,157 \pm 14$ USD, which was 5.86 % higher than the hospital cost for the NP patients with appendicitis ($1,093 \pm 1$ USD). Table 5 presents the differences in the adjusted costs and LOS between the LIP and NP

patients stratified by various determinants. The coefficients in the multiple linear regression models represent the differences in specific outcomes between the target and reference groups. For example, the cost for the male LIP patients was higher by 37 ± 13 USD ($p = 0.004$) than the cost for the male NP patients. After multivariate adjustment, the adjusted costs for the female LIP patients were significantly higher than the costs for the female NP patients (96 ± 14 USD, $p < 0.001$) for the 30-to-44-year,

Table 4 Descriptive statistics of the sample population for LIP and NP patients with appendicitis from Taiwan's NHIRD (2000–2011)

Year	SUM	Normal population		Low-income population	
		n	%	n	%
2000	27,048	26,839	99.23 %	209	0.77 %
2001	27,941	27,677	99.06 %	264	0.94 %
2002	27,480	27,188	98.94 %	292	1.06 %
2003	25,099	24,819	98.88 %	280	1.12 %
2004	24,828	24,540	98.84 %	288	1.16 %
2005	23,686	23,401	98.80 %	285	1.20 %
2006	23,057	22,728	98.57 %	329	1.43 %
2007	23,122	22,831	98.74 %	291	1.26 %
2008	23,140	22,807	98.56 %	333	1.44 %
2009	23,365	23,013	98.49 %	352	1.51 %
2010	23,239	22,855	98.35 %	384	1.65 %
2011	22,586	22,212	98.34 %	374	1.66 %
Sum	294,591	290,910	98.75 %	3,681	1.25 %

The total number of patients (294,544) was smaller than the sum of the number of NP and LIP patients (294,591) because some patients belonged to different SES groups when they were readmitted to the hospital at different times

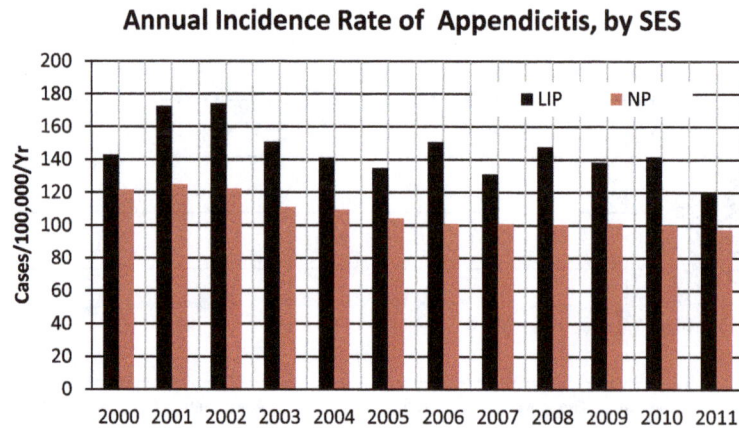

Fig. 5 Annual incidence of appendicitis in Taiwan according to socioeconomic status (2000–2011)

45-to-59-year, and 60 years and older age groups (144 ± 17, 274 ± 31, and 234 ± 48 USD, $p < 0.001$, respectively) and in the patients with perforated appendicitis (133 ± 2 USD, $p < 0.001$). The adjusted LOS for the male LIP patients was significantly longer than the LOS for the male NP patients (0.57 ± 0.009, $p < 0.001$) in the 45-to-59-year and 60 years and older age groups (1.39 ± 0.19 and 1.83 ± 0.26, $p < 0.001$, respectively) and in the patients with perforated appendicitis (0.68 ± 0.15, $p < 0.001$) (Table 5).

Temporal trends from 2000 to 2011

From 2000 to 2011, with the exception of a slightly higher incidence in 2001 compared to 2000, a clear downward trend was observed for the overall annual incidence of appendicitis. In 2000, the incidence was 121.41 per 100,000 per year (95 % CI: 114.58–128.23), and in 2011, the incidence was 97.24 per 100,000 per year (95 % CI: 91.14–103.35), reflecting a decrease of

19.9 % during the 12-year study period. Similar temporal trends were also observed regarding the incidence of acute appendicitis and primary appendectomy, with decreases from 2000 to 2011 of 19.2 % and 20.1 %, respectively. The overall incidence trend for perforated appendicitis displayed a gradual decrease from 2000 to 2009 and increased from 2009 to 2011 (Fig. 7).

Discussion

Previous studies have provided various definitions of appendicitis. For example, several studies have lumped patients undergoing appendectomy with patients diagnosed with appendicitis [22, 23, 1]. David et al. [3] proposed that a patient with a positive primary appendectomy was considered to have acute appendicitis; thus, these terms were used interchangeably in their studies. Lee et al. [8] defined appendicitis as acute appendicitis (K35), other appendicitis (K36), and unspecified appendicitis (K37) according to the

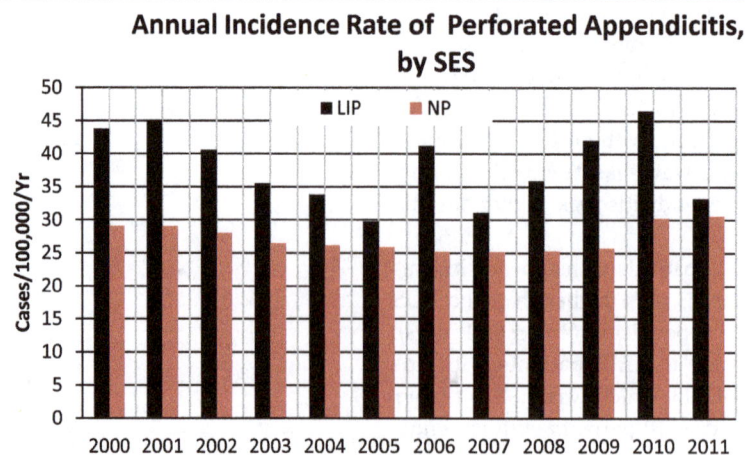

Fig. 6 Annual incidence of perforated appendicitis in Taiwan according to socioeconomic group (2000–2011)

Table 5 Subgroup analysis with a multiple linear regression analysis to compare the differences in hospital costs (USD) and LOS (days) between LIP and NP patients

Stratified variables	Hospital cost (USD)			LOS (days)		
	SES (LIP versus NP)			SES (LIP versus NP)		
	Coefficient	SE	P	Coefficient	SE	P
Gender						
Male	37	13	0.004	0.57	0.09	< 0.001
Female	96	14	< 0.001	0.19	0.08	0.013
Age (years)						
0–14 y/o	−40	18	0.031	−0.20	0.12	0.086
15–29 y/o	45	11	< 0.001	0.02	0.07	0.819
30–44 y/o	144	17	< 0.001	0.34	0.06	< 0.001
45–59 y/o	274	31	< 0.001	1.39	0.19	< 0.001
60 y/o or more	234	48	< 0.001	1.83	0.26	< 0.001
Perforated appendicitis						
No	37	8	< 0.001	0.26	0.05	< 0.001
Yes	133	25	< 0.001	0.68	0.15	< 0.001

A multivariate analysis was conducted after adjusting for age, gender, hospital level, and comorbidities

LIP low-income population *NP* normal population *SE* standard error

ICD-10. The definition used in the present study was similar to that defined by Lee et al., where a diagnosis of appendicitis was used regardless of whether the patient underwent an appendectomy. This definition can easily distinguish between appendicitis, acute appendicitis, and appendectomy but may slightly increase the incidence of appendicitis compared to other definitions.

In this study, the overall incidence of appendicitis was 107.76 per 100,000 per year (95 % CI: 101.33–114.19), which is consistent with the previously reported values of 75 to 120 per 100,000 per year in Western populations [1, 23, 3, 22, 24, 5, 6] but lower than a value in a South Korean population (227.1 per 100,000 per year) [8]. An epidemiological feature of appendicitis is the marked incidence variation according to age and gender. For both genders, the highest rates were observed in participants aged 15 to 29 years; this finding differed slightly from several previous studies that reported the highest incidence in participants aged 10 to 19 years [3, 22, 8]. In addition, the incidence of appendicitis was higher in male patients, with an overall male-to-female ratio of 1.14:1. This ratio is lower than the ratios reported in a previous study [3], which ranged from 2.2:1 to 3.3:1. In several previous studies [3, 25], the incidence of appendicitis declined with age in adults; however, in our study, although the incidence of appendicitis declined

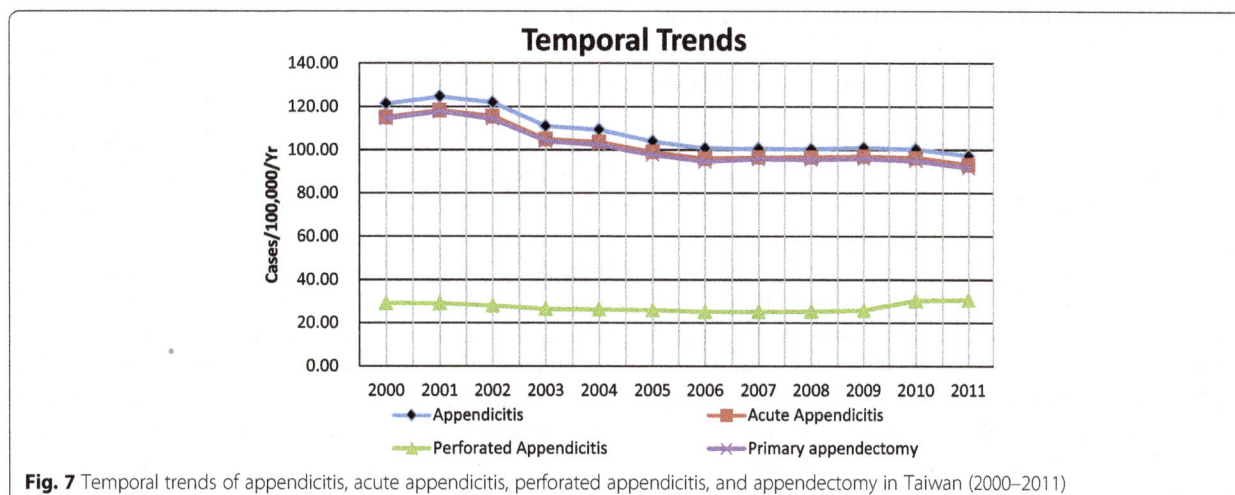

Fig. 7 Temporal trends of appendicitis, acute appendicitis, perforated appendicitis, and appendectomy in Taiwan (2000–2011)

from the age of 15 to 55 years, the incidence increased after 55 years for both genders, suggesting that the risk of appendicitis increases with age after 55 years. Other studies have also suggested an increased incidence in the 60 year and above population. For example, Roger et al. [23] reported an increased incidence of perforating acute appendicitis in the 60 year and above population for people of Asian or African descent (as shown in Figs. 3–4 in [23]). Lee et al. [8] reported an increased incidence in the 55–79-year-old male population (Fig. 1 in [8]). In general, the age patterns for the incidence of appendicitis varied by country; the reason remains unexplained and requires further in-depth study via clinical trials.

The overall incidence of appendicitis was decreased by approximately 20 % from 2000 to 2011. A declining trend of appendicitis has been reported in several previous studies [3, 26, 22, 5, 27], but the reasons for the trend remain unclear. David et al. [3] summarized several possible explanations that have been proposed by previous studies, including nutritional and dietary changes [28], the increased use of antibiotics [29], improvements in SES [30], and changes in patterns of infectious disease and immunity [26]. All of these explanations may be relevant for the declining incidence of appendicitis in Taiwan, but no causal associations have been demonstrated. Contrary to the declining trends, other studies have also reported an increasing trend for the incidence of appendicitis [6, 31, 8] and a constant incidence of appendicitis [8, 32].

During the observation period, the proportion of patients undergoing laparoscopic appendectomy (LA) (19.54 %) was lower than that of patients receiving open appendectomy (OA) for appendicitis. There may be three reasons for why only a small amount of patients underwent LA. First, some surgeons had a doubling in the utilization of laparoscopy for appendectomy between 1999 and 2003 [33], and some surgeons were not very skilled at LA surgery when it was first introduced to Taiwan. Second, many patients were unwilling to try new surgical options; although LA is a standard operation, OA is more conventional than LA. Finally, changes in the NHI payment policy may have had a significant impact on the selection of LA for patients in Taiwan. The claims for appendicitis were processed by case payments before December 31, 2009. Thus, some of the material costs of LA were not covered by the NHI payment. This portion of hospital expenses may have required payment by the patients themselves, which led to some patients not selecting LA for economic reasons. Fortunately, the payment claims for appendicitis were changed to Taiwan Diagnosis Related Groups (Tw-DRGs) since January 1, 2010, and all LA costs have been included in the NHI payment system. Although the overall proportion of patients undergoing LA was lower than that of patients undergoing OA in our research phase, the frequency of LA

increased over time, from 0 % in 2000 to 54.77 % in 2011 (data not shown).

A multilevel analysis using HLM was performed using data from 294,544 patients to assess the odds ratio of the occurrence of perforated appendicitis. As shown in Table 3, male, younger, and elderly patients were at increased risk of being diagnosed with perforated appendicitis. In addition, the analysis revealed that the risk of perforated appendicitis was significantly greater for the LIP patients and for patients who were readmitted for complications. As shown in Fig. 2, the perforation ratio was correlated with age, with the highest ratio in elderly and young patients. A similar phenomenon, which is referred to as the "J-shaped" trend, has also been reported in several previous studies [3, 8, 34, 35]; our study revealed a V-shaped trend. David et al. [3] stated that this pattern reflects both the increased diagnostic difficulty and the less timely surgical intervention for persons in these extreme age groups.

Clear seasonal variation was observed in the incidences of appendicitis, acute appendicitis, and appendectomy for both genders; the incidences increased in the summer season and decreased in the winter season. This pattern has been observed in several previous studies [3, 22, 24, 8, 11]. Wei et al. [11] analyzed the relationship between the incidence of appendicitis and climatic factors, including ambient temperature, relative humidity, atmospheric pressure, rainfall, and hours of sunshine; they reported a positive correlation between ambient temperature and the incidence of appendicitis. Kaplan et al. [36] reported a significant effect of air pollution on the incidence of appendicitis in the summer season. Although several factors may contribute to the seasonal variation in the incidences of appendicitis and appendectomy, no single causative factor has been identified [23, 3, 8]. In addition, the present study observed a slight but consistent increase in the incidence of perforated appendicitis in the summer season, which is inconsistent with several previous studies [37, 8].

The incidences of appendicitis (34.99 %) and perforated appendicitis (40.40 %) for the LIP patients were significantly higher than those for the NP patients. The reason for this pattern remains unexplained and requires further in-depth study, and clinical trials should be conducted to determine the reasons for such differences in risk. Moreover, the present study revealed that the mean LOS for the LIP patients with appendicitis was higher than the LOS for the NP patients. This finding may be attributable to three factors. First, the LIP patients may have resided in more remote areas than the NP patients, thereby requiring additional travel to obtain medical care [15]. Treatment delays related to travel may increase disease severity when patients finally arrive at a hospital, thereby necessitating a longer LOS. This may also explain the higher incidence of perforated appendicitis that was observed in the LIP patients compared to the NP patients. Second, poor financial conditions may reduce quality of life; therefore, the constitution of LIP patients may be weaker than that of NP patients, which may require a longer recovery time after an appendectomy. Finally, because health care provisions in Taiwan do not require LIP patients to pay for hospital costs, LIP patients may not consider the limitations of higher costs for a longer LOS.

The NHIB has established a uniform system to control the quality of medical services and coding. When the medical services provided to beneficiaries by contracted medical care institutions are deemed to be incompatible with the provisions of the NHI Act by the Professional Peer Review Committee, the expenses thereof are borne by the contracted medical care institutions themselves. Otherwise, the Disputes Settlement Board, which was established under the NHI scheme, settles disputes that arise in cases that were approved by the insurer and in cases that were claimed by the insured, group insurance applicants, or contracted medical care institutions [38, 39, 13, 40]. Based on the above, the data acquisition quality of the present study can be considered reliable. However, the present data are still subject to limitations.

One limitation is common to other administrative and claimed database-based studies: we could not review individual patient medical records that contained clinical data, and all of the information was in the form of numbers or codes. Without reviewing the individual medical records of each patient to ensure that the records were coded precisely, there could be deviations between the codes and the actual severity of the disease. Nonetheless, because the same database has been applied in many other fields of study with numerous high-impact publications, we believe that this population-based national claims database can be recognized as reliable [41]. The other limitation is that the information regarding gender was missing for 4,030 records of patients with appendicitis between the years 2000 and 2004 (958 records in 2000, 955 records in 2001, 879 records in 2002, 816 records in 2003, and 422 records in 2004). Information regarding gender was absent for one record in both 2006 and 2010 but was complete for all other years. The missing information regarding gender did not affect the calculation of the overall incidence, which was unrelated to the gender of the participants, but certain deviations are possible when comparing the incidence in male and female patients at various ages. To resolve this problem, we calculated the number of records for male and female patients in each age group, and the number of male patients was then divided by the number of female patients to obtain the male-to-female ratio. Subsequently, the records of the same age groups without information regarding gender were randomly assigned to the male or female groups according to the obtained gender ratio.

This solution retained the total number of records and ensured that the male-to-female ratio was relatively accurate; nevertheless, some deviation still persisted, which is a limitation of our study.

Conclusions

The present study shows that the incidence of appendicitis in Taiwan is consistent with several previous studies on Western populations but lower than the reported value of a South Korean population. The results also show that appendicitis is more common in males and that the appendicitis rate is higher in the summer months than in the winter months. The incidences of appendicitis, acute appendicitis, and primary appendectomy decreased annually, whereas the incidence of perforated appendicitis did not exhibit a clear trend. The above patterns are consistent with the results of several previous studies. However, the highest incidence of appendicitis was found in persons aged 15 to 29 years, which is different than the highest incidence in the 10-to-19-year group that was obtained in previous studies. A crucial finding was that the overall incidence of appendicitis for the LIP patients was 34.99 % higher than the overall incidence for the NP patients, and the incidence of perforated appendicitis was 40.40 % higher in the LIP than in the NP patients, indicating a significant negative effect of lower SES on the incidence and management of appendicitis and appendectomy.

Abbreviations

LIP: Low-income population; NP: Normal population; SES: Socioeconomic status; NHI: National Health Insurance; NHIB: National Health Insurance Bureau; NHIRD: National Health Insurance Research Database; LOS: Length of hospital stay; HLM: Hierarchical linear modeling; DD: Inpatient expenditures by admissions; DO: Details of inpatient orders; CD: Ambulatory care expenditures by visits; OO: Details of ambulatory care orders; IRB: Institutional review board; CI: Confidence interval; ANOVA: Analysis of Variance; AOR: Adjusted odds ratio; SPSS: Statistical package for the social sciences.

Competing interests
All authors declare that they have no conflicts of interest, including directorships, stock holding or contracts.

Author contributions
The study was designed by KBL and NPY; the data were collected and analyzed by KRL and RHP; the initial draft of the manuscript was written by CLC and KBL; and the accuracy of the data and analyses was assured by YHL, KRL and CHH. All authors participated in the preparation of this manuscript and approved the final version. All authors have read and approved the final manuscript. KBL, KRL, NPY, and CLC contributed equally to this study.

Acknowledgements
The authors would like to thank the Innovation Center for Big Data and Digital Convergence of Yuan Ze University for supporting the study. The authors also thank Yu-Tzuen Lu and Yu-Zhen Lin for their advice and generous help. This study was partially supported by the Ministry of Science and Technology, MOST 104-2218-E-155-004 and MOST104-3115-E-155-002.

Author details
[1]School of Computer & Information Engineering, Xiamen University of Technology, Xiamen 361024, China. [2]Department of Computer Science and Engineering, Yuan Ze University, Taoyuan 32003, Taiwan. [3]Management Center, Keelung Hospital, Ministry of Health and Welfare, Keelung 20147, Taiwan. [4]Institute of Public Health, National Yang-Ming University, Taipei

11221, Taiwan. [5]Department of Information Management, Yuan Ze University, Taoyuan 32003, Taiwan. [6]Innovation Center for Big Data and Digital Convergence, Yuan Ze University, Taoyuan 32003, Taiwan. [7]Section of Cardiology, Cardiovascular Center, Far Eastern Memorial Hospital, New Taipei City, Taiwan. [8]Department of Obstetrics & Gynecology, Taoyuan General Hospital, Ministry of Health and Welfare, Taoyuan, Taiwan.

References

1. Blomqvist HL P, Nyrén O, Ekbom A. Appendectomy in Sweden 1989–1993 assessed by the Inpatient Registry. J Clin Epidemiol. 1998;51(10):859–65.
2. Paajanen H, Gronroos JM, Rautio T, Nordstrom P, Aarnio M, Rantanen T, et al. A prospective randomized controlled multicenter trial comparing antibiotic therapy with appendectomy in the treatment of uncomplicated acute appendicitis (APPAC trial). BMC Surg. 2013;13:3. doi:10.1186/1471-2482-13-3.
3. David G, Addiss NS, Barbara S, Fowler BS, Tauxe RV. The Epidemiology of Appendicitis and Appendectomy in the United States. Am J Epidemiol. 1990;132(5):910–25.
4. Ilves I, Fagerstrom A, Herzig KH, Juvonen P, Miettinen P, Paajanen H. Seasonal variations of acute appendicitis and nonspecific abdominal pain in Finland. World J Gastroenterol. 2014;20(14):4037–42. doi:10.3748/wjg.v20.i14.4037.
5. Aarabi S, Sidhwa F, Riehle KJ, Chen Q, Mooney DP. Pediatric appendicitis in New England: epidemiology and outcomes. J Pediatr Surg. 2011;46(6):1106–14. doi:10.1016/j.jpedsurg.2011.03.039.
6. Buckius MT, McGrath B, Monk J, Grim R, Bell T, Ahuja V. Changing epidemiology of acute appendicitis in the United States: study period 1993–2008. J Surg Res. 2012;175(2):185–90. doi:10.1016/j.jss.2011.07.017.
7. Rai R, D'Souza RC, V V, Sudarshan SH, P.S A, Pai. J R, et al. An Evaluation of the Seasonal Variation in Acute Appendicitis. J Evol Med Dental Sci. 2014;3(2):257–60. doi:10.14260/jemds/2014/1818.
8. Lee JH, Park YS, Choi JS. The Epidemiology of Appendicitis and Appendectomy in South Korea: National Registry Data. J Epidemiol. 2010;20(2):97–105. doi:10.2188/jea.JE20090011.
9. Huang T-H, Huang YC, Tu C-W. Acute appendicitis or not: Facts and suggestions to reduce valueless surgery. J Acute Med. 2013;3(4):142–7. doi:10.1016/j.jacme.2013.10.003.
10. Chao PW, Ou SM, Chen YT, Lee YJ, Wang FM, Liu CJ, et al. Acute appendicitis in patients with end-stage renal disease. J Gastrointesti Surg. 2012;16(10):1940–6. doi:10.1007/s11605-012-1961-z.
11. Wei PL, Chen CS, Keller JJ, Lin HC. Monthly variation in acute appendicitis incidence: a 10-year nationwide population-based study. J Surg Res. 2012;178(2):670–6. doi:10.1016/j.jss.2012.06.034.
12. Wang CC, Tu CC, Wang PC, Lin HC, Wei PL. Outcome comparison between laparoscopic and open appendectomy: evidence from a nationwide population-based study. PLoS One. 2013;8(7):e68662. doi:10.1371/journal.pone.0068662.
13. Wei P-L, Liu S-P, Keller JJ, Lin H-C. Volume-Outcome Relation for Acute Appendicitis:Evidence from a Nationwide Population-Based Study. PLoS One. 2012;7(12):1–5. doi:10.1371/journal.pone.0052539.t001.
14. Yu CW, Juan LI, Wu MH, Shen CJ, Wu JY, Lee CC. Systematic review and meta-analysis of the diagnostic accuracy of procalcitonin, C-reactive protein and white blood cell count for suspected acute appendicitis. Br J Surg. 2013;100(3):322–9. doi:10.1002/bjs.9008.
15. Huang N, Yip W, Chang HJ, Chou YJ. Trends in rural and urban differentials in incidence rates for ruptured appendicitis under the National Health Insurance in Taiwan. Public Health. 2006;120(11):1055–63. doi:10.1016/j.puhe.2006.06.011.
16. Liu TL, Tsay JH, Chou YJ, Huang N. Comparison of the perforation rate for acute appendicitis between nationals and migrants in Taiwan, 1996–2001. Public Health. 2010;124(10):565–72. doi:10.1016/j.puhe.2010.05.009.
17. Yeh CC, Wu SC, Liao CC, Su LT, Hsieh CH, Li TC. Laparoscopic appendectomy for acute appendicitis is more favorable for patients with comorbidities, the elderly, and those with complicated appendicitis: a nationwide population-based study. Surg Endosc. 2011;25(9):2932–42. doi:10.1007/s00464-011-1645-x.
18. Lin K-B, Chan C-L, Yang N-P, Lai RK, Liu Y-H, Zhu S-Z et al. Epidemiology of appendicitis and appendectomy for the low-income population in Taiwan, 2003–2011. BMC Gastroenterology. 2015;15(1). doi:10.1186/s12876-015-0242-1.
19. Taiwan NHI Information for the public: essential data of ensured affair. [Available at : http://www.nhi.gov.tw/webdata/webdata.aspx?menu=17&menu_id=661&WD_ID=689&webdata_id=805]. Assessed 5 Feb 2015.
20. Ministry of Health and Welfare, Taiwan Social Assistance Act. http://law.moj.gov.tw/LawClass/LawAll.aspx?PCode=D0050078. Assessed 5 Feb 2015.
21. Diez-Roux AV. Multilevel analysis in public health research. Annu Rev Public Health. 2000;21:171–92. doi:10.1146/annurev.publhealth.21.1.171.
22. Mohammed Al-Omran MMM, Robin ML. Epidemiologic features of acute appendicitis in Ontario, Canada. Can J Surg. 2003;46(4):263–8.
23. Roger Luckmann PD. The Epidemiology of Acute Appendicitis in California: Racial, Gender, and Seasonal Variation. Epidemiology. 1991;2(5):323–30.
24. Noudeh YJ, Sadigh N, Ahmadnia AY. Epidemiologic features, seasonal variations and false positive rate of acute appendicitis in Shahr-e-Rey, Tehran. Int J Surg. 2007;5(2):95–8. doi:10.1016/j.ijsu.2006.03.009.
25. OSR MD. Appendicitis-a study of incidence, death rates and consumption of hospital resources. Postgrad Med J. 1984;60:341–5.
26. Barker D. Acute appendicitis and dietary fibre: an alternative hypothesis. Br Med J. 1985;290:1125–7.
27. Raguveer-Saran MKKN. The falling incidence of appendicitis. Br J Surg. 1980;67(9):681.
28. Arnbjornsson EAN-G, Westin SI. Decreasing incidence of acute appendicitis with special reference to the consumption of dietary fiber. Acta Chir Scand. 1982;148:461–4.
29. Noer T. Decreasing incidence of acute appendicitis. Acta Chir Scand. 1975;141:431–2.
30. Palumbo L. Appendicitis: Is it on the wane? Am J Surg. 1969;98:702–3.
31. Oguntola AS, Adeoti ML, Oyemolade TA. Appendicitis: Trends in incidence, age, sex, and seasonal variations in South-Western Nigeria. Ann Afr Med. 2010;9(4):213–7. doi:10.4103/1596-3519.70956.
32. Susan M, Bernard JMS, Anne G, Ebi KL, Isabelle R. The Potential Impacts of Climate Variability and Change on Air Pollution-Related Health Effects in the United States. Environ Health Perspect. 2001;109(2):199–209.
33. Nguyen NT, Zainabadi K, Mavandadi S, Paya M, Stevens CM, Root J, et al. Trends in utilization and outcomes of laparoscopic versus open appendectomy. AmJ Surg. 2004;188(6):813–20. doi:10.1016/j.amjsurg.2004.08.047.
34. Koepsell TDIT, Farewell VT. Factors affecting perforation in acute appendicitis. Surg Gynecol Obstet. 1981;153:508–10.
35. Scher KSCJ. Appendicitis: factors that influence the frequency of perforation. South Med J. 1980;73:1561–3.
36. Kaplan GG, Dixon E, Panaccione R, Fong A, Chen L, Szyszkowicz M, et al. Effect of ambient air pollution on the incidence of appendicitis. Can Med Assoc J. 2009;181(9):591–7. doi:10.1503/cmaj.082068.
37. Deng Y, Chang DC, Zhang Y, Webb J, Gabre-Kidan A, Abdullah F. Seasonal and day of the week variations of perforated appendicitis in US children. Pediatr Surg Int. 2010;26(7):691–6. doi:10.1007/s00383-010-2628-z.
38. Yang NP, Deng CY, Chou YJ, Chen PQ, Lin CH, Chou P, et al. Estimated prevalence of osteoporosis from a Nationwide Health Insurance database in Taiwan. Health Policy. 2006;75(3):329–37. doi:10.1016/j.healthpol.2005.04.009.
39. Yang NP, Chen HC, Phan DV, Yu IL, Lee YH, Chan CL, et al. Epidemiological survey of orthopedic joint dislocations based on nationwide insurance data in Taiwan, 2000–2005. BMC Musculoskelet Disord. 2011;12:253. doi:10.1186/1471-2474-12-253.
40. Yang NP, Chan CL, Chu D, Lin YZ, Lin KB, Yu CS, et al. Epidemiology of hospitalized traumatic pelvic fractures and their combined injuries in Taiwan: 2000–2011 National Health Insurance data surveillance. BioMed Res Intl. 2014;2014:878601. doi:10.1155/2014/878601.
41. Cheng HT, Wang YC, Lo HC, Su LT, Soh KS, Tzeng CW et al. Laparoscopic appendectomy versus open appendectomy in pregnancy: a population-based analysis of maternal outcome. Surgical endoscopy. 2014. doi:10.1007/s00464-014-3810-5.

6

Laparoscopic surgery in abdominal trauma

Kyoung Hoon Lim[1,2]*, Bong Soo Chung[2], Jong Yeol Kim[2] and Sung Soo Kim[2]

Abstract

Introduction: Laparoscopic surgery has greatly improved surgical outcome in many areas of abdominal surgery. But many concerns of safety have limited its application in abdominal trauma. We hypothesized that laparoscopy could be safe and efficacious in treatment of patients with abdominal trauma, and reduce the laparotomy related complications (i.e. wound infection, pain, or long hospital stay) as avoiding unnecessary laparotomy.

Methods: From January 2006 to August 2012, a total of 111 patients underwent emergent surgical exploration (laparoscopic, 41; open laparotomy, 70) in Andong General Hospital. Of the 41 patients subjected to laparoscopy, 30 patients had suffered blunt trauma, the remaining 11 patients had sustained penetrating trauma. 31 patients were treated exclusively by laparoscopy and 10 patients underwent laparoscopy-assisted surgery.

Results: The conversion rate was 18%. Major complication was none without postoperative mortality. Comparing laparoscopic surgery with open laparotomy, lesser wound infection, early gas passage, and shorter hospital stay. Otherwise operative times were similar, and neither approach was complicated by missed injury or postoperative intra-abdominal abscess.

Conclusions: Laparoscopic surgery can be performed safely whether injuries are blunt or penetrating, given hemodynamic stability and proper technique. Patients may thus benefit from the shorter hospital stays, greater postoperative comfort (less pain), quicker recoveries, and low morbidity/mortality rates that laparoscopy affords.

Keywords: Laparoscopy, Therapeutic laparoscopy, Blunt abdominal trauma, Penetrating abdominal trauma

Introduction

Laparoscopy has greatly improved surgical outcomes in many areas of elective abdominal surgery. In acute care surgery, laparoscopy is becoming widely accepted and used with significant advantages in the majority of ACS patients in certain centers with specific experience and laparoscopic skills [1]. However, a number of safety issues have limited its application in abdominal trauma [2]. Due to a high rate of missed injuries, laparoscopy was not well-received for diagnostic evaluation of trauma to the abdomen. However, equipment improvements over time and growing experience on the part of surgeons have overcome former misgivings with respect to penetrating abdominal injuries. Laparoscopy has being slowly attempted as a diagnostic tool for such patients, provided

they are hemodynamically stable [3,4]. Under these circumstances, laparoscopic surveillance has been shown to reduce the negative laparotomy rate [5-8]. On the other hand, its utility in patients sustaining blunt abdominal trauma has received only minor attention [9], and the therapeutic role of laparoscopy in trauma patients is still evolving. It was our contention that laparoscopy could be safe and efficacious in both diagnosis and treatment of patients with abdominal trauma, eliminating unnecessary laparotomies and the risks attached.

Methods

Medical records from the trauma registry at Andong General Hospital were reviewed retrospectively between January, 2006 and August, 2012. A total of 111 patients required surgical exploration for abdominal trauma in this time frame. For patients with penetrating injuries, breach of the peritoneum was grounds for surgical exploration. In patients with blunt injuries, those with

* Correspondence: drlimkh@naver.com
[1]Department of Surgery, Kyungpook National University Hospital, School of Medicine, Kyungpook National University, 50, Samduk-dong 2ga, Jung-gu, Daegu, South Korea
[2]Andong General Hospital, Department of Surgery, Andong, South Korea

unexplained free fluid/air by computed tomography (CT) or worrisome clinical signs and symptoms (ie, evidence of peritoneal irritation, tachycardia, and leukocytosis) were typically evaluated surgically. Five surgeons, each well-trained in colorectal, upper gastrointestinal, or hepatobiliary laparoscopy, performed the collective procedures. Laparoscopy was used at the discretion of the attending trauma surgeon, regardless of the nature of trauma (blunt or penetrating), but hemodynamic stability was mandatory. Therefore, to match two groups, 15 patients that had preoperative hemodynamic instability were excluded in the open group.

Demographic and clinical data retrieved included the type of injury, hemodynamic status on admission, indication for surgery, operative findings, therapeutic procedures performed, need for conversion (to laparotomy), Injury Severity Score (ISS), Sum of abdominal Abbreviated Injury Scale (AIS), presence of peritonitis, operative time, postoperative complications, and mortality. Complications of note were wound infection (requiring delayed closure), anastomotic leak, bleeding with reoperation, missed injury, and postoperative intra-abdominal abscess development. Written informed consent was obtained from the patient for publication of this report and any accompanying images.

Laparoscopic techniques
Initially, a 10-mm trocar was inserted via infraumbilical incision. A pneumoperitoneum was then created, using carbon dioxide to induce and maintain (at 12 mmHg) pressure. A 0-degree angle, 10-mm laparoscope was generally used for abdominal exploration. Two additional 5-mm laparoscopic ports were also placed under direct vision at right iliac fossa and at right upper quadrant (paramedial area), with mirror-image ports on the left as needed (Figure 1). Upon insertion of the laparoscope, a search for blood, bile, or intestinal contents was done. Standard examination included inspection of the spleen and liver for bleeding, a check for hollow viscus injury from stomach to rectum, and assessment of small bowel from Treitz's ligament to ileocecal valve. Using atraumatic bowel graspers, small bowel and mesentery were elevated and appraised in segments. By crossing the graspers, the reverse sides were similarly viewable [10] (Figure 2). This approach was repeated until reaching ileocecal valve, at which point colon was inspected from cecum to rectum. Ultimately, the lesser sac was pierced (through gastrocolic ligament), allowing visualization of posterior gastric wall and most of pancreas (body and tail).

Any bowel perforations detected were simply sutured (3–0 vicryl or silk) or closed by linear stapling (endo-GIA®) in the course of the procedure (Figure 3). If segmental resection was needed, a mini-laparotomy was performed by extending the umbilical port to permit

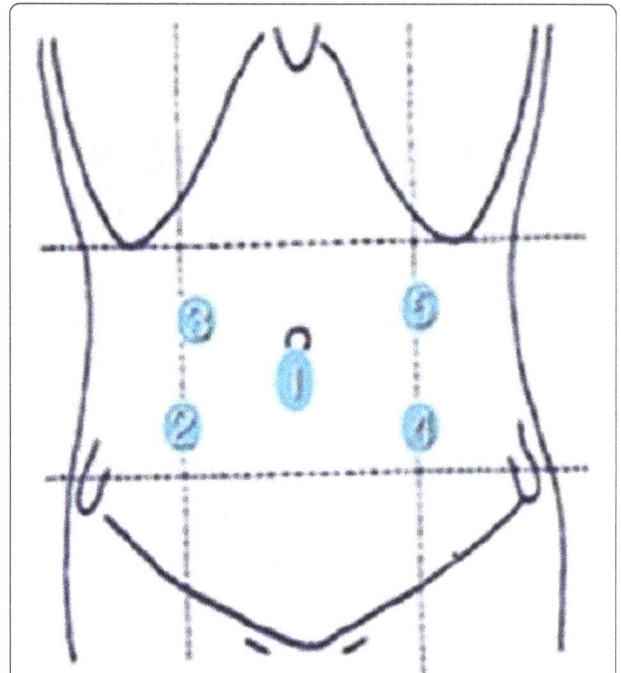

Figure 1 Laparoscopic trocar entries in abdominal trauma. ① Umbilical port for laparoscope (10-mm). ② Working port, right iliac fossa (5-mm or 12-mm). ③ Paramedial assist port, right upper quadrant (5-mm). ④ Optional port (5-mm). ⑤ Optional port (5-mm or 12-mm).

laparoscopy-assisted extracorporeal surgery. Bleeding from torn mesentery was controlled by suture ligation or cauterization (Ligasure® or Harmonic scalpel®) (Figure 4). For large volumes of spilled soilage or hematoma (mostly clots) not amenable to aspiration by conventional mode of endo-suction, evacuation was achieved by direct insertion of a silastic tube through a 12-mm port (Figure 5).

Statistical analysis
Statistical analysis relied on standard windows software (SPSS v20, Chicago, IL), expressing group variables as mean ± standard deviation. Student's t-test was applied to independent samples of continuous variables, whereas

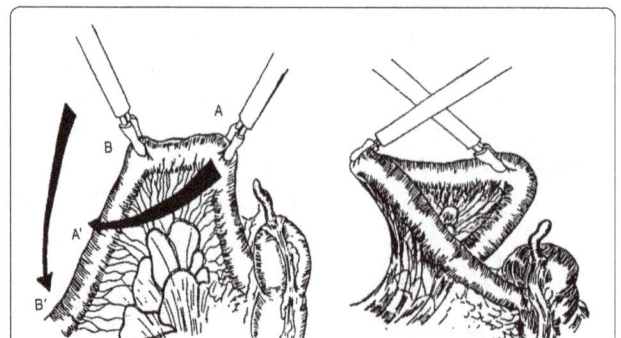

Figure 2 Elevation of small bowel via atraumatic graspers, with twisting to inspect both aspects of bowel wall and mesentery [10].

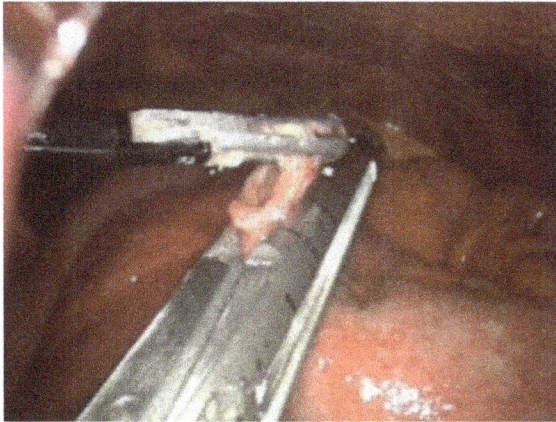

Figure 3 Stapling of perforated small bowel.

chi-square or Fisher's exact test was used for categorical values. Statistical significance was set at $p < 0.05$.

Results

In a 7-year period, 111 patients underwent surgery for abdominal trauma. Of these, 41 patients (36.9%) retained the hemodynamic stability required for a laparoscopic procedure and subsequent analysis. Laparoscopy alone was sufficient in 31 (75.6%) instances, whereas 10 patients underwent laparoscopy-assisted procedures. The other 70 patients (63.1%) were treated by open laparotomy, including any conversions (Figure 6). 15 patients of open laparotomy were excluded due to hemodynamic instability for the comparison between laparoscopy and open laparotomy. Therefore, we analyzed laparoscopic group (n = 41) and open group (n = 55).

Causes of abdominal trauma

Of the 41 patients subjected to laparoscopy, 30 patients (73.2%) had suffered blunt trauma, largely as a consequence of traffic accidents. The remaining 11 patients had sustained penetrating trauma, primarily stab injuries (Table 1).

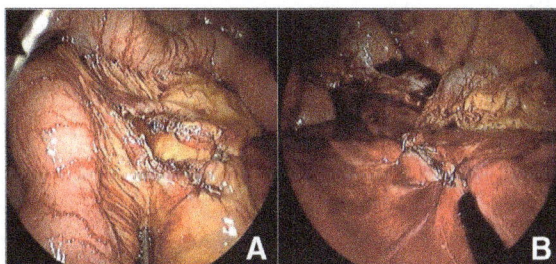

Figure 4 Control of bleeding from mesenteric tears.
A. Cauterization by Ligasure, **B**. Suturing of torn mesentery.

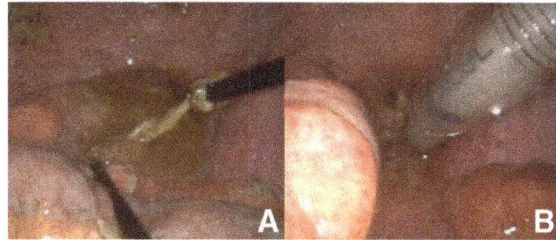

Figure 5 Methods of evacuation. A. Large particulate intestinal contents defying conventional endo-sucton, **B**. complete evacuation of large particles via silastic tube, directly inserted through 12-mm port.

Injured organs

With blunt trauma, small bowel perforation was most common, followed by torn mesentery. Three patients suffering penetrating trauma also had colon or small bowel perforations. Hemoperitoneum often resulted from injuries of omentum, mesentery, abdominal wall, or spleen (Table 2).

Methods of operation

In the 31 patients treated exclusively through laparoscopy, simple closures with suture or stapling (endo-GIA®) sufficed for 13 patients, whereas 11 patients required hemostasis using Ligasure®, Harmonic scalpel®, or suture. If segmental resection was needed for multiple perforations or transection of bowel or for intestinal ischemic changes due to mesenteric tearing, a laparoscopy-assisted mini-laparotomy was performed (Table 3).

Conversion to open laparotomy

The rate of conversion to open laparotomy was 18% (9/50). In early attempts, three laparoscopic procedures were done for diagnosis only. Reasons for conversion were uncontrolled bleeding, voluminous hematoma or spilled bowel contents, massive adhesions from prior surgery, and poor visibility due to edematous bowel (Table 4).

Comparisons between laparoscopic and open surgery

Comparing laparoscopic surgery with open laparotomy (excluding 15 patients with hemodynamic instability), The parameters presenting severity (ISS, Sum of abdominal AIS, and the presence of peritonitis) were not different between two groups. Wound infection necessitating delayed closure occurred with significantly greater frequency after open laparotomy, and other temporal parameters (time to passage of gas and hospital stay) of open laparotomy were prolonged. Otherwise, respective operative times were similar, and neither approach was complicated by missed injury or postoperative intra-abdominal abscess (Table 5).

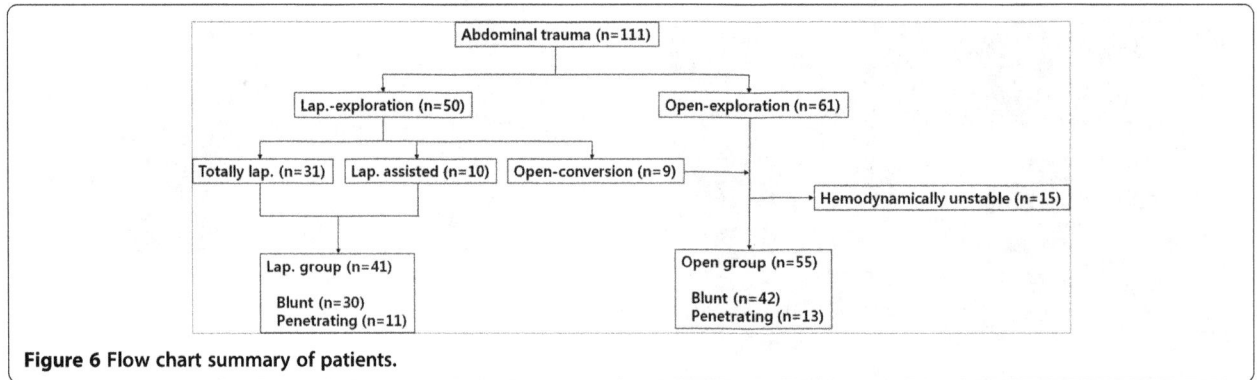

Figure 6 Flow chart summary of patients.

Discussion

It is generally upheld that patients who undergo laparoscopy, rather than conventional open surgery, are privy to quicker recovery, less pain, and faster resumption of normal daily routines [11,12]. Laparoscopy is thus a universal choice for elective abdominal surgery. However, a number of concerns have limited its application in abdominal trauma.

Until recently, the presence of peritonitis was a perceived contraindication for laparoscopy, based on the theoretical risk of malignant hypercapnia and toxic shock syndrome. The presumptive risk of malignant hypercapnia implies greater carbon dioxide absorption in the presence of severe intra-abdominal infection and inflammation of the peritoneum; and the danger of toxic shock syndrome is based on potential passage of bacteria and toxins into circulation, due to increased intraperitoneal pressure [13,14]. However, numerous reports of successful outcomes in duodenal and colonic perforation [15-17] soon followed the ground-breaking laparoscopic treatment of a perforated peptic ulcer with peritonitis [18,19]. Unfortunately, treatment of traumatic peritonitis and hemoperitoneum is where laparoscopic surgery has lagged. We have found the above concerns unwarranted with either approach.

Two publications in the 1920s were the first to suggest use of laparoscopy in diagnosing traumatic hemoperitoneum or for detecting blood from traumatic rupture of a viscus [20]. However, the modern concept of diagnostic laparoscopy for trauma was proffered in the 1960s by Heselson [21-23], who reported a series of 68 victims of trauma. In this cohort, laparoscopy was performed to detect hemoperitoneum, penetration of parietal peritoneum, and injury to abdominal organs. Thus the safety, efficacy, and economic benefits of laparoscopy, such as reduced hospitalization time and avoidance of unnecessary laparotomies, were demonstrated. Although infrequently reported, laparoscopy has also served as a therapeutic tool in selected trauma scenarios [24,25], to include the following: autotransfusion of hemoperitoneum [26]; stapling or suturing of small-intestinal wounds; stapling or suturing of stomach and diaphragmatic injuries [24]; splenorrhaphy, hepatorrhaphy, cautery, and topical hemostasis of spleen and liver injuries [24,25,27,28]; laparoscopy-assisted sigmoid

Table 1 Causes of trauma in patients undergoing surgical intervention

Causes of abdominal trauma	Laparoscopic	Open
Blunt trauma	30 (73.2)	42 (76.4)
Traffic accident	23 (56.2)	33 (60.0)
Fall	3 (7.3)	5 (9.1)
Work-related injury	3 (7.3)	2 (3.6)
Violence	1 (2.4)	2 (3.6)
Penetrating trauma	11 (26.8)	13 (23.6)
Stab injury	10 (24.4)	13 (23.6)
Gunshot	1 (2.4)	0 (0)

Table 2 Injured organs stratified by injury type

Injured organs	Laparoscopic	Open
Blunt trauma	30 (73.2)	42 (76.4)
Small bowel	19 (46.3)	27 (49.1)
Mesentery	7 (17.1)	10 (18.2)
Omentum	2 (4.9)	0 (0)
Spleen, liver	2 (4.9)	2 (3.6)
Colon	0 (0)	2 (3.6)
Bladder	0 (0)	1 (1.9)
Penetrating trauma	11 (26.8)	13 (23.6)
Omentum	3 (7.3)	1 (1.8)
Mesentery	2 (4.9)	5 (9.1)
Abdominal wall	2 (4.9)	0 (0)
Colon	2 (4.9)	1 (1.8)
Spleen, liver	1 (2.4)	2 (3.6)
Small bowel	1 (2.4)	4 (7.3)

Table 3 Operative procedures in patients undergoing surgery

Operative procedures	Patients (%)
Exclusively laparoscopic	31 (75.6)
Simple closure (suture, endo-GIA)	13 (31.7)
Bleeding control (suture, Ligasure®)	11 (26.8)
Irrigation & drainage (liver, spleen, pancreas)	4 (9.8)
Examination only (stab injury)	2 (4.9)
Loop colostomy	1 (2.4)
Laparoscopy-assisted (mini-laparotomy)	10 (24.4)
Segmental resection of small bowel	10 (24.4)
Open laparotomy	55 (100)
Simple closure (suture)	25 (45.5)
Bleeding control	18 (32.7)
Segmental resection of small bowel	11 (20.0)
Loop colostomy	1 (1.8)

Table 5 Open laparotomy and laparoscopic surgery comparison by outcomes

	Open (n = 55)	Laparoscopic (n = 41)	p-value
Age	57.2 ± 15.6	53.8 ± 15.7	0.296
ISS	9.07 ± 2.8	9.32 ± 3.6	0.708
Sum of abdomen AIS	3.16 ± 0.9	3.17 ± 1.4	0.977
Presence of peritonitis	35 (64%)	23 (56%)	0.529
Operative time (min)	97.2 ± 31.0	91.2 ± 34.6	0.374
Gas passage (day)	2.98 ± 0.9	2.44 ± 0.9	0.006
Hospital stay (day)	17.58 ± 12.7	11.5 ± 5.3	0.004
Complications			
Wound infection	5	0	0.000
Postoperative abscess	0	0	-
Mortality	0	0	-

colostomy [29]; and application of Ligaclips® to control mesenteric bleeding [30].

When first used for trauma, laparoscopy resulted in high rates of missed injury (41-77%), generating considerable criticism [31]. One of the most serious concerns was its lack of consistency in detecting small bowel damage [4,31,32], which is the main reason surgeons still hesitate today; but because these studies involved both prospective and retrospective analyses and procedures were not standardized, the data are difficult to interpret. In addition, the learning curve of laparoscopic surgery was ignored in early evaluations, and subjective preferences do seem to drive decisions during laparoscopy. One prior report underscored the reliability of laparoscopy as a tool for evaluating traumatic injuries, when used for specific indications and with appropriate technique [24,33,34]. Choi [10] and Kawahara, et al. [8] devised systematic laparoscopic explorations of the abdomen that resulted in no missed injuries. In accordance with the method of Choi, we found it relatively easy to effectively inspect all abdominal organs, without missing an injury.

The primary limitation of laparoscopic intervention is the poor visibility conferred by excessively edematous

Table 4 Reasons for converting to open laparotomy

Reasons for open conversion	Patients
Diagnostic laparoscopy only	3
Uncontrolled bleeding	2
Voluminous hematoma	1
Adhesions from prior surgery	1
Soilage in large amount	1
Edematous bowel (poor visibility)	1

bowel or uncontrolled active bleeding at presentation. These are the major motivations for conversion to open laparotomy. Edema of the bowel is a time-dependent process. Thus, patients presenting shortly after the traumatic event are more easily managed through laparoscopy, whereas lengthier time intervals usually portend severe intestinal edema. Not only is the laparoscopic window obscured by edematous bowel, but traction injury is more likely to occur during manipulation. One patient in our study was converted to open laparotomy on the basis of intestinal edema. On admission, sedation should be administered for the mechanical ventilation required by respiratory failure due to massive lung contusion, so the initial evaluation of abdomen was omitted, unfortunately. finally, bowel perforation was overlooked initially and was detected three days later after reducing a sedative.

Another cause of open conversion is the spillage of large-sized particulates that cannot be aspirated via the usual mode of endo-suction. However, we were able to achieve complete evacuation in this event by direct insertion of a silastic tube through a 12-mm port. Subsequently, our fears of postoperative intra-abdominal abscess never materialized. A fair number of our open conversions stemmed from trial-and-error in early experience, contributing to an open conversion rate of 18% (9/50). In three patients, the laparoscopies were done for diagnostic purposes only. Two patients with uncontrolled splenic bleeding were converted, as well as two others where large volumes of hematoma and spilled soilage were encountered. With more experience, these conversions very well could have been avoided.

Traumatic abdominal injury is traditionally subject to open exploration and remains a challenge for the general surgeon, especially with respect to controlling wound-related complications. Wound complications still play a major role in lengthy hospital stays and may lead to other delayed morbidities. Our aim was to extend the benefits of minimally invasive surgery to traumatic abdominal injury, thereby decreasing postoperative complications. Indeed, wound infections requiring delayed closure were limited to five patients following open laparotomy. By comparison, none of the patients undergoing laparoscopy suffered a wound complication.

Various temporal parameters (ie, time to passage of gas and hospital stay) were also comparatively better with laparoscopy, although some qualification is needed. Hospital stay was difficult to determine as a function of abdominal surgery in a setting of combined injuries (musculoskeletal, cerebrovascular, pulmonary, etc.). Therefore, we defined hospital stay by points at which oral intake was possible and wound healing was complete.

In conclusion, although we disclose that this study was many limitations caused by selection bias and retrospective study, laparoscopy gradually has being accepted as a diagnostic and/or treatment modality for penetrating abdominal injuries in patients that are hemodynamically stable. The relative rates of morbidity/mortality, postoperative complications, and missed injury are low and compare favorably with an open approach. However, laparoscopic surgery can be performed safely whether injuries are blunt or penetrating, given hemodynamic stability and proper technique. Patients may thus benefit from the shorter hospital stays, greater postoperative comfort (less pain), quicker recoveries, and low morbidity/mortality rates that laparoscopy affords.

Abbreviations
CT: Computed tomography; ISS: Injury severity score; AIS: Abbreviated injury scale.

Competing interests
The authors declare that they have no competing interests.

Authors' contributions
KHL as lead investigator made substantial contributions to conception, design, collection of data and management of patients; BSC, JYK, and SSK managed patients. All authors read and approved the final manuscript.

References
1. Di Saverio S. Emergency laparoscopy: a new emerging discipline for treating abdominal emergencies attempting to minimize costs and invasiveness and maximize outcomes and patients' comfort. J Trauma Acute Care Surg. 2014;77:338–50.
2. Rossi P, Mullins D, Thal E. Role of laparoscopy in the evaluation of abdominal trauma. Am J Surg. 1993;166:707–10. discussion 710–701.
3. Fabian TC, Croce MA, Stewart RM, Pritchard FE, Minard G, Kudsk KA. A prospective analysis of diagnostic laparoscopy in trauma. Ann Surg. 1993;217:557–64. discussion 564–555.
4. Ivatury RR, Simon RJ, Stahl WM. A critical evaluation of laparoscopy in penetrating abdominal trauma. J Trauma. 1993;34:822–7. discussion 827–828.
5. Simon RJ, Rabin J, Kuhls D. Impact of increased use of laparoscopy on negative laparotomy rates after penetrating trauma. J Trauma. 2002;53:297–302. discussion 302.
6. Chol YB, Lim KS. Therapeutic laparoscopy for abdominal trauma. Surg Endosc. 2003;17:421–7.
7. Murray JA, Demetriades D, Asensio JA, Cornwell 3rd EE, Velmahos GC, Belzberg H, et al. Occult injuries to the diaphragm: prospective evaluation of laparoscopy in penetrating injuries to the left lower chest. J Am Coll Surg. 1998;187:626–30.
8. Kawahara NT, Alster C, Fujimura I, Poggetti RS, Birolini D. Standard examination system for laparoscopy in penetrating abdominal trauma. J Trauma. 2009;67:589–95.
9. Kaban GK, Novitsky YW, Perugini RA, Haveran L, Czerniach D, Kelly JJ, et al. Use of laparoscopy in evaluation and treatment of penetrating and blunt abdominal injuries. Surg Innov. 2008;15:26–31.
10. Choi GS. Systematized laparoscopic surgery in abdominal trauma. J Korean Surg Soc. 1998;54:492–500.
11. Druart ML, Van Hee R, Etienne J, Cadiere GB, Gigot JF, Legrand M, et al. Laparoscopic repair of perforated duodenal ulcer. A prospective multicenter clinical trial. Surg Endosc. 1997;11:1017–20.
12. Lau WY, Leung KL, Kwong KH, Davey IC, Robertson C, Dawson JJ, et al. A randomized study comparing laparoscopic versus open repair of perforated peptic ulcer using suture or sutureless technique. Ann Surg. 1996;224:131–8.
13. Diebel LN, Wilson RF, Dulchavsky SA, Saxe J. Effect of increased intra-abdominal pressure on hepatic arterial, portal venous, and hepatic microcirculatory blood flow. J Trauma. 1992;33:279–82. discussion 282–273.
14. Maddaus MA, Ahrenholz D, Simmons RL. The biology of peritonitis and implications for treatment. Surg Clin North Am. 1988;68:431–43.
15. Katkhouda N, Mouiel J. A new technique of surgical treatment of chronic duodenal ulcer without laparotomy by videocoelioscopy. Am J Surg. 1991;161:361–4.
16. Regan MC, Boyle B, Stephens RB. Laparoscopic repair of colonic perforation occurring during colonoscopy. Br J Surg. 1994;81:1073.
17. O'Sullivan GC, Murphy D, O'Brien MG, Ireland A. Laparoscopic management of generalized peritonitis due to perforated colonic diverticula. Am J Surg. 1996;171:432–4.
18. Nathanson LK, Easter DW, Cuschieri A. Laparoscopic repair/peritoneal toilet of perforated duodenal ulcer. Surg Endosc. 1990;4:232–3.
19. Mouret P, Francois Y, Vignal J, Barth X, Lombard-Platet R. Laparoscopic treatment of perforated peptic ulcer. Br J Surg. 1990;77:1006.
20. Short AR. The uses of coelioscopy. Br Med J. 1925;2:254–5.
21. Heselson J. The value of peritoneoscopy as a diagnostic Aid in abdominal conditions. Cent Afr J Med. 1963;31:395–8.
22. Heselson J. Peritoneoscopy; a review of 150 cases. S Afr Med J. 1965;39:371–4.
23. Heselson J. Peritoneoscopy in abdominal trauma. S Afr J Surg. 1970;8:53–61.
24. Zantut LF, Ivatury RR, Smith RS, Kawahara NT, Porter JM, Fry WR, et al. Diagnostic and therapeutic laparoscopy for penetrating abdominal trauma: a multicenter experience. J Trauma. 1997;42:825–9. discussion 829–831.
25. Chen RJ, Fang JF, Lin BC, Hsu YB, Kao JL, Kao YC, et al. Selective application of laparoscopy and fibrin glue in the failure of nonoperative management of blunt hepatic trauma. J Trauma. 1998;44:691–5.
26. Smith RS, Meister RK, Tsoi EK, Bohman HR. Laparoscopically guided blood salvage and autotransfusion in splenic trauma: a case report. J Trauma. 1993;34:313–4.
27. Hallfeldt KK, Trupka AW, Erhard J, Waldner H, Schweiberer L. Emergency laparoscopy for abdominal stab wounds. Surg Endosc. 1998;12:907–10.
28. Smith RS, Fry WR, Morabito DJ, Koehler RH, Organ Jr CH. Therapeutic laparoscopy in trauma. Am J Surg. 1995;170:632–6. discussion 636–637.
29. Namias N, Kopelman T, Sosa JL. Laparoscopic colostomy for a gunshot wound to the rectum. J Laparoendosc Surg. 1995;5:251–3.
30. VanderKolk WE, Garcia VF. The use of laparoscopy in the management of seat belt trauma in children. J Laparoendosc Surg. 1996;6:S45–9.
31. Villavicencio RT, Aucar JA. Analysis of laparoscopy in trauma. J Am Coll Surg. 1999;189:11–20.
32. Becker HP, Willms A, Schwab R. Laparoscopy for abdominal trauma. Chirurg. 2006;77:1007–13.

7

Risk factors for delayed neuro-surgical intervention in patients with acute mild traumatic brain injury and intracranial hemorrhage

Fu-Yuan Shih[1†], Hsin-Huan Chang[1†], Hung-Chen Wang[1*], Tsung-Han Lee[1], Yu-Jun Lin[1], Wei-Che Lin[3], Wu-Fu Chen[1], Jih-Tsun Ho[1] and Cheng-Hsien Lu[2*]

Abstract

Background: Mild traumatic brain injury (TBI) patients with initial traumatic intracranial hemorrhage (tICH) and without immediate neuro-surgical intervention require close monitoring of their neurologic status. Progressive hemorrhage and neurologic deterioration may need delayed neuro-surgical intervention. This study aimed to determine the potential risk factors of delayed neuro-surgical intervention in mild TBI patients with tICH on admission.

Methods: Three hundred and forty patients with mild TBI and tICH who did not need immediate neuro-surgical intervention on admission were evaluated retrospectively. Their demographic information, clinical evaluation, laboratory data, and brain CT was reviewed. Delayed neuro-surgical intervention was defined as failure of non-operative management after initial evaluation. Risk factors of delayed neuro-surgical intervention on admission were analyzed.

Results: Delayed neuro-surgical intervention in mild TBI with tICH on initial brain CT accounted for 3.8 % (13/340) of all episodes. Higher WBC concentration, higher initial ISS, epidural hemorrhage (EDH), higher volume of EDH, midline shift, and skull fracture were risk factors of delayed neuro-surgical intervention. The volume of EDH and skull fracture is independent risk factors. One cubic centimeter (cm3) increase in EDH on initial brain CT increased the risk of delayed neurosurgical intervention by 16 % ($p = 0.011$; OR: 1.190, 95 % CI:1.041–1.362).

Conclusions: Mild TBI patients with larger volume of EDH have higher risk of delayed neuro-surgical interventions after neurosurgeon assessment. Longer and closer neurological function monitor and repeated brain image is required for those patients had initial larger EDH. A large-scale, multi-centric trial with a bigger study population should be performed to validate the findings.

Keywords: Risk factor, Mild traumatic brain injury, Surgical intervention

Background

Mild traumatic brain injury is a common presentation at the emergency department. Brain CT is the standard diagnostic tool for detecting the intracranial condition of patients with acute TBI. The incidence of associated intracranial abnormalities is 0.7–20 % [1–4]. Some patients with large intracranial hematoma will undergo surgical management initially following guidelines for the surgical management of traumatic brain injury [5]. Repeat brain CT scans after admission and monitoring the neurologic status [6, 7] are used for the early detection of progressive hematoma and increasing intracranial hypertension (IICP) [6, 8–10] in patients without initially surgical intervention. Surgical intervention is used for evacuation of the hematoma and failure of medical treatment of IICP. Several studies have focused on risk factors of intracranial lesion and delayed hemorrhage and

* Correspondence: m82whc@gmail.com;
†Equal contributors
[1]Departments of Neurosurgery, Chang Gung University College of Medicine, Kaohsiung, Taiwan
[2]Departments of Neurology, Chang Gung University College of Medicine, Kaohsiung, Taiwan
Full list of author information is available at the end of the article

intensive care unit (ICU) monitoring to prevent poor outcome of mild TBI patients [1–4, 6]. Few studies have given attention to the risk of surgical intervention [11] after initial neurosurgeon assessment. Because there is a need for better delineation of potential risk factors and clinical features in this specific subgroup, this study aimed to analyze the clinical features, neuro-imaging findings, and measurements to determine the potential risk factors predictive of surgical intervention in patients with mild TBI and tICH on admission.

Methods

Study design

This is a single center retrospective study. Three hundred and forty adult patients (age: 15–75 years) with acute TBI and tICH on initial brain CT admitted within 24 h after onset of acute TBI to Kaohsiung Chang Gung Memorial Hospital, a 2715-bed acute-care teaching medical center in southern Taiwan providing both primary and tertiary referral care, were enrolled. The tICH included epidural hemorrhage (EDH), subdural hemorrhage (SDH), intraparenchymal hemorrhage (IPH), and subarachnoid hemorrhage (SAH). All patients received complete medical and neurologic examinations, and brain CT. Neurosurgeon would be consulted to assessment of neuro-surgical intervention at ER. Neuro-radiologists correlated the neuro-imaging findings. The hospital's Institutional Review Committee on Human Research approved the study.

The diagnosis of acute TBI was confirmed by clinical history and brain CT. Patients were excluded if they had: 1) penetrating head injury or gunshot wound; 2) moderate-to-severe TBI (Glasgow Coma Score <13); 3) no tICH found on initial brain CT; 4) immediate neuro-surgical intervention on admission; and 5) only chronic intracranial hemorrhage in the initial brain CT.

The criteria for non-operative management [11] were primarily based on the clinical and radiographic findings upon admission, including alert mental status, absent lateralizing signs, basal cistern effacement or obliteration, and midline shift <5 mm. Initial neuro-surgical intervention was defined as an operation done immediately while the patient was at the emergency department. Delayed neuro-surgical intervention was defined as an operation done after the failure of non-operative management.

Clinical assessment

The patients' demographic information, mechanism of injury, initial vital signs, Glasgow Coma Score (GCS), complete physical and neurologic examination, laboratory data, and ISS [12] were all assessed. The patients underwent brain CT scan shortly after arriving at the ER. Repeat brain CT scans were performed for any clinical deterioration (e.g., acute-onset focal neurologic deficits, seizures, status epilepticus, or progressively disturbed consciousness) and as routine post-neurosurgical procedure. The principal investigator reviewed all of the initial and follow-up CT scans. In equivocal cases, a second observer made the review. Both were blinded to the laboratory results at the time of clinical and radiologic assessment.

The criteria for TBI-associated early coagulopathy included the presence of thrombocytopenia (platelet count <100,000/ml) and/or elevated international normalized ratio >1.2 and/or prolonged activated partial thromboplastin time >36 s at admission [13, 14]. Early hypotension was defined as systolic blood pressure <90 mmHg and/or diastolic pressure <40 mmHg, documented at the ER [15]. A neurosurgeon evaluated the acute TBI patients and decided on initial neuro-surgical intervention or non-operative management. Neurologic deterioration was defined as a GCS score decline ≥2, acute-onset focal neurologic deficits, seizures, or signs of progressive increased intracranial pressure (IICP). A second brain CT, taken for neurologic deterioration or upon the neurosurgeon's request, was categorized as improved, worsened, or unchanged, as Sifri mentioned in 2004 [16].

Neurosurgical intervention was defined as placement of craniotomy or craniectomy with or without an intracranial pressure monitor. Patients with intracranial pressure monitor placed were excluded in the neurosurgical group.

Statistical analysis

Data were expressed as median (inter-quartile range [IQR]). Statistical significance was set at $p < 0.05$. Categorical variables were compared using the Chi-square test or Fisher's exact test, as appropriate, while continuous variables were assessed by the Mann–Whitney U test. Correlation analysis using the Spearman rank test explored the relationship between age, GCS on admission, and ISS on admission.

Stepwise logistic regression analysis was used to evaluate the relationship between significant variables and therapeutic outcomes, with adjustments made for other potential confounding factors. Variables with zero cell count in a 2-by-2 table were eliminated from logistic analysis and only variables with strong association with poor outcome ($p < 0.05$) were included in the final model. The receiver operating characteristic (ROC) curve analysis was used to estimate an optimal cut-off value for volume of tICH on admission. The areas under the ROC curves were calculated for each parameter and compared. All of the statistical analyses were conducted using the SPSS software package, version 12.0 (Chicago, IL, USA). Statistical significance was set at $p = 0.05$.

Results

Baseline characteristics of the study patients

Of the 347 patients with acute mild TBI and tICH admitted, six underwent immediately surgical intervention and one underwent ICP monitor insertion due to orthopedic surgery. Thus, 340 patients with acute mild TBI and tICH were finally included. Based on their characteristics on admission (Table 1), there were 203 males (59.7 %) and 137 females (40.3 %). Their median age was 50 years (range: 16–75 years). Eighteen patients (5.3 %) had an initial GCS score of 13, 66 (19.4 %) had an initial GCS score of 14, and 256 (74.6 %) had an initial GCS score of 15. The most common mechanism of injury was vehicle accident (75.3 %). Hypertension and diabetes mellitus were the two most common underlying diseases. The median ISS was 10 and the median ICU and hospital stay were one and 8 days, respectively.

Table 1 Summary of admission characteristics of patients with mild TBI and tICH

Patient demographics	No. of patients
Total patients	340
Median age, years (IQR)	50 (32, 60.75)
Male: female (%)	203 (59.7 %):137 (40.3 %)
GCS score on admission (%)	
13	18 (5.3 %)
14	66 (19.4 %)
15	256 (74.6 %)
Mechanism of injury (%)	
Assault	7 (2 %)
Fall	73 (21.5 %)
Traffic accident	260 (75.3 %)
ISS score on admission (IQR)	10 (9, 16)
Anti-platelet and/or warfarin therapy (%)	13 (3.8 %)
Underlying disease (%)	
Hypertension	91 (26.8 %)
Diabetes mellitus	51 (15.0 %)
Old cerebral vascular accident	9 (2.6 %)
Coronary artery disease	8 (2.4 %)
Arrhythmia	6 (1.8 %)
Liver cirrhosis	5 (1.5 %)
Chronic kidney disease	7 (2.1 %)
Renal failure	5 (1.5 %)
Median ICU stay in days (IQR)	1 (0, 3)
Median hospital stays (IQR)	8 (5,12)

Abbreviations: *TBI* traumatic brain injury; *tICH* traumatic intracranial hemorrhage; *GCS* Glasgow Outcome Scale; *ICU* intensive care unit; *IQR* inter-quartile range

Brain imaging results

The patient characteristics in terms of tICH in the brain CT (Table 2) revealed that 222 (65.3 %) patients had single intracranial hemorrhage. EDH, subarachnoid hemorrhage (SAH), midline shift, skull fracture, and volume of EDH were significantly different between the groups of delayed and no surgical intervention. The median volume of EDH was 30.98 ml higher than volume of SDH and contusive hemorrhage. 6/26 (18.8 %) patients with EDH would undergo delayed surgical intervention. SAH was the most common type of hemorrhage in mild TBI. A few of patients had intra-ventricular hematoma but one third needed delayed surgical intervention. Skull fracture was the most common non-hemorrhagic lesion seen on initial brain CT. Midline shift was highest among patients who underwent delayed surgical intervention.

Neurologic deterioration, secondary brain CT, hospital event, and outcome of hospitalization

Recorded hospital events, secondary brain CT, and outcomes (Table 3) demonstrated that 25 patients (7.3 %) had neurologic deterioration that was significantly different between groups with delayed and those without surgical intervention. Fourteen patients (4.1 %) had GCS decline, two (0.6 %) had focal weakness, six (1.8 %) had seizures, and six (1.8 %) had signs of progressive IICP. The decline in GCS and the signs in progressive IICP were significantly different between the delayed and no surgical intervention groups.

In this series, 166 patients received a second brain CT during hospitalization. The result of patients with secondary CT were improved (33/166, 19.9 %), unchanged (99/166, 59.6 %), and worsened (34/166, 20.5 %).

The 13 patients who received delayed neurosurgical intervention included nine with neurologic deterioration and enlarged tICH, three with signs of progressive IICP and unchanged tICH, and one with enlarged tICH on regular brain CT follow-up without neurologic deterioration. The median time of surgical intervention after injury was 67.7 (11.7, 130.9) hours.

Three patients died during hospitalization and the overall mortality rate is 0.9 %. One died due to progressive hemorrhage but the family refused surgery. One died because of pneumonia with severe sepsis and another was due to endocarditis. Seven patients had a respiratory event (2.1 %) and two had a cardiac event (0.6 %). One had respiratory failure with ventilator support and two had myocardial infarction. The mean hospitalization days were 12 an 8 days in patients with delayed neurosurgical intervention and without it.

Risk factors of surgical intervention in mild TBI

Risk factors of failure of non-operative management in patients with acute mild TBI and tICH (Table 2) were

Table 2 Comparison of acute mild TBI with tICH patients who needed delayed neuro-surgical and non-surgical intervention on admission

	Delayed neuro-surgical intervention n = 13	Non-neurosurgical intervention n = 327	p value	OR	95 % CI
Median age, years, (IQR)	43(25, 49)	50(32, 61)	0.082		
Male/female (%)	9 (69 %)/4 (31 %)	194 (59 %)/133 (41 %)	0.573	0.648	0.196–2.149
GCS at presentation, Median (IQR)	15(14, 15)	15(15, 15)	0.189		
13 (%)	2 (15.4 %)	16 (4.9 %)			
14 (%)	3 (23.1 %)	63 (19.3 %)			
15 (%)	8 (61.5 %)	248 (75.8 %)			
Anti-platelet and/or warfarin therapy	1 (7.7 %)	12 (3.7 %)	0.403	2.188	0.263–18.222
Statin therapy	0	6 (1.8 %)	1.000		
Hypotension	0	4 (1.2 %)	1.000		
Blood test					
WBC count (1000/mL), Median (IQR)	15.00 (12.4, 17.05)	11.7 (8.80, 17.05)	0.023		
RBC count (1000/mL), Median (IQR)	4.74 (4.075, 5.945)	4.59 (4.26, 4.98)	0.401		
Hemoglobin, Median (IQR)	14.10 (12.85, 14.90)	13.60 (12.30, 15.00)	0.606		
Coagulopathy	0	10 (3.1 %)	1.000		
Underlying diseases					
Hypertension (%)	2 (15.4 %)	89 (27.2 %)	0.526	0.484	0.105–2.228
Diabetes mellitus (%)	2 (15.4 %)	49 (15.0 %)	1.000	1.028	0.221–4.780
Old cerebral vascular accident	0	9 (2.8 %)	1.000		
Coronary artery diseases	0	8 (2.4 %)	1.000		
Arrhythmia	0	6 (1.8 %)	1.000		
Liver cirrhosis	0	5 (1.5 %)	1.000		
Chronic renal disease	0	7 (2.1 %)	1.000		
Renal failure	0	5 (1.5 %)	1.000		
ISS score, Median (IQR)	16 (15, 17.5)	10 (9, 16)	0.005		
Single intracranial hemorrhage (%)	6 (46.2 %)	216 (66.1 %)	0.149		
Multiple intracranial hemorrhage (%)	7 (53.8 %)	111 (33.9 %)	0.149		
Type of intracranial hemorrhage					
EDH (%)	6 (46.2 %)	26 (8.0 %)	≤0.001	9.923	3.105–31.708
SDH (%)	6 (46.2 %)	159 (48.6 %)	1.000	0.906	0.298–2.753
IPH (%)	6 (46.2 %)	105 (32.1 %)	0.366	1.812	0.594–5.526
SAH (%)	3 (23.1 %)	178 (54.4 %)	0.044	0.251	0.068–929
IVH (%)	1 (33.4 %)	2 (0.6 %)	0.111	13.542	1.147–159.876
Midline shift (%)	5 (33.4 %)	10 (3.1 %)	≤0.001	19.813	5.495–71.435
Skull fracture (%)	11 (14.3 %)	66 (20.2 %)	≤0.001	21.750	4.707–100.510
Pneumocranium (%)	0	32 (9.8 %)	0.621		
Volume of hemorrhage in initial brain CT					
Volume of EDH, Median (IQR)	30.98 (9.68, 46.86)	2.20 (0.67, 6.71)	≤0.001		
Volume of SDH, Median (IQR)	4.56 (1.13, 17.83)	1.32 (0.15, 5.38)	0.092		
Volume of IPH, Median (IQR)	2.33 (0.11, 7.3)	0.59 (0.11, 2.53)	0.657		

Abbreviations: *TBI* traumatic brain injury; *tICH* traumatic intracranial hemorrhage; *N* number of cases; *IQR* inter-quartile range; *OR* odds ratio; *CI* confidence interval; *EDH* epidural hemorrhage; *SDH* subdural hemorrhage; *IPH* intraparenchymal hemorrhage; *SAH* sub-arachnoid hemorrhage; *IVH* intraventricular hemorrhage; *GCS* Glasgow Outcome Scale

Table 3 Summary of hospital events, secondary brain computed tomography, and outcome

	Delayed neuro-surgical intervention n = 13	Non-surgical intervention n = 327	Total (%) n = 340	p value
Neurologic deterioration	12	13	25 (7.3)	≤0.001
GCS decline	7	7	14 (4.1)	≤0.001
Focal weakness	1	1	2 (0.6)	0.075
Seizure	1	5	6 (1.8)	0.210
Progressive IICP signs	4	2	6 (1.8)	≤0.001
Secondary brain CT				
Improved	0	33	33 (19.9)	0.073
Unchanged	3	96	99 (59.6)	0.007
Worsened	10	24	34 (20.5)	≤0.001
Respiratory event	0	7	6 (1.8)	1.000
Cardiac event	0	2	2 (0.6)	1.000
Time of surgical intervention, hours, Mean (IQR)	67.7 (31.5, 125)			
Mean Hospitalization days, Median (IQR)	12 (11, 28)	8 (4, 12)		≤0.001

Abbreviations: GCS Glasgow Coma Score; *IICP* increased intracranial pressure; *IQR* inter-quartile range; *OR* odds ratio; *CI* confidence interval

higher WBC count, EDH, larger volume of EDH, midline shift, skull fracture, and higher initial ISS ($p < 0.05$). After stepwise logistic regression, only the volume of EDH was independently associated with delayed neuro-surgical intervention. A cut-off value of 9.3 ml EDH on admission had 83.3 % sensitivity and 84.6 % specificity for predicting delayed neuro-surgical intervention. Furthermore, an increase of one cubic centimeter (cm [3]) in EDH on initial brain CT increased the risk of delayed surgical intervention by 16.0 % ($p = 0.011$; OR: 1.190, 95 % CI: 1.041–1.362). The area under the curve for volume of EDH was 0.917 (95 % CI: 0.797–1.000). Using the ROC curves of the detailed prediction model, for a linear predictor score of 1.67, sensitivity was 83.3 % and specificity was 84.6 % for delayed neuro-surgical intervention. With increased volume of epidural hemorrhage, the sensitivity of the model to detect very positive finding decreased, while the specificity of the model increased. All hematoma >26 ml needed neurosurgical evacuation.

Discussion

Patient with acute mild TBI constitute a significant number of patients in the emergency department. Regular follow-up brain CT, monitoring in the intensive care unit, and financial difficulties have all been discussed. Surgical intervention is the most important consideration. In the current study, the failure rate of non-operative management is 3.8 % (13/340). Such figures are consistent with those of five recent studies, with a range of 1–8.7 % [6, 10, 17–19]. The rate and number of patients with acute mild TBI undergoing neurosurgical intervention is low. The rate of craniotomy is 0.9–5.8 % and ICP monitor insertion is 0.2–2.9 %. In 2009, Bee et

al. reported the largest number and rate of neurosurgical intervention in mild TBI with tICH [6]. Thomas et al. reported the largest number of patient with mild TBI with tICH [10]. Their number of neurosurgical intervention was 18 and 14, respectively. Both studies focused on repeat brain CT, progressive hemorrhage, and ICU monitor. We identified the risk of factors of mild TBI with initial tICH and delayed neurosurgical intervention including volume of EDH.

In the initial brain CT, only volume of EDH was the risk of delayed neuro-surgical intervention. The median volume of EDH was larger than volume of SDH and IPH. Patients can tolerate the larger volume of EDH without neurologic deficit than others of hemorrhage. Chen et al. reported that an EDH volume >30 ml, thickness >15 mm, and midline shift >5 mm tended to require surgery [20]. In this series, there is no successful non-operative management in patients with EDH >26 ml on initial brain CT. All of them had signs of progressive IICP during non-operative management. Moreover, any increase of one cubic centimeter (cm [3]) increased the presence of delayed neurosurgical intervention by 16.0 % ($p = 0.011$; OR: 1.190, 95 % CI: 1.041–1.362). Larger volume of initial EDH tended to have higher risk of delayed neuro-surgical management.

Previous reports found that progressive hemorrhage occurred in approximately 15–28 % of patients with acute mild TBI [6, 16, 21]. Most developed early (within one day after the injury) during the clinical course [22–24]. In this study, 20.5 % of patients had larger hematoma seen in following up brain images. The median time of repeated brain CT is 65.9 (10.1, 128.4) hours in delayed neurosurgical intervention. Most patients (12/13, 92.3 %) had neurologic deficit. The median time of neurologic deterioration and neurosurgical intervention was 51.8 (9.9, 92.9) hours and 67.7 (31.5, 125) hours in delayed neuro-surgical intervention.

In the current study, neurologic deterioration in acute mild TBI accounts for 7.3 % (25/340) of all episodes, including 48 % (12/25) who underwent neuro-surgical intervention. The study by Sifri et al. had 161 patients with mild traumatic brain injury and intracranial bleed on initial cranial CT. Due to abnormal neurologic findings on repeat CT scan, 6 % of these patients underwent emergency craniotomy [17]. In another study, 3.7 % (21/565) had acute neurologic deterioration and 29 % (6/21) led to neuro-surgical or medical intervention [18]. Washington et al. reported 321 patients with mild TBI and abnormal head CT, including four patients (1 %) with neurologic decline and three who underwent neurosurgical intervention [19]. In the present series, there was a higher incidence of neurologic deterioration in the delayed neuro-surgical intervention group.

In terms of laboratory data, higher WBC count is a risk of delayed neurosurgical intervention. Leukocytosis is associated with the severity of injury and outcome [25, 26]. Although the mechanism is still controversial, catecholamines increase the leukocyte count by releasing marginated cells into the circulating pool. Corticosteroids increase the neutrophil count by releasing cells from the storage pool in the bone marrow. In this study, leukocytosis is significantly different in the two groups of non-operative management and delayed neurosurgical intervention. There were thirteen patients received anticoagulation therapy in our study, but only ten patients had coagulopathy at the time of injury. However, no patient with coagulopathy needs delayed neurosurgical intervention. In our clinical practice, we corrected those patients with coagulopathy as soon as possible after intracranial hemorrhage was diagnosed. Furthermore, we only enrolled patients with mild traumatic brain injury. This could be why no patient with coagulopathy needs delayed neurosurgical intervention in this study.

This study has several limitations. First, the study is retrospective. Second, following brain images during non-operative management are irregular, and that could be a confounding factor. The real rate of progressive intracranial hemorrhage is also unknown. Lastly, there is the short-term follow-up period and relatively small sample size. A larger cohort is necessary to generate more powerful conclusions and to refine predictors of neuro-surgical interventions.

Conclusions

Larger volume of EDH on initial brain CT had higher risk of delayed neuro-surgical intervention after neurosurgeon assessment. Longer and closer neurological function monitor and repeated brain image is required for those patients had initial larger EDH. A large-scale, multi-centric trial with a bigger study population should be performed to validate the findings.

Abbreviations
aPTT: activated partial thromboplastin time; BP: blood pressure; ROC: receiver operating characteristic; EDH: epidural hemorrhage; ER: emergency room; GCS: Glasgow Coma Score; ICU: intensive care unit; IICP: increased intracranial pressure; SAH: subarachnoid hemorrhage; SDH: subdural hemorrhage; TBI: traumatic brain injury; tICH: traumatic intracranial hemorrhage.

Competing interest
None of the authors have any commercial association, such as consultancies, stock ownership, or other equity interests or patent-licensing arrangements that may influence this study.

Authors' contributions
SFY and CHH participated in the design of the study and drafted the manuscript. Wang HC, LYJ, LTH, HJT, and CWF participated in the sequence alignment and clinical evaluation of patients. WHC and LWC interpreted the imaging studies. SFY and WHC performed the statistical analysis. WHC and LCH conceived the study, participated in its design and coordination, and helped draft the manuscript. All authors read and approved the final manuscript.

Acknowledgements
The authors thank all of the subjects who participated in this study and Dr. Gene Alzona Nisperos for editing and reviewing the manuscript for English language considerations.

Author details
[1]Departments of Neurosurgery, Chang Gung University College of Medicine, Kaohsiung, Taiwan. [2]Departments of Neurology, Chang Gung University College of Medicine, Kaohsiung, Taiwan. [3]Departments of Radiology, Kaohsiung Chang Gung Memorial Hospital and Chang Gung University College of Medicine, Kaohsiung, Taiwan.

References
1. Bordignon KC, Arruda WO. CT scan findings in mild head trauma: a series of 2,000 patients. Arq Neuropsiquiatr. 2002;60:204–10.
2. Holmes JF, Hendey GW, Oman JA, et al. Epidemiology of blunt head injury victims undergoing ED cranial computed tomographic scanning. Am J Emerg Med. 2006;24:167–73.
3. Mower WR, Hoffman JR, Herbert M, et al. Developing a decision instrument to guide computed tomographic imaging of blunt head injury patients. J Trauma. 2005;59:954–9.
4. Haydel MJ, Preston CA, Mills TJ, Luber S, Blaudeau E, DeBlieux PM. Indications for computed tomography in patients with minor head injury. N Engl J Med. 2000;343:100–5.
5. Bullock MR, Chesnut R, Ghajar J, et al. Surgical management of acute epidural hematomas. Neurosurgery. 2006;58:S7–15. discussion Si-iv.
6. Bee TK, Magnotti LJ, Croce MA, et al. Necessity of repeat head CT and ICU monitoring in patients with minimal brain injury. J Trauma. 2009;66:1015–8.
7. Nishijima DK, Sena MJ, Holmes JF. Identification of low-risk patients with traumatic brain injury and intracranial hemorrhage who do not need intensive care unit admission. J Trauma. 2011;70:E101–7.
8. Park HK, Joo WI, Chough CK, Cho CB, Lee KJ, Rha HK. The clinical efficacy of repeat brain computed tomography in patients with traumatic intracranial haemorrhage within 24 hours after blunt head injury. Br J Neurosurg. 2009;23:617–21.
9. Stein SC, Fabbri A, Servadei F. Routine serial computed tomographic scans in mild traumatic brain injury: when are they cost-effective? J Trauma. 2008;65:66–72.
10. Thomas BW, Mejia VA, Maxwell RA, et al. Scheduled repeat CT scanning for traumatic brain injury remains important in assessing head injury progression. J Am Coll Surg. 2010;210:824–30. 31–2.

11. Patel NY, Hoyt DB, Nakaji P, et al. Traumatic brain injury: patterns of failure of nonoperative management. J Trauma. 2000;48:367–74. discussion 74–5.

12. Baker SP, O'Neill B, Haddon Jr W, Long WB. The injury severity score: a method for describing patients with multiple injuries and evaluating emergency care. J Trauma. 1974;14:187–96.

13. Lozance K, Dejanov I, Mircevski M. Role of coagulopathy in patients with head trauma. J Clin Neurosci. 1998;5:394–8.

14. Kuo JR, Chou TJ, Chio CC. Coagulopathy as a parameter to predict the outcome in head injury patients–analysis of 61 cases. J Clin Neurosci. 2004;11:710–4.

15. Chen H, Guo Y, Chen SW, et al. Progressive epidural hematoma in patients with head trauma: incidence, outcome, and risk factors. Emerg Med Int. 2012;2012:134905.

16. Sifri ZC, Livingston DH, Lavery RF, et al. Value of repeat cranial computed axial tomography scanning in patients with minimal head injury. Am J Surg. 2004;187:338–42.

17. Sifri ZC, Homnick AT, Vaynman A, et al. A prospective evaluation of the value of repeat cranial computed tomography in patients with minimal head injury and an intracranial bleed. J Trauma. 2006;61:862–7.

18. Velmahos GC, Gervasini A, Petrovick L, et al. Routine repeat head CT for minimal head injury is unnecessary. J Trauma. 2006;60:494–9. discussion 9–501.

19. Washington CW, Grubb Jr RL. Are routine repeat imaging and intensive care unit admission necessary in mild traumatic brain injury? J Neurosurg. 2012;116:549–57.

20. Chen TY, Wong CW, Chang CN, et al. The expectant treatment of "asymptomatic" supratentorial epidural hematomas. Neurosurgery. 1993;32:176–9. discussion 9.

21. Stippler M, Smith C, McLean AR, et al. Utility of routine follow-up head CT scanning after mild traumatic brain injury: a systematic review of the literature. EMJ. 2012;29:528–32.

22. Oertel M, Kelly DF, McArthur D, et al. Progressive hemorrhage after head trauma: predictors and consequences of the evolving injury. J Neurosurg. 2002;96:109–16.

23. Ashkenazi E, Constantini S, Pomeranz S, Rivkind AI, Rappaport ZH. Delayed epidural hematoma without neurologic deficit. J Trauma. 1990;30:613–5.

24. Radulovic D, Janosevic V, Djurovic B, Slavik E. Traumatic delayed epidural hematoma. Zentralbl Neurochir. 2006;67:76–80.

25. Rovlias A, Kotsou S. The blood leukocyte count and its prognostic significance in severe head injury. Surg Neurol. 2001;55:190–6.

26. Gurkanlar D, Lakadamyali H, Ergun T, Yilmaz C, Yucel E, Altinors N. Predictive value of leucocytosis in head trauma. Turk Neurosurg. 2009;19:211–5.

8

Surgical management of AAST grades III-V hepatic trauma by Damage control surgery with perihepatic packing and Definitive hepatic repair–single centre experience

Krstina Doklestić[1], Branislav Stefanović[1], Pavle Gregorić[1], Nenad Ivančević[1], Zlatibor Lončar[1], Bojan Jovanović[2], Vesna Bumbaširević[2], Vasilije Jeremić[1], Sanja Tomanović Vujadinović[3], Branislava Stefanović[2], Nataša Milić[4] and Aleksandar Karamarković[1*]

Abstract

Background: Severe liver injury in trauma patients still accounts for significant morbidity and mortality. Operative techniques in liver trauma are some of the most challenging. They include the broad and complex area, from damage control to liver resection.

Material and method: This is a retrospective study of 121 trauma patients with hepatic trauma American Association for Surgery of Trauma (AAST) grade III–V who have undergone surgery. Indications for surgery include refractory hypotension not responding to resuscitation due to uncontrolled hemorrhage from liver trauma; massive hemoperitonem on Focused assessment by ultrasound for trauma (FAST) and/or Diagnostic peritoneal lavage (DPL) as well as Multislice Computed Tomography (MSCT) findings of the severe liver injury and major vascular injuries with active bleeding.

Results: Non-survivors have significantly higher AAST grade of liver injury and higher Injury Severity Score (ISS) ($p = 0.000$; $p = 0.0001$). Non-survivors have significant hypotension on arrival and lower Glasgow Coma Scale (GCS) on admission ($p = 0.000$; $p = 0.0001$). Definitive hepatic repair was performed in 62(51.2 %) patient. Damage Control, liver packing and planned re-laparotomy after 48 h were used in 59(48.8 %). There was no statistically significant difference in terms of the surgical approach. There was significant difference in the amount of red blood cells (RBC) transfusion in the first 24 h between survivors and non-survivors ($p = 0.001$). Overall mortality rate was 33.1 %. Regarding complications non-survivors had significantly prolonged bleeding and higher rate of Acute respiratory distress syndrome (ARDS) ($p = 0.0001$; $p = 0.0001$), while survivors had significantly higher rate of pleural effusion ($p = 0.0001$).

Conclusion: All efforts in the treatment of severe liver injuries should be directed to the rapid and effective control of bleeding, because uncontrollable hemorrhage is the cause of early death and it requires massive blood transfusion, all of which contributes to the late fatal complication.

Keywords: Liver trauma, Damage control surgery (DCS), Hemorrhage, Exsanguinating trauma patients, Mortality

* Correspondence: alekara@sbb.rs
[1]Faculty of Medicine, University of Belgrade and Clinical Center of Serbia, Clinic for Emergency Surgery, University of Belgrade, Serbia, Pasteur Str.2, Belgrade 11000, Serbia
Full list of author information is available at the end of the article

Introduction

Despite the great advances in surgical treatment and resuscitation of trauma patients with liver injuries in the last decades, severe liver trauma still accounts for significant morbidity and mortality [1–4]. Major liver injury is the leading cause of death in patients with abdominal trauma, and their treatment continues to challenge surgeons [5, 6]. The main cause of early liver injury-related death is uncontrolled bleeding, and it is associated with a mortality rate of 50–54 % in the first 24 h after admission, with 80 % of operative deaths [1, 2, 5].

Early diagnosis of the extent of liver trauma with adequate treatment adapted to the severity of the injury and the physiological condition of the patient, may result in significant reduction of morbidity and mortality [5]. Hemodynamic stability is key for diagnostic and therapeutic approach to the severe liver injuries. The diagnosis of hepatic trauma starts simultaneously with reanimation, immediately after admission, which implies targeted clinical examination, laboratory blood tests, abdominal ultrasound (Focused assessment with sonography for trauma, FAST) followed by Multislice Computed Tomography (MSCT) [6–10]. Elevation of the serum aspartate aminotransferase (AST) and alanine aminotransferase (ALT) is the laboratory indicator of liver injury [9].

Menagment of a severe trauma patient involves systematic sequence of actions [8–15]. Haemodynamically unstable patients with major liver injuries require rapid manoeuvers to control bleeding [10]. Accordingly, exsanguinating patients require substantial blood transfusions [11]. Uncontrolled bleeding leads to new adverse events that announce catastrophe–coagulopathy, as a result of depletion and dilution of coagulation factors, acidosis, and hypothermia [10, 11]. The decision for an emergency laparotomy is usually based upon the presence of the "lethal triad" with coagulopathy, acidosis and hypothermia [5, 11]. Surgical treatment in bleeding liver trauma is required in cases of progressive hemodynamic instability due to hemorrhage shock [11]. Operative techniques in liver trauma are some of the most challenging. They include the broad and complex area from Damage control surgery (DCS) to the liver resection [2, 5]. Surgical control of bleeding is the main goal in damage control strategy as well as the prevention of biliary complications which are specific for liver injuries. In unstable patients with severe physiological derangement surgical procedures such as direct vessel repair of juxtahepatic venous injuries and early perihepatic packing with the correction of hypothermia, coagulopathy, and acidosis may lead to improved outcome [5, 10, 11].

The purpose of this study was to determine the predictors of morbidity and mortality in trauma patients that underwent surgery for severe hepatic injury, as well as to identify a better approach for exsanguinating patients.

Materials and methods

This is the retrospective study of 121 trauma patients with severe hepatic trauma, who have been admitted and operated at Clinic of Emergency Surgery, Clinical Center of Serbia, Belgrade, from November 2008 to January 2015. This study has been performed with the approval of the Ethics Committee of the Clinical Centre of Sebia with a reference number 1533/21.

Severe liver injuries were graded according to the American Association for the surgery of Trauma (AAST) - Organ Injury Scale (OIS) as liver trauma grades III, IV and V [1, 4]. Hemodynamically stable patients who had AAST grade I-II liver injury, treated by Non Operative Management (NOM) were not included in study.

Upon arrival at the emergency room of the trauma patient with uncontrolled hemorrhage, the main goal was identification of the sources of bleeding, followed by prompt bleeding control and resuscitation in order to restore tissue perfusion and to achieve haemodynamic stability. After complete, targeted and very fast clinical examination, Focused assessment with sonography for trauma (FAST) is the first tool used as to see the presence of free fluid (means hemoperitoneum) and associated solid organ injury. In hemodynamically unstable Diagnostic peritoneal lavage (DPL) was performed following a negative FAST scan in the setting of blunt abdominal trauma for rapid diagnosis of abdominal injury requiring emergency laparotomy. Initial MSCT of thorax and abdomen in order to determine the severity of the liver trauma and the presence of associated injuries, was done in haemodynamic stable patients. Shock was defined as a systolic blood pressure of <90 mmHg. Glasgow Coma Scale (GCS) used for evaluation the severity of associated CNS and head injury, by measuring three parameters (motor response, verbal response and eye opening response) range was from 0 (brain death) to the maximum score of 15 for normal cerebral function. The Injury Severity Score (ISS) as an anatomical scoring system providing an overall score for trauma patients with multiple injuries. Each injury is assigned an Abbreviated Injury Scale (AIS) score and is allocated to one of the six body regions (Head, Face, Chest, Abdomen, Extremities (including Pelvis), External). The ISS score takes values from 0 to 75 (lethal injury).

Indications for emergency laparotomy within 30 min uppon trauma patients arrival included: uncontrolled bleeding from liver trauma with positive FAST and/or DPL (hemoperitoneum: blood at initial aspiration or a red blood cell count in the lavage fluid was >100.000/mm^3); MSCT findings of the massive hemoperitoneum and severe liver trauma with major hepatic vein/VCI laceration, complex perihilar injuries with active bleeding presented as extravasations of intravenous contrast; and hemorrhagic shock with refractory hypotension not responding to initial resuscitation. Laparotomy was performed through midline incision searching for intraperitoneal bleeding, liver trauma, associated abdominal injury and intestinal perforations that call for emergency repair. Blood from the peritoneal cavity was sucked out, folowed by emergency care of intraperitoneal haemorrhage and control of the sources of contamination. Inflow vascular control was employed as Pringle maneuver under vascular clamp before proceeding of liver parenchymal and vascular repair. Direct liver repair techniques have been used as extensive suture (hepatorrhaphy), hepatotomy with selective vascular ligation, selective right hepatic artery (RHA) ligation, resectional de'bridement and liver resection. Major resection was used only to control extensive laceration of liver and extensive devitalized liver tissue.

In exsanguinating patients with severe physiological derangement (lethal triade) due to exsanguinating liver injuries we used strategy of Damage Control Surgery (DCS). Exsanguination presented the extreme blood loss caused by traumatic complex liver injuries and major blood vessels, with an initial blood loss of >40 % of the entire blood volume. Indications for DCS were:

- Metabolic acidosis (lactic acid level >5 mmol/L, pH <7.2, base deficit >14)
- Hypothermia (core hypothermia <34 °C)
- Coagulopathy (PT and PTT >2 times normal)

Initial emergency laparotomy was the first step of the damage control: fast and limited surgical intervention in order to control life-threatening hemorrhage and control of contamination. We performed perihepatic packing (packing of the liver) with approximately 4–6 abdominal swabs to provide liver compression and bleeding control. Abdominal swabs were never placed directly into the liver laceration and bleeding blood vessels were suture/ligated prior to liver packing. After liver packing, the abdomen was closed temporarily. From operating theater patient was transferred to the Intensive Care Unit (ICU) for ICU resuscitation and correction of acidosis, coagulopathy, hypothermia, including antibiotic with broad-spectrum aerobic and anaerobic coverage in all patients (DCS II step). Indications for red blood cell (RBC) transfusion included acute blood loss greater than 1500 mL, or 30 percent of blood volume, or hemoglobin level <9 g/dl. Massive transfusion was defined as transfusion of ten or more RBC products within 24 h. The third step in DCS was a planed re-laparotomy and definitive reconstruction. Removal of perihepatic packing and definitive surgical procedure was performed after 48 h when the patient's temperature has been normalized, shock has been corrected, and the International Normalized Ratio (INR) was less than 1.5.

Data were collected in terms of age, sex, blood pressure on arrival, mechanism of trauma, AAST grades of liver injury, ISS due to severe associated injuries, management and outcome. Types of surgical procedures, RBC transfusion (ml) within first 24 h, Intensive Care Unit (ICU) stay and hospital length of stay were recorded. Liver-related complications were considered to include prolonged massive bleeding (more than 100 ml/h on abdominal drain) despite the surgical control of bleeding, liver failure, bile leak, bile fistula and liver abscess. Biliary leak was defined as any drainage through the abdominal catheter with bilirubin content 2× higher than the plasma levels. The Acute Respiratory Distress Syndrome (ARDS) was defined on three mutually exclusive categories based on degree of hypoxemia: mild (200 mm $Hg < PaO_2/FIO_2 \leq 300$ mm Hg), moderate (100 mm Hg < $PaO_2/FIO_2 \leq 200$ mm Hg), and severe ($PaO_2/FIO_2 \leq$ 100 mm Hg) and four ancillary variables for severe ARDS: radiographic severity with bilateral infiltrates, respiratory system compliance (≤ 40 mL/cm H_2O), positive end-expiratory pressure (≥ 10 cm H_2O), and corrected expired volume per minute (≥ 10 L/min). Mortality was defined as death within 30 days of hospitalization. Early trauma-related mortality was defined when death occurred within the first 48 h.

Statistical analysis

Data were analyzed using methods of descriptive and analytical statistics. The methods of descriptive statistics were: measures of central tendency (mean and median), measures of variability (standard deviation and interquartile range) and the relative numbers. The methods of analytical statistics were: identification methods of empirical distributions, methods to assess the significance of differences and Student's t test and rank sum test for numerical variables depending on the normality of distribution and Chi-square and Fisher's test for categorical variables. Univariate and multivariate logistic regression analysis were used to determine the prognostic factors of mortality with 95 % confidence intervals (CI). For survival analysis was used Kaplan Meier's survival analysis and Cox's Proporción hazardous model. A $p < 0.05$ was considered statistically significant.

Results

The general characteristics of all 121 patients with severe liver trauma who were included in our study with comparison between the survivors and non-survivors summarizes in Table 1. In this study 81(66.9 %) patients survived, while 40(33.1 %) of them died. In this study there were 90(74.4 %) males and 31(25.6 %) females (Table 1). Blunt hepatic injury was the leading mechanism of trauma, seen in 98(80.9 %) patients (Table 1). Road traffic accident was the leading cause of blunt

Table 1 Comparison between clinical characteristics in survivors and non-survivors

Variable	Survivors	Non-survivors	Total	p
	(n = 81)	(n = 40)	(n = 121)	
Male sex[a]	61(75.3 %)	29(72.5 %)	90(74.4 %)	>0.05
Age[b]	35.78 ± 18.54	43.34 ± 12.26	41.36 ± 17.80	>0.05
Penetrating liver injury[a]	16(19.7 %)	7(17.5 %)	23 (19.0 %)	>0.05
Blunt hepatic injury[a]	65 (80.2 %)	33(82.5 %)	98(80.9 %)	>0.05
Associated injury>2 body regions[a]	70(86.4 %)	38(95.0 %)	108(89.2 %)	>0.05

[a]Data are expressed as number of patients and percentages (n, %), [b]Data are presented as Mean ± Standard Deviation

trauma recorded in 80 (66.1 %) patients, and among them were 37(30.6 %) drivers, 36 (29.7 %) pedestrians and 7(5.8 %) passengers (data not shown). The remaining 10 (8.2 %) patients with blunt liver trauma were injured by falling from a roof and eight were hiting by assailant (6.6 %). Pentrating liver injury was recorded in 23 (19.0 %), with equal distribution between the groups: 15(19.0 %) suffered stab wounds, while 8(6.6 %) injured by firearms (Fig. 1). A total of 108(89.2 %) had liver trauma associated with injury >2 body regions, there was no difference between survivors and non-survivors (Table 1). Total of 82(67.8 %) patients had a ISS>34 (Table 2).

In this study there was 42(34.7 %) patients with liver trauma AAST III, 53(43.8 %) AAST IV and 26(21.5 %) patients with liver trauma AAST V including 4(3.3 %) retrohepatic vena cava and 10(8.3 %) major hepatic veins injury (Table 2). There was a significant difference between survivors 49(60.5 %) with ISS>34 and non-survivors 33(82.5 %) with ISS>34 (p = 0.0001) (Table 2). In comparison with the survivors, non-survivors have significantly higher liver AAST grade of injury: there was a statistical significance for the AAST III and AAST V (p = 0.001; p = 0.0001), while the AAST IV showed the same distribution (p > 0.05) (Table 2). Non-survivors

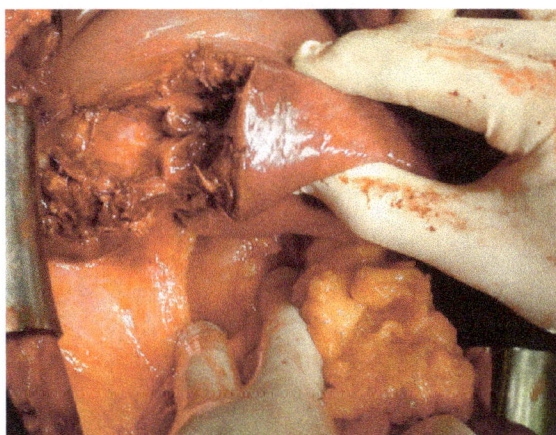

Fig. 1 Intraoperative finding in penetrating liver injury. A 36 year old male suffered a penetrating abdominal injury (stab wound to the right upper abdomen) with AAST grade IV liver injury. Non-anatomic liver resection was performed

showed significant hypotension on arrival (p = 0.0001) and lower GCS (p = 0.0001) (Table 2). Non-survivors needed significalntly more RBC units transfusions (p = 0.001) (Table 2). Non-survivors had significantly higher serum AST and ALT level within first 24 h (p = 0.010; p = 0.033) (Table 2).

There was no statistically significant difference in the application of surgical approach (p= > 0.05) (Table 3). Range of blood removed from peritoneal cavity was 500–1500 ml. Definitive hepatic repair was performed in 62(51.2 %) patients (Table 3). Liver resection was performed in 12(9.9 %) patients: non-anatomic resection in 6(4.9 %) patients and major resection (≥3 Couinauds segments) in 6(4.9 %) (Fig. 1, 2). DCS with perihepatic packing and planned re-laparotomy after 48 h was used in 59(48.8 %) (Table 3). In DC strategy we used different additional procedures in combination with liver packing (Fig. 3).

Most common non-related liver complications were: right-sided exudative pleural effusion in 24(19.8 %) patients, ARDS in 20(16.5 %) and pneumonia in 12(9.9 %) (Table 4). As liver-related complications we recorded: prolonged hemorrhage in 18(14.9 %), bile leak 21(17.3 %), biloma 12(9.9 %), liver abscess 2(1.6 %) and liver failure 1(0.8 %) (Table 4). Regarding complications non-survivors had a significantly prolonged bleeding and higher rate of ARDS (p = 0.0001, for all) (Table 4). Survivors had a significantly higher biloma (p = 0.014) and pleural effusion (p = 0.0001) (Table 4). Eleven (9.0 %) of all patients required re-operation during hospitalization: 9(7.4 %) due to prolonged bleeding and 2(1.6 %) due to uncontrolled bile fistula (Table 4). Other complications were treated with non-surgical approach, in one case the liver failure, patients had associated severe brain and lung injury.

Mortality was 33.1 %. We recorded statistical significance in terms of ICU and hospital stay (p = 0.001; p = 0.001) (Table 5). The early trauma-related mortality within the first 24 h after admission was noted in 35 % (Table 5). The cause of mortality in "early period" was massive prolonged bleeding. Among non-survivals 62.5 % died within the first 7 days (Table 5). Patients died in the further course of hospitalization due to late respiratory complications: ARDS and pneumonia.

Table 2 Comparison between clinical characteristics in survivors and non-survivors at arrival time and within first 24 h

Variable	Survivors (n = 81)	Non-survivors (n = 40)	Total (n = 121)	p
Liver AAST grade III[a]	37(45.7 %)	5(12.5 %)	42(34.7 %)	0.001
Liver AAST grade IV[a]	37(45.7 %)	16(40.0 %)	53(43.8 %)	>0.05
Liver AAST grade V[a]	7(8.6 %)	19(47.5 %)	26(21.5 %)	0.0001
ISS`34 (arrival)[a]	49(60.5 %)	33(82.5 %)	82(67.8 %)	0.0001
Systolic blood pressure ≤90 mmHg (arrival)[a]	28(34.6 %)	34(85.0 %)	62(51.2 %)	0.0001
GCS`9 (arrival)[a]	4(4.9 %)	25(62.5 %)	29(23.9 %)	0.0001
AST(U/L) within first 24 h[b]	454.09 ± 130.3	1405.22 ± 605.10	820.32 ± 315.12	0.010
ALT(U/L) within first 24 h[b]	505.13 ± 270.626	905.79 ± 412.385	675.32 ± 189.34	0.033
RBC transfusion (ml) within first 24 h[b]	1500.31 ± 607.46	5810.63 ± 2817.31	2510.03 ± 817.21	0.001

[a]Data are expressed as number of patients and percentages (n, %), [b]Data are presented as Mean ± Standard Deviation, *AAST* American Association for Surgery of Trauma, *GCS* Glasgow Coma Scale, *ISS* Injury Severity Score, *RBC* Red blood cell

Discusson

In hemodynamically unstable patients with hemorrhage from major liver injury and massive hemoperitoneum on abdominal imaging, the strategy and techniques for bleeding control can be extremely demanding and complex. We presented the results of surgical treatment of 121 trauma patients with severe bleeding liver injuries.

Since Pringle's publication of inflow vascular control on liver, the primary focus of trauma surgeons was to find the best way to achieve hemo-stasis, bile-stasis and infection control in hepatic injuries [15–23]. Today the focus of trauma surgeons is selection of appropriate patients for operative management, who are the candidates for surgery and when to operate [7, 8]. The general contraindications for none-operative management of liver trauma included the hemodynamic instability, extravasations of intravenous contrast on abdominal imaging, expanding hematoma and grade IV and V liver injury [6, 7]. According to the study conducted by Coimbra et al. nonoperative management has been accepted as treatment of choice only for stable patients with low grade of injury [23]. Fang et al. study of 214 patients with a hepatic injury showed that the independent predictors for the surgical treatment even in hemodynamically stable patients included intraperitoneal contrast extravasation and hemoperitoneum in six compartments on CT scan [22]. FAST is able to sensitively detect hemoperitoneum presented as free fluid in the abdomen and pelvis, but its numerous limitations have been recognized [8, 24]. MSCT is the imaging modality of choice in evaluating hemodynamically stable patients with suspected hepatic injury [7, 22]. Abdominal CT accurately defines the morphology and extent of the hepatic trauma, identifies associated visceral injuries and depicts the amount of hemoperitoneum [7, 25]. It is important to know that life-threatening liver injuries can be detected by MSCT with high sensitivity.

In this study indications for emergency laparotomy were: hemorrhage shock on admission, refractory hemodynamic instability, signs of haemoperitoneum on ultrasound, MSCT

Table 3 Surgical procedures for hepatic hemorrhage control in complex liver trauma

Variable	Survivors (n = 81)	Non-survivors (n = 40)	Total (n = 121)	p
Damage control surgery[a]	39(48.1 %)	20(50.0 %)	59(48.8 %)	>0.05
DCS-perihepatic packing + direct parenchyma suture[a]	21(25.9 %)	10(25.0 %)	31(25.6 %)	
DCS-perihepatic packing + liver resection[a]	4(4.9 %)	4(10.0 %)	8(6.6 %)	
DCS-perihepatic packing + RHA ligation[a]	1(1.2 %)	1(2.5 %)	2(1.6 %)	
DCS-perihepatic packing + direct vessel repair[a]	13(16.0 %)	5(12.5 %)	18(14.8 %)	
Definitive hepatic repair[a]	42(51.8 %)	20(50.0 %)	62(51.2 %)	>0.05
Direct parenchyma suture + hemostatic fibrin gel[a]	15(18.5 %)	5(12.5 %)	20(16.5 %)	
Hepatotomy + direct vessel repair, vascular ligation and debridement[a]	23(28.4 %)	5(12.5 %)	28(23.1 %)	
Non-anatomic liver resection[a]	2(2.5 %)	4(10.0 %)	6(4.9 %)	
Major liver resections[a]	2(2.5 %)	4(10.0 %)	6(4.9 %)	
Selective RHA ligation[a]	0(0.0 %)	2(5.0 %)	2(1.6 %)	

[a]Data are expressed as number of patients and percentages (n, %), *DCS* Damage control surgery, *RHA* Right hepatic artery

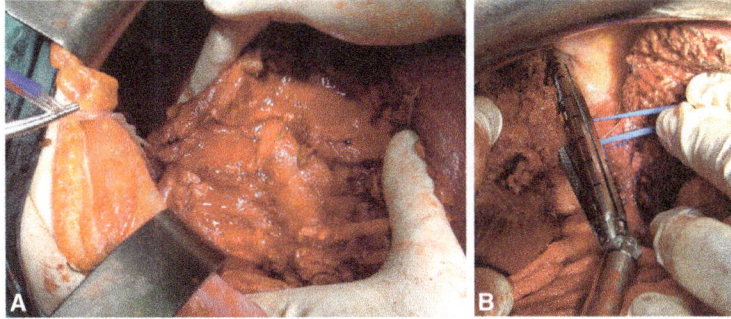

Fig. 2 Intraoperative findings in blunt liver trauma. Road traffic accident was the cause of trauma in 40 year old driver with AAST grade V blunt liver injury (**a**). Right hepatectomy: transection of right Glissonean pedicle using endo-GIA vascular stapling device (**b**)

findings of the severe liver trauma with contrast extravasation which indicate active hemorrhage. It is important to know that life-threatening liver injuries can be detected by MSCT with high sensitivity. The operative management of liver injuries requires the use of some of the most complex surgical techniques, including extensive hepatotomy with selective deep vessel ligation, hepatorrhaphy, selective hepatic artery ligation, non-anatomic resection and debridement and hepatectomy [6, 7]. The surgical treatments of severe liver injuries in this study were definitive procedure (hepatorrhaphy, hepatotomy with vascular ligation, debridement, selective hepatic artery ligation, liver resection) and DCS with liver packing. The incidence of trauma patients requiring liver packing varies from 5 to 62 % in the literature [6, 21, 26]. We performed perihepatic packing in 48.8 % patients. It is important to recognize that liver packing will not control arterial bleeding and that any bleeding artery should be suture/ligated prior to liver packing. A precise perihepatic packing technique starting with a Pringle manoeuvre and complete liver mobilization, with systematized placement of packs. Strategies for haemorrhage control are more efficient when DCS is associated with appropriate additional strategies such as an effective fluid resuscitation/transfusion protocols, a carefully selected angioembolization and an accurate ICU critical care [13, 19, 27]. According to the Asensio results, improvements in outcome can be achieved using damage control strategy to control hepatic bleeding in

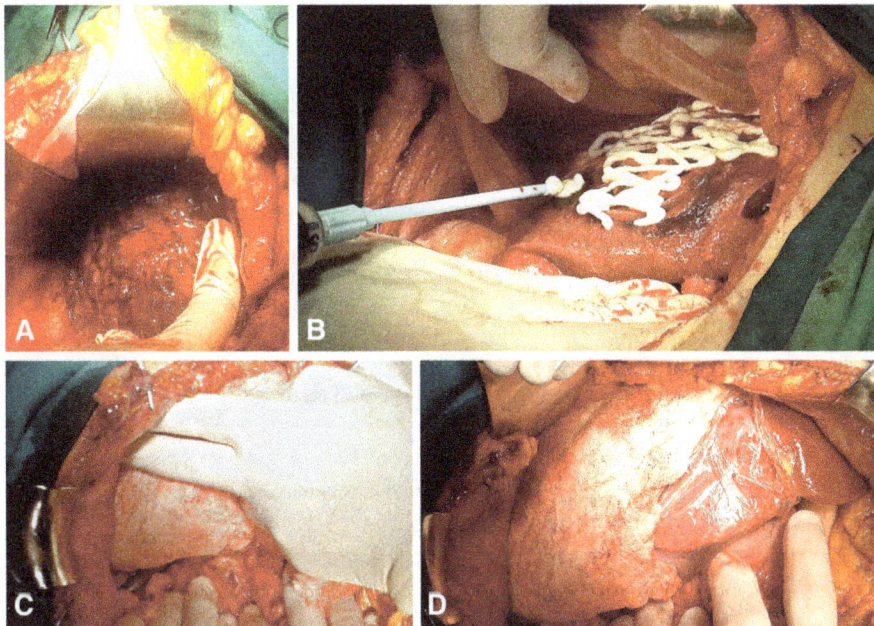

Fig. 3 Damage Control Surgery in blunt liver trauma (DCS I –Initial laparotomy). A 41 year old exsanguinating man with AAST grade V blunt liver injury (**a**). In order to control life-threatening hemorrhage emergency laparotomy was followed by direct liver vessel repair with bleeding vessels sutured prior to liver packing and hemostatic fibrin gel on liver surface (**b**). We performed liver packing with four abdominal swabs to provide liver compression (**c**, **d**)

Table 4 Postoperative complications in survivors and non-survivors

Variable	Survivors (n = 81)	Non-survivors (n = 40)	Total (n = 121)	p
Re-operations[a]	7(8.6 %)	4(10.0 %)	11(9.0 %)	>0.05
Prolonged bleeding[a]	5(6.2 %).	13(32.5 %)	18(14.9 %)	0.0001
Bile fistula[a]	16(19.7 %)	5(12.5 %)	21(17.3 %)	>0.05
Bilom[a]	10(12.3 %)	2(5.0 %)	12(9.9 %)	0.014
Liver abscess[a]	2(2.5 %)	0(0.0 %)	2(1.6 %)	>0.05
Liver failure[a]	0(0.0 %)	1(2.5 %)	1(0.8 %)	>0.05
ARDS[a]	9(11.1 %)	11(27.5 %)	20(16.5 %)	0.0001
Pneumonia[a]	8(9.9 %)	4(10.0 %)	12(9.9 %)	>0.05
Pleural effusion[a]	24(29.6 %)	0(0.0 %)	24(19.8 %)	0.0001

[a]Data are expressed as number of patients and percentages (n,%), *ARDS* Acute respiratory distress syndrome, *MODS* Multiple organ dysfunction syndrome

patients with severe liver injuries and compromised physiological stage [6]. However, interventional radiology with embolization may play an important role in cases of liver packing followed by re-bleeding. Angiography and angioembolization were not used in our study group which is the limitation of this study. Although this surgical technique was not a predictor of outcome in our study, the question is whether the use of DCS in combination with angioembolization for emergency control bleeding, would contribute to the lower rate of complications and deaths in this study. The reported survival rate associated with packing increased up to 65.5 % as reported by Peitzman et al [2]. Outcome could be improved by combining of venous bleeding control by liver packing and arterial haemorrhage control with angioembolization [2, 5, 6, 28].

Over half of patients surviving grade III–V liver injuries will be at risk for the development of complications [29]. Liver-related complications occur in approximately 20–45 % of patients and include hemorrhage, hemobilia, arteriovenous fistula, pseudo-aneurysm, biloma, bile leak and abscess formation [5, 10, 27, 29]. MSCT and ultrasaund was used in diagnosing specific post- traumatic postoperative complications such as hepatic or perihepatic abscesses or bilomas. Postoperative prolonged hemorrhage can be associated with coagulopathy [5, 10, 27, 29]. While blood transfusion is necessary because of massive bleeding in trauma, it carries many complications [29, 30].

Table 5 Postoperative ICU stay, hospital stay and survival time

Variable	Survivors (n = 81)	Non-survivors (n = 40)	p
ICU stay[a](days)	2 (1–6)	8.5 (2–18)	0.001
Hospital stay[a] (days)	30 (15–90)	10 (4–30)	0.001
Died within the first 24 h	/	14(35 %)	
Died within the first 7 days	/	25(62.5 %)	

[a]ICU and hospital stay are presented by median range

Complex hepatic injuries have a high mortality rate (8,36,38). Our study shows that non-survivors had higher AAST grade of injury, higher AST and ALT level, significant hypotension, higher ISS score and lower GCS on arrival; and significalntly more RBC units transfusions within the first 24 h. Early liver injury-related death is typically secondary to uncontrolled bleeding (20–60 %), which is worsened with attendant coagulopathy, whereas late mortality is usually secondary to multiorgan failure (MOF), Acute Respiratory Distress Syndrom (ARDS) in 27(32.1 %), and Multiple Organ Dysfunction Syndrome (MODS) [6, 29–31]. Previous studies have shown that increased risk of ARDS and MODS has been associated with massive transfusion, which can itself contribute to coagulopathy [30]. In blunt liver trauma mortality also appears to be higher in older patients, those with higher grade injuries, and those with hemodynamic instability on presentation [29–31]. In a series of 144 patients with grade III–V hepatic injuries, uncontrollable bleeding from the liver injury and associated severe splenic injury favors early laparotomy and damage control strategy [31]. Asensio and colleagues showed that predictors of mortality in grade IV–V injuries are related to severe bleeding and include blood loss, number of red cell units transfused, hypothermia, acidosis, and dyasrhythmia [6].

Conclusion

Prolonged bleeding and amount of blood transfusions are statistically significant predictors of mortality in severe hepatic trauma. All efforts in the treatment of trauma patients with complex liver injuries AAST grade III–V should be directed to the rapid and effective control of liver hemorrhage and taking care of all associated life-threatening injuries.

Abbreviations
DCS: Damage control surgery; OIS: Organ injury scale; AAST: American association for surgery of trauma; FAST: Focused assessment by ultrasound for trauma; ICU: Intensive care unit; MSCT: Multislice computed tomography; DPL: Diagnostic peritoneal lavage; AST: Aspartate transaminase; ALT: Alanine aminotransferase; ARDS: Acute respiratory distress syndrome.

Competing interests
The authors declare that they have no competing interests.

Author' contributions
Krstina Doklestić, Aleksandar Karamarković and Branislav Stefanović contributed equally to this work and designed the study. All authors were involved in management and follow-up of the patient. Vasilije Jeremić, Zlatibor Lončar, Bojan Jovanović, Vesna Bumbaširević, Sanja Tomanović Vujadinović, and Branislava Stefanović performed the research. Pavle Gregorić, Nenad Ivančević and Nataša Milić participated in the design of the study and performed the statistical analysis. Aleksandar Karamarković and Krstina Doklestić wrote the paper. Branislav Stefanović proof-read the manuscript, reviewed the corrections and revised the manuscript. All authors read and approved the final manuscript.

Author details

[1]Faculty of Medicine, University of Belgrade and Clinical Center of Serbia, Clinic for Emergency Surgery, University of Belgrade, Serbia, Pasteur Str.2, Belgrade 11000, Serbia. [2]Faculty of Medicine, University of Belgrade and Clinical Center of Serbia, Department for Anesthesiology, University of Belgrade, Serbia, Belgrade, Serbia. [3]Faculty of Medicine, University of Belgrade and Clinical Center of Serbia, Clinic for Physical and Rehabilitation Medicine, Clinical Center of Serbia, Belgrade, Serbia. [4]Faculty of Medicine and Institute for Medical Statistics and Informatics, University of Belgrade, Belgrade, Serbia.

References

1. Tinkoff G, Esposito TJ, Reed J, Kilgo P, Fildes J, Pasquale M, et al. American Association for the Surgery of Trauma organ injury scale I: spleen, liver and kidney, validation based on the National Trauma Data Bank. J Am Coll Surg. 2008;207:646–55.

2. Peitzman AB, Richardson JD. Surgical treatment of injuries to the solid abdomi-nal organs: a 50-year perspective from the Journal of Trauma. J Trauma. 2010;69:1011–21.

3. Moore EE, Cogbill TH, Jurkovich GJ, Shackford SR, Malangoni MA, Champion HR. Organ injury scaling: spleen and liver (1994 revision). J Trauma. 1995;38:323–4.

4. Asensio JA, Roldán G, Petrone P, Rojo E, Tillou A, Kuncir E, et al. Operative management and outcomes in 103 AAST-OIS Grades IV and V complex hepatic injuries: Trauma Surgeons still need to operate, but angioembolization helps. J Trauma. 2003;54:647–54.

5. Piper GL, Peitzman AB. Current management of hepatic trauma. Surg Clin North Am. 2010;90:775–85.

6. Asensio JA, Petrone P, Garcia-Nunez L, Kimbrell B, Kuncir E. Multidisciplinary approach for the management of complex hepatic injuries AAST-OIS grades IV–V: a prospective study. Scand J Surg. 2007;96:214–20.

7. Petrowsky H, Raeder S, Zuercher L, Platz A, Simmen HP, Puhan MA, et al. A quarter century experience in liver trauma: a plea for early computed tomography and conservative management for all hemodynamically stable patients. World J Surg. 2012;2:247–54.

8. Natarajan B, Gupta PK, Cemaj S, Sorensen M, Hatzoudis GI, Forse RA. FAST scan: is it worth doing in hemodynamically stable blunt trauma patients? Surgery. 2010;148:695–700. discussion 700-1.

9. Srivastava AR, Kumar S, Agarwal GG, Ranjan P. Blunt abdominal injury: serum ALT-A marker of liver injury and a guide to assessment of its severity. Injury. 2007;38:1069–74.

10. Richardson JD, Franklin GA, Lukan MD, Carrillo EH, Spain DA, Miller FB, et al. Evolution in the management of hepatic trauma: a 25-year perspective. Ann Surg. 2000;232:324–30.

11. Holcomb JB. Damage control resuscitation. J Trauma. 2007;62:S36–7.

12. Cotton BA, Gunter OL, Isbell J, Au BK, Robertson AM, Morris Jr JA, et al. Damage control hematology: the impact of a trauma exsanguination protocol on survival and blood product utilization. J Trauma. 2008;64:1177–82. discussion 1182-3.

13. Hess JR, Holcomb JB, Hoyt DB. Damage control resuscitation: the need for specific blood products to treat the coagulopathy of trauma. Transfusion. 2006;46:685–6.

14. Maegele M, Lefering R, Yucel N, Tjardes T, Rixen D, Paffrath T, et al. Early coagulopathy in multiple injury: an analysis from the German Trauma Registry on 8724 patients. Injury. 2007;38:298–304.

15. Asensio JA, McDuffie L, Petrone P, Roldán G, Forno W, Gambaro E, et al. Reliable variables in the exsanguinated patient which indicate damage control and predict outcome. Am J Surg. 2001;182:743–56.

16. Holcomb JB, Jenkins D, Rhee P, Johannigman J, Mahoney P, Mehta S, et al. Damage control resuscitation: directly addressing the early coagulopathy of trauma. J Trauma. 2007;62(2):307–10.

17. Spahn DR, Bouillon B, Cerny V, Coats TJ, Duranteau J, Fernández-Mondéjar E, et al. Management of bleeding and coagulopathy following major trauma: an updated European guideline. Crit Care. 2013;17(2):R76. doi:10.1186/cc12685.

18. Holcomb JB, Wade CE, Michalek JE, Chisholm GB, Zarzabal LA, Schreiber MA, et al. Increased plasma and platelet to red blood cell ratios improves

outcome in 466 massively transfused civilian trauma patients. Ann Surg. 2008;248:447–58.

19. Klein HG, Spahn DR, Carson JL. Red blood cell transfusion in clinical practice. Lancet. 2007;370(9585):415–26.

20. Pringle JH. Notes on the arrest of hepatic haemorrhage due to trauma. Ann Surg. 1908;48:541–8.

21. Sitzmann JV, Spector SA, Jin X, Barquist E, Koniaris LG. A technique for emergency liver packing. J Gastrointest Surg. 2005;9:284–7.

22. Fang JF, Wong YC, Lin BC, Hsu YP, Chen MF. The CT risk factors for the need of operative treatment in initially hemodynamically stable patients after blunt hepatic trauma. J Trauma. 2006;61:547–54.

23. Coimbra R, Hoyt DB, Engelhart S, Fortlage D. Nonoperative management reduces the overall mortality of grades 3 and 4 blunt liver injuries. Int Surg. 2006;91(5):251–7.

24. Williams SR, Perera P, Gharahbaghian L. The FAST and E-FAST in 2013: trauma ultrasonography: overview, practical techniques, controversies, and new frontiers. Crit Care Clin. 2014;30(1):119–50.

25. Christe A, Ross S, Oesterhelweg L, Spendlove D, Bolliger S, Vock P, et al. Abdominal trauma–sensitivity and specificity of postmortem noncontrast imaging findings compared with autopsy findings. J Trauma. 2009;66(5):1302–7.

26. Nicol AJ, Hommes M, Primrose R, Navsaria PH, Krige JE. Packing for control of hemorrhage in major liver trauma. World J Surg. 2007;31:569–74.

27. Baldoni F, Di Saverio S, Antonacci N, Coniglio C, Giugni A, Montanari N, et al. Refinement in the technique of perihepatic packing: a safe and effective surgical hemostasis and multidisciplinary approach can improve the outcome in severe liver trauma. Am J Surg. 2011;201(1):e5–14.

28. Mohr AM, Lavery RF, Barone A, Bahramipour P, Magnotti LJ, Osband AJ, et al. Angiographic embolization for liver injuries: low mortality, high morbidity. J Trauma. 2003;55(6):1077–81.

29. Bala M, Gazalla SA, Faroja M, Bloom AI, Zamir G, Rivkind AI, et al. Complications of high grade liver injuries: management and outcomewith focus on bile leaks. Scand J Trauma Resusc Emerg Med. 2012;20:20.

30. Li Petri S, Gruttadauria S, Pagano D, Echeverri GJ, Di Francesco F, Cintorino D, et al. Surgical management of complex liver trauma: a single liver transplant center experience. Am Surg. 2012;78(1):20–5.

31. Leppäniemi AK, Mentula PJ, Streng MH, Koivikko MP, Handolin LE. Severe hepatic trauma: nonoperative management, definitive repair, or damage control surgery? World J Surg. 2011;35(12):2643–9.

Resuscitative endovascular balloon occlusion of the aorta for uncontrollable nonvariceal upper gastrointestinal bleeding

Hidefumi Sano[1], Junya Tsurukiri[1]*, Akira Hoshiai[1], Taishi Oomura[1], Yosuke Tanaka[1] and Shoichi Ohta[2]

Abstract

Background: Although resuscitative endovascular balloon occlusion of the aorta (REBOA) in various clinical settings was found to successfully elevate central blood pressure in hemorrhagic shock, this intervention is associated with high mortality and may represent a last-ditch option for trauma patients. We conducted a retrospective study of patients with nonvariceal upper gastrointestinal bleeding (UGIB) who underwent REBOA to identify the effectiveness of REBOA and reviewed published literatures.

Methods: REBOA were performed by trained acute care physicians in the emergency room and intensive care unit. The deployment of balloon catheters was positioned using ultrasonography guidance. Collected data included clinical characteristics, hemorrhagic severity, blood cultures, metabolic values, blood transfusions, REBOA-related complications and mortality. A literature search using PUBMED to include "aortic occlusion" and "gastrointestinal bleeding" was conducted.

Results: REBOA was attempted in eight patients among 140 patients with UGIB and median age was 66 years. Systolic blood pressure significantly increased after REBOA (66 ± 20 vs. 117 ± 45 mmHg, $p < 0.01$) and the total occlusion time of REBOA was 80 ± 48 min. Strong positive correlations were found between total occlusion time of REBOA and lactate concentration (Spearman's $r=0.77$), clinical Rockwall score (Spearman's $r=0.80$), and age (Spearman's $r=0.88$), respectively.

Conclusion: REBOA can be performed with a high degree of technical success and is effective at improving hemodynamic in patients with UGIB. Correlations between total occlusion time and high lactate levels, clinical Rockall score, and age may be important for successful use of REBOA.

Background

Uncontrollable hemorrhage is a main cause of death in patients with hemorrhagic shock admitted to the emergency department (ED) or intensive care unit (ICU), and trauma and nonvariceal upper gastrointestinal bleeding (UGIB) are the most common causes of massive hemorrhage in acute care setting [1, 2]. Although main aim of resuscitation is to stop the source of hemorrhage and restore hemodynamics, persistent hemorrhage can be rapidly fatal. The options for impending cardiac collapse are resuscitative thoracotomy and aortic clamping immediately performed in such cases [3].

A recent systematic review of REBOA in various clinical settings was found to successfully elevate central blood pressure in hemorrhagic shock [4]. Although, REBOA is increasingly used as an alternative to resuscitative thoracotomy, a recent report suggested that REBOA was associated with increased mortality and may represent a last-ditch option for trauma patients with hemodynamic instability in Japan [5]. However, there are no satisfactory reports regarding the effectiveness of REBOA among patients with UGIB. Therefore, we conducted a retrospective study of patients with UGIB who underwent REBOA at a single emergency center to evaluate the effectiveness of REBOA. In addition, we reviewed the published literature to provide a summary of the experience data.

---

* Correspondence: junya99@tokyo-med.ac.jp
[1]Emergency and Critical Care Medicine, Tokyo Medical University Hachioji Medical Center, 1163 Tatemachi, Hachioji, Tokyo 193-0998, Japan
Full list of author information is available at the end of the article

Methods

Patients

The ethics committee of Tokyo Medical University Hachioji Medical Center approved the design of this retrospective study. UGIB patients with suspected hemorrhagic shock who subsequently underwent REBOA in the ER or who were admitted to our intensive care unit (ICU) and subsequently developed hemorrhagic shock and underwent REBOA in the ICU were enrolled in this study between September 2011 and April 2015. Patients with a systolic blood pressure (SBP) <90 mmHg or a shock index (SI; ratio of heart rate to SBP) ≥1.0 were considered to be in shock. We excluded patients aged <15 years and those who had cardiac arrest on admission or were diagnosed with any terminal disease during the study period.

Intervention

Patients with hemorrhagic shock in the transient- and non-response groups were considered to be hemodynamically unstable on the basis of their response to an initial fluid resuscitation with 1 L of Ringer's lactate. Although it is important to administer blood and blood products as soon as possible for trauma or non-trauma shock patients, the preparation of blood or blood products takes time in Japan, at least in our hospital. Consequently, the empirical transfusion of blood and blood products was initiated as soon as possible. REBOA was initiated by one or two acute care physicians in patients showing hemodynamic instability and an inability to remain normotensive following resuscitation. In our department, one acute care physician (TJ) was trained for ≥1 year as a member of the endovascular team in the Radiology Department of another university hospital, whereas all other acute care physicians in our ER performed REBOA under the guidance of TJ.

For the REBOA procedure, a 10 Fr. Intra-aortic balloon occlusion (IABO) catheters (BLOCK BALLOON™; Senko Medical Instrument, Tokyo, Japan) or 7 Fr. IABO catheters (RESCUE BALLOON®; Tokai Medical Products, Tokyo, Japan) have been available in our ER and ICU. These are a double lumen balloon catheter with a stainless steel styled. For percutaneous deployment of IABO catheters, all necessary guidewires, sharps and introducers are packaged together in the kit. An acute care physician first inserts 7 Fr. or 10 Fr. sheath into the femoral artery using the Seldinger method. After insertion of the femoral artery sheath, the IABO catheter was placed into the aorta and REBOA was performed. IABO catheter was placed into the aorta, with selection of the aortic zone for occlusion according to the recommendations of Stannard et al. under ultrasonography guidance [6]. Placement of the balloon is normally performed in Zone I (proximal of the aorta, origin of the left subclavian artery to the celiac artery) in patients with suspected UGIB. IABO catheter positioning was performed under ultrasonography guidance before REBOA placement and confirmed by portable chest radiography in ER (Fig. 1) [7].

Data collection

The following characteristics were noted from the charts and radiographs of the patients with hemodynamic instability: age, sex, vital signs, Acute Physiology and Chronic Health Evaluation (APACHE) II score, hemorrhagic severity, blood cultures, metabolic and coagulation values [pH, lactate concentration, base excess (BE), prothrombin time, and activated partial thrombin time], blood transfusion, REBOA-related complications and mortality. Hemorrhagic severity was evaluated using SI and severity of UGIB was evaluated at the onset using the Glasgow-Blatchford bleeding score (GBS), clinical Rockall score (CRS) and AIMS65 score [8]. In patients admitted to ER or ICU, blood cultures and metabolic and coagulation values were measured at the beginning of resuscitative interventions. Markers of end-organ dysfunction included serum aspartate transaminase (AST), blood urea nitrogen (BUN), creatinine, potassium, sodium, total bilirubin, lactate dehydrogenase (LDH), and creatine kinase (CK) as described in previous reports thoroughly reviewed by two acute care

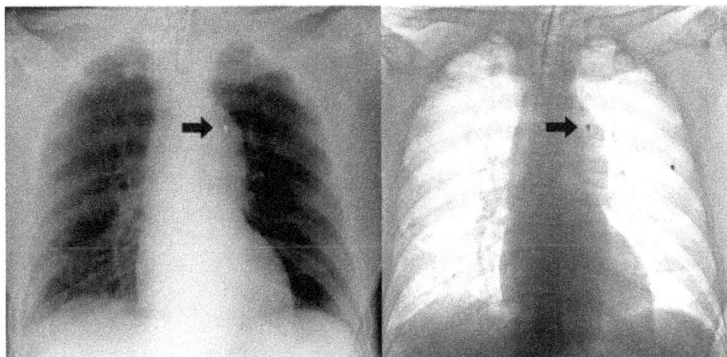

Fig. 1 Placement of the balloon is performed in Zone I (Patient 5). The tip of IABO catheter (arrow)

Table 1 Clinical characteristics of the patients

Variables	Patient 1	Patient 2	Patient 3	Patient 4	Patient 5	Patient 6	Patient 7	Patient 8
Age (y)	69	36	83	64	78	69	50	79
Sex	male	male	male	male	male	male	male	male
Body temperature (°C)	35.5	36.2	36.8	37.3	36.0	37.0	36.1	35.7
Hemodynamics								
Shock index	2.3	0.8	2.1	2	0.8	1.7	1.1	1.3
SBP pre-REBOA (mmHg)	60	90	96	54	41	63	61	–
SBP post REBOA (mmHg)	97	111	206	74	82	112	140	–
ΔSBP (mmHg)	37	21	110	20	41	49	79	–
APACHE II	22	7	26	31	22	26	21	30
Severity of upper gastrointestinal bleeding								
Glasgow Blatchford bleeding score	17	7	19	11	14	13	12	17
Clinical Rockall score	3	3	4	3	5	3	2	3
AIM 65 score	3	0	4	3	2	5	0	2
Initial blood values								
White blood cell count (/μL)	12900	13600	24000	17300	9120	10600	11500	7170
Hemoglobin (g/dL)	5.5	14.8	11.2	7.3	5	5.3	8.8	6.1
Hematocrit (%)	16	44	31	21	15	16	26	19
Platelet connt (×10^4/μL)	11.9	34.6	9.3	36.8	17.3	12.2	36	22.9
BUN (mg/dL)	18.7	21.1	62.1	8.2	44.1	13.9	46.9	32.0
Lactate (mmol/L)	11.1	1.3	9.6	5.6	15.8	6.6	63	15.0
pH	7.25	7.36	7.38	6.94	7.35	7.24	7.30	6.96
Base excess (mmol/L)	0.1	–2.5	–11.5	–14.5	–14.6	–9.3	–9.4	–21.8
Prothrombin time (%)	51	113	64	62	83	51	105	62
APTT (sec)	64.5	30.1	35.3	240	64.3	123.9	33.4	–
Diagnosis	Gastric ulcer	Gastric ulcer	Duodenum ulcer	Anastomotic bleeding	Duodenum ulcer	Left gastric artery aneurysm	Duodenum ulcer	Esophageal cancer
Definitive hemostatic control	endoscopy	endoscopy	endoscopy	AE	AE (failed endoscopy)	AE (failed endoscopy)	AE (failed endoscopy)	AE
CPA during procedures	no	no	no	yes	no	yes	no	no

Table 1 Clinical characteristics of the patients (Continued)

Blood and blood product transfusion within 24 h (mL)

PRBC	1400	280	1960	2520	1960	2800	3080	1680
FFP	1200	0	1200	1680	2160	1920	1920	720
Re-bleeding	no	no	no	no	yes	yes	no	no
REBOA								
Total occlusion time (min)	57	20	140	54	145	95	50	Failure
REBOA-related complication	none	none	none	none	none	none	none	none
Outcome within 30 days	Alive	Alive	Alive	Alive	Died < 24 h	Alive	Alive	Died < 24 h

SBP systolic blood pressure, REBOA resuscitative endovascular balloon occlusion of the aorta, APACHE acute physiology and chronic health evaluation, BUN blood urea nitrogen, APTT activated partial thrombin time, AE angioembolization, CPA cardiopulmonary arrest, PRBC packed red blood cells, and FFP fresh-frozen plasma

physicians (SH and TJ) [9, 10]. These values were measured within 12 h after definitive hemostasis. The REBOA-related complications included vessel injuries (i.e., aortic dissection, rupture, perforation, pseudo-aneurysm, and arteriovenous fistula), groin hematoma, embolization, air emboli, peripheral ischemia, and organ dysfunction.

Literature search
A literature search using PUBMED to include "aortic occlusion" and "gastrointestinal bleeding" was conducted. Original articles and case reports published in English language were reviewed, and follow-up references listed were further investigated.

Statistical analyses
Data from all eligible patients were analyzed. Continuous variables are shown as mean values with standard deviation in text and median and interquartile range in Tables. Between-group differences were statistically assessed using the Mann–Whitney U test for continuous variables, paired t test for continuous dependent variables and the Fisher's exact test for categorical variables. The Spearman correlation coefficient was used to identify correlations between the evaluated parameters. All statistical analyses were performed using Prism version 6.0a statistical software (GraphPad Software, San Diego, CA, USA). Categorical variables were calculated as the ratio (percentage) of the frequency of occurrence. A probability (p) value of > 0.05 was considered statistically significant.

Results
Demographics and clinical characteristics
REBOA was attempted in eight patients among 140 patients with UGIB. The mean age was 66 ± 16 years, and all of the patients were male. The mean SI, GBS, CRS, AIMS65 score and APACHE II were 1.5 ± 0.6, 16 ± 4, 3 ± 1, 2 ± 2, and 23 ± 7, respectively. The demographics and clinical characteristics of all patients are shown in Table 1. Placement of the IABO catheter failed in one patient aged 79 years with severe aortic calcifications. Definitive hemostasis was endoscopy in 3 cases, anigo-embolization (AE) in 2 cases, and AE after failed endoscopy in 3 cases, respectively. The total occlusion time of REBOA was 80 ± 48 min in this study. The mean volume of packed red blood cells, fresh frozen plasma and Ringer's lactate administered during the resuscitation were 2000 ± 949 mL, 1440 ± 733 mL, and 4000 ± 2363 mL, respectively. The mortality rates within 24 h and 30 days were 15 % each. No REBOA-related complications were encountered.

Changes in acute care management with REBOA
Systolic blood pressure was significantly higher after initiating of REBOA (66 ± 20 vs. 117 ± 45 mmHg, $p < 0.01$). Heart rate, lactate concentration, and BE were not

significantly different between before and after REBOA. Initial serum concentration of AST, BUN, creatinine, CK, potassium, sodium, total bilirubin, white blood cell counts, and C-reactive response were not significantly different compared with those after completion of hemostasis. The serum concentration of LDH following REBOA was significantly higher than that before REBOA (227 ± 154 vs. 595 ± 406 IU/L, $p=0.04$) (Table 2).

Correlations between total occlusion time and vital indicators
Strong positive correlations were found between total occlusion time and lactate concentration (Spearman's $r=0.77$, $p=0.04$), CRS (Spearman's $r=0.80$, $p=0.03$), and age (Spearman's $r=0.88$, $p < 0.01$), respectively (Fig. 2).

Discussion
REBOA is an adjunct procedure designed to sustain the circulation until definitive hemostasis is obtained.

Upon review of the existing literature, it was evident that there are only a very limited number of publications related to REBOA treatment for UGIB, and only four case references were retrieved. We identified 4 published reports involving 4 patients (1 patient per 1 report) with hemodynamic instability caused by UIGB. Among them, 2

Table 2 Comparison of the vital indicators between before and after REBOA

Vital indicators, median (IQR)	Before REBOA ($n=7$)	After REBOA ($n=7$)
Systolic blood pressure (mmHg)	61 (57–77)	111 (90–126)*
Heart rate (beat/min)	126 (112–131)	123 (113–127)
White blood cells (/µL)	12100 (11050–14250)	16600 (13950–17900)
Hemoglobin (g/dL)	7.3 (5.4–10)	9.7 (8.7–10.6)
Platelet ($\times 10^4$/µL)	17.3 (12.1–35.3)	10.3 (7.2–13.6)
Prothrombin time (%)	64 (57–94)	56 (50–70)
Lactate (mmol/L)	3.2 (2.9–6.0)	5.4 (4.3–7.0)
Base excess (mmol/L)	−11.5 (−14.6 - −8.7)	−3.1 (−4.8 - −1.4)
Blood urea nitrogen (mg/dL)	21.1 (16.3–45.5)	30.8 (16.6–38.8)
Creatinine (mg/dL)	0.97 (0.90–1.03)	1.14 (0.83–1.29)
Aspartate transaminase (U/L)	14 (11.5–43.5)	101 (64.5–608)
Total bilirubin (mg/dL)	0.40 (0.35–0.6)	0.60 (0.45–0.80)
Potassium (mmol/L)	4.0 (3.8–4.1)	3.5 (3.5–4.2)
Sodium (mmol/L)	138 (135–139)	137 (136–141)
Creatine kinase (U/L)	56 (47–80)	263 (109–620)
Alkaline phosphatase (U/L)	191 (153–197)	137 (104–249)
Lactate dehydrogenase (U/L)	158 (123–285)	411 (328–862)*
C reactive protein (mg/dL)	1.61 (0.55–2.64)	1.07 (0.70–3.55)

IQR interquartile range, REBOA, resuscitative endovascular balloon occlusion of the aorta; * = $p < 0.05$ vs. Before REBOA

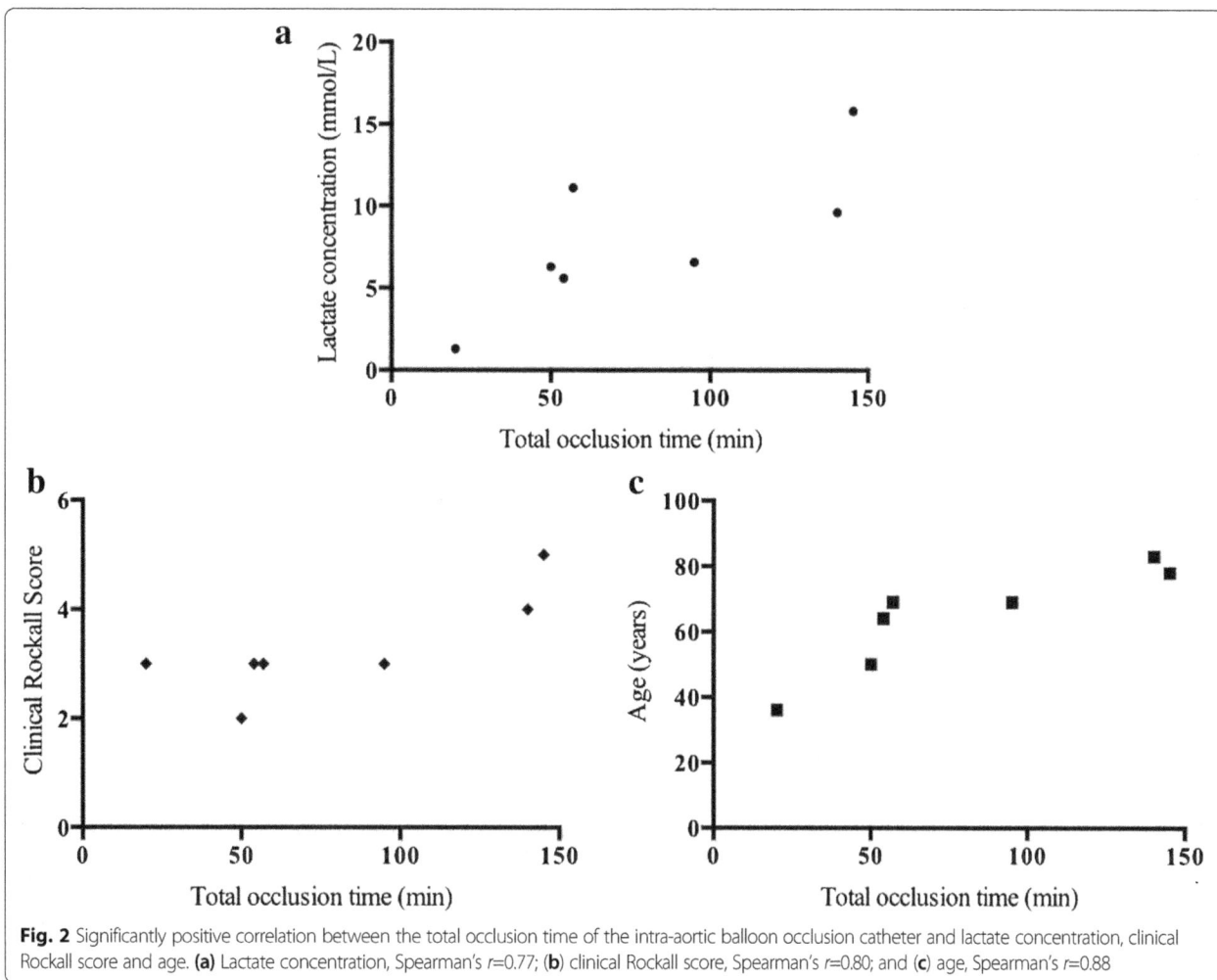

Fig. 2 Significantly positive correlation between the total occlusion time of the intra-aortic balloon occlusion catheter and lactate concentration, clinical Rockall score and age. (**a**) Lactate concentration, Spearman's r=0.77; (**b**) clinical Rockall score, Spearman's r=0.80; and (**c**) age, Spearman's r=0.88

patients underwent REBOA for duodenum ulcers, one child for aorta-esophageal fistula, and one for unknown UGIB [11–14]. Table 3 showed the clinical characteristics. Placement of the balloon was in Zone I without fluoroscopy and hemodynamics have improved in all cases. There was no REBOA-related complication and the mortality rate was 25 %. To the best of our knowledge, the present study represents the first retrospective study to evaluate the utility of REBOA among patients with UGBI.

In the present study, our trained acute care physicians could achieve REBOA procedures in the ED/ICU with a high degree of technical success. Blood pressure following REBOA did significantly increased compared with that before REBOA, and no significant differences detected between patients with UGIB in terms of almost all markers of end-organ dysfunction. A recent study reported a REBOA duration of >90 min in an animal model of hemorrhage-induced organ dysfunction, particularly that of the kidneys and liver. Our results were consistent with those reported by Markov et al. [9]. We also found clinically significant correlations between the total occlusion time of REBOA

and lactate concentration and CRS measured at the beginning of resuscitation among patients with UGIB. Conventionally, these parameters are used to confirm a suspected massive hemorrhage and permit the earlier achievement of hemostasis or administration of massive transfusion if required [15]. Thus, it is very important to shorten the time from ED arrival to initiation of hemostatic procedures before hemodynamic collapse as much as possible. Although endoscopic treatment for UGIB is generally acceptable, it can be difficult to achieve complete hemostasis in some patients with a high lactate concentration and/or CRS. Excessive hemorrhage may rapidly become fatal and can be challenging to secure. In addition, it makes maintaining a visual field during endoscopy difficult. These complications result in significant time delays during procedures. In the present study, one patient (Patient No. 2) who had a transient response to initial resuscitation had his systolic blood pressure decrease to 80 mmHg. It was then decided to place an IABO catheter prior to endoscopic treatment, and an IABO catheter was promptly inserted at ED. His blood pressure subsequently increased

Table 3 Literature review

	Author	Year of publication	Study type	Number of patient	Age (years)	Sex	Diagnosis	CPA	Sheath (Fr)	Insertion method	Use fluoroscopy	Position (Zone)	Intervals for REBOA (min)	Hemodynamics (SBP)	Complications	Definitive hemostatic control	Outcome
1	Low et al. [11]	1986	case series	1	NA	NA	mesenteric thrombosis	yes	11.5	cutdown	no	NA	NA	improved	NA	NA	Dead
2	Karkos et al. [12]	2001	case report	1	36	female	duodenum ulcer	no	NA	cutdown	no	I	30	70 → 140 mmHg	none	surgery	Alive
3	Hill et al. [13]	2010	case report	1	9	female	aortoesophageal fistula	yes	7	percutaneous	no	I	NA	improved	none	stent graft	Alive
4	Shigesato et al. [14]	2015	case report	1	79	female	duodenum ulcer	yes	9	percutaneous	no	I	150	40 → 240 mmHg	none	surgery	Alive

CPA cardiopulmonary arrest, *REBOA* resuscitative endovascular balloon occlusion of the aorta, *SBP* systolic blood pressure

following balloon inflation, and he underwent endoscopic treatment at ED. The bleeding vessel was visualized from the ulcer at the gastric angle, and the bleeding was arrested using balloon inflation. We believe that this case denotes the effectiveness of a balloon-assisted hemostatic technique in decreasing bleeding to secure a visual field and to reduce the volume of blood transfusion.

The immediately availability of an IABO catheter and the earlier introduction of REBOA have enabled us to sustain the circulation as an adjunct procedure until definitive hemostasis is attained. A formal algorithm that is utilized in a prospective manner is essential for UGIB treatment (endoscopy, AE, and surgery) and may shorten the occlusion time of REBOA. In the present study, one patient (Patient No. 5) with failed endoscopic hemostasis died within 24 h; the total occlusion time was 145 min. Although, REBOA for 60 min was reportedly to be well tolerated in an animal model of uncontrolled hemorrhagic shock, a recent report has suggested that partial REBOA could increase the survival time to 180 min while maintaining central blood pressure and carotid blood flow [10, 16]. In future, this method may be helpful for successful use of REBOA in patients with a high lactate concentration and a high CRS.

The major complications observed with REBOA included vessel injuries (i.e. aortic dissection, rapture and perforation), embolization, and peripheral ischemia. Recent reports have reported no vessel injuries caused by an IABO catheter or inflated balloon in trauma patients [17]. We routinely use ultrasonography to guide positioning of the IABO catheter during procedures and evaluate balloon placement using portable radiography after catheter deployment and there was no REBOA-related complications. Giuliani et al. support this result in the study showing that ultrasonography alone is safe and accurate as fluoroscopy for positioning and deployment of an IABO catheter [7].

However, this study has several limitations, particularly the small number of evaluated patients. Second, this was not a randomized, controlled trial because in the acute care setting, it is difficult to perform a randomized trial in a single emergency center. Furthermore, use of a propensity score is not suitable for a small sample size. Thus, large multi-institutional studies are essential for further evaluating the utility of REBOA against UGIB. Third, patients were allocated to REBOA use and treatments according to the decision of the attending lead acute care physicians, and this should be considered when interpreting our outcomes. Although patient selection was carefully performed, we believe the number of patients could have been greater. Consequently, our methods may be evaluated and incorporated into future studies to optimize the criteria for patient selection. Finally, application of this approach in other emergency centers may be limited by a lack of resources.

Conclusion

Immediate availability of an IABO catheter device can perform REBOA in ER and ICU and achieve a high degree of technical success. Temporary aortic balloon occlusion is effective at improving hemodynamics and perfusion in patients with UGIB. Furthermore, the correlations of total occlusion time and high clinical Rockall score, as the most relevant one, lactate levels, and advanced age may be important for successful use of REBOA. Formal prospective study is warranted to clarify the role of this adjunct procedure in UGIB treatment.

Abbreviations
AE: angio-embolization; APACHE: acute physiology and chronic health evaluation; AST: aminotransferases; BE: base excess; BUN: blood urea nitrogen; CK: creatine kinase; CRS: clinical rockall score; ED: emergency department; GBS: Glasgow-Blatchford bleeding score; IABO: intra-aortic balloon occlusion; LDH: lactate dehydrogenase; REBOA: resuscitative endovascular balloon occlusion of the aorta; SBP: systolic blood pressure; SI: shock index; UGIB: upper gastrointestinal bleeding.

Competing interests
None. This manuscript has not been published previously and is not under consideration for publication elsewhere.

Authors' contributions
SH and TJ: conceived and designed the study, collected date and data interpretation. HA, OT and TY: data interpretation. OS: data interpretation and final approval of the version to be submitted. All authors read and approved the final manuscript.

Acknowledgments
The authors would like to thank Enago (www.enago.jp) for the English language review.

Author details
[1]Emergency and Critical Care Medicine, Tokyo Medical University Hachioji Medical Center, 1163 Tatemachi, Hachioji, Tokyo 193-0998, Japan. [2]Emergency and Disaster Medicine, Tokyo Medical University, 6-7-1 Nishi-shinjuku, Shinjuku, Tokyo 160-0023, Japan.

References
1. Dries DJ. The contemporary role of blood products and components used in trauma resuscitation. Scand J Trauma Resusc Emerg Med. 2010;18:63. doi: 10.1186/1757-7241-18-63.
2. Baracat F, Moura E, Bernardo W, Pu LZ, Mendonça E, Moura D, et al. Endoscopic hemostasis for peptic ulcer bleeding: systematic review and meta-analyses of randomized controlled trials. Surg Endosc. 2015. Epub ahead of print.
3. Rabinovici R, Bugaev N. Resuscitative thoracotomy: an update. Scand J Surg. 2014;103:112–9.
4. Morrison JJ, Galgon RE, Jansen JO, Cannon JW, Rasmussen TE, Eliason JL. A systematic review of the use of resuscitative endovascular balloon occlusion of the aorta in the management of hemorrhagic shock. J Trauma Acute Care Surg. 2016;80:324–34. doi:10.1097/TA.0000000000000913.
5. Norii T, Crandall C, Terasaka Y. Survival of severe blunt trauma patients treated with resuscitative endovascular balloon occlusion of the aorta compared with propensity score-adjusted untreated patients. J Trauma Acute Care Surg. 2015;78:721–8. doi:10.1097/TA.0000000000000578.
6. Stannard A, Eliason JL, Rasmussen TE. Resuscitative endovascular balloon occlusion of the aorta (REBOA) as an adjunct for hemorrhagic shock. J Trauma. 2011;71:1869–72. doi:10.1097/TA.0b013e31823fe90c.
7. Guliani S, Amendola M, Strife B, Morano G, Elbich J, Albuquerque F, et al. Central aortic wire confirmation for emergent endovascular procedures: as

fast as surgeon-performed ultrasound. J Trauma Acute Care Surg. 2015;79: 549–54. doi:10.1097/TA.0000000000000818.

8.   Jung SH, Oh JH, Lee HY, Jeong JW, Go SE, You CR, et al. Is the AIMS65 score useful in predicting outcomes in peptic ulcer bleeding? World J Gastroenterol. 2014;20:1846–51. doi:10.3748/wjg.v20.i7.1846.

9.   Markov NP, Percival TJ, Morrison JJ, Ross JD, Scott DJ, Spencer JR, et al. Physiologic tolerance of descending thoracic aortic balloon occlusion in a swine model of hemorrhagic shock. Surgery. 2013;153:848–56. doi:10.1016/j. surg.2012.12.001.

10. Scott DJ, Eliason JL, Villamaria C, Morrison JJ, Houston 4th R, Spencer JR, et al. A novel fluoroscopy-free, resuscitative endovascular aortic balloon occlusion system in a model of hemorrhagic shock. J Trauma Acute Care Surg. 2013;75:122–8.

11. Low RB, Longmore W, Rubinstein R, Flores L, Wolvek S. Preliminary report on the use of the percluder occluding aortic balloon in human beings. Ann Emerg Med. 1986;15:1466–9.

12. Karkos CD, Bruce IA, Lambert ME. Use of the intra-aortic balloon pump to stop gastrointestinal bleeding. Ann Emerg Med. 2001;38:328–31.

13. Hill SJ, Zarroug AE, Ricketts RR, Veeraswamy R. Bedside placement of an aortic occlusion balloon to control a ruptured aorto-esophageal fistula in a small child. Ann Vasc Surg. 2010;24:822.e7–9. doi:10.1016/j.avsg.2009.12.016.

14. Shigesato S, Shimizu T, Kittaka T, Akimoto H. Intra-aortic balloon occlusion catheter for treating hemorrhagic shock after massive duodenal ulcer bleeding. Am J Emerg Med. 2015;33:473.e1–2. doi:10.1016/j.ajem.2014.01.024.

15. Bozkurt S, Köse A, Arslan ED, Erdoğan S, Uçbilek E, Cevik I, et al. Validity of modified early warning, Glasgow Blatchford, and pre-endoscopic Rockall scores in predicting prognosis of patients presenting to emergency department with upper gastrointestinal bleeding. Scand J Trauma Resusc Emerg Med. 2015;23:109. doi:10.1186/s13049-015-0194-z.

16. Russo RM, Williams TK, Grayson JK, Lamb CM, Cannon JW, Clement NF, et al. Extending the golden hour: partial resuscitative endovascular balloon occlusion of the aorta (P-REBOA) in a highly lethal swine liver injury model. J Trauma Acute Care Surg. 2016;80:372–80. doi:10.1097/TA.0000000000000940.

17. Brenner ML, Moore LJ, DuBose JJ, Tyson GH, McNutt MK, Albarado RP, et al. A clinical series of resuscitative endovascular balloon occlusion of the aorta for hemorrhage control and resuscitation. J Trauma Acute Care Surg. 2013; 75:506–11. doi:10.1097/TA.0b013e31829e5416.

10

Factors affecting morbidity and mortality in traumatic colorectal injuries and reliability and validity of trauma scoring systems

Nurettin Ay[1*], Vahhaç Alp[2], İbrahim Aliosmanoğlu[3], Utkan Sevük[4], Şafak Kaya[5] and Bülent Dinç[6]

Abstract

Background and aim: This study aims to determine the factors that affect morbidity and mortality in colon and rectum injuries related with trauma, the use of trauma scoring systems in predicting mortality and morbidity.

Patients and methods: Besides patient demographic characteristics, the mechanism of injury, the time between injury and surgery, accompanying body injuries, admittance Glasgow coma scale (GCS), findings at surgery and treatment methods were also recorded. With the obtained data, the abbreviated injury scale (AIS), injury severity score (ISS), revised trauma score (RTS) and trauma-ISS (TRISS) scores of each patient were calculated by using the 2008 revised AIS.

Results: Of the patients, 172 (88.7 %) were male, 22 (11.3 %) were female and the mean age was 29.15 ± 12.392 (15–89) years. The morbidity of our patients were 32 % and mortality were 12.4 %. ISS ($p < 0.001$), RTS ($p < 0.001$), and the TRISS ($p < 0.001$) on mortality were found to be significant. TRISS ($p = 0.008$), the ISS ($p < 0.001$), the RTS ($p = 0.03$), the trauma surgery interval (TSI, $p < 0.001$) were observed to have significant effects on morbidity.

Regression analysis showed that the ISS (OR 1.1; CI 95 % 1.01–1.2; $p = 0.02$), the RTS (OR 0.37; CI 95 % 0.21–0.67; $p = 0.001$) had significant effects on mortality. While the effects of TSI (OR 5.3; CI 95 % 1.5–18.8; $p = 0.01$) on morbidity were found to be significant.

Conclusion: Predicting mortality by using scoring systems and close postoperative follow up of patients in the risk group may ensure decreases in the rates of morbidity and mortality.

Keywords: Trauma, Colorectal, TRISS, RTS, ISS

Introduction

Colorectal injuries are rare in trauma patients and are associated with increased mortality. These injuries constitute 1 % of all trauma patients [1]. Most colonic and rectal injuries occur following penetrating trauma and injury from blunt trauma is uncommon [2]. The mortality associated with colonic trauma has decreased considerably over the last half century; from 40 % during World War II to 1–3 % over the last several decades [3]. Common postoperative complications include systemic complications such as pneumonia, sepsis and complications specific to

abdominal surgery such as surgical site infection, intraabdominal abscess, and abdominal sepsis [4].

Staging according to the severity of injury is necessary for the management of trauma and as well as a basic requirement for clinical trials [5]. Trauma scoring systems try to translate the severity of injury into a number. The scores enable physicians to translate different severity of injuries into a common language [6]. Quantitative characterizations of injury are essential for research and meaningful evaluation of patient outcome, quality improvement, and prevention programs [6, 7]. For this purpose, many anatomical and physiological scoring systems are created [8]. There are around 50 scoring systems published for the classification of trauma patients [6]. Some of these scoring systems are new injury severity score (NISS), AIS, ISS, GCS, RTS and TRISS [9]. This study aims to determine the

* Correspondence: nurettinay77@hotmail.com
[1]Diyarbakır Gazi Yaşargil Education and Research Hospital, Transplantation Center, Diyarbakır, Turkey
Full list of author information is available at the end of the article

factors that affect morbidity and mortality in colon and rectum injuries related to trauma, to utilize trauma scoring systems for predicting mortality and morbidity.

Materials and methods

Between January 2005 and December 2010, all the patients who were operated on for blunt or penetrating abdominal injury at Dicle University Faculty of Medicine Hospital were evaluated retrospectively. One ninety four patients with colorectal injury were included in the study.

After the initial evaluation of the patients in the emergency room, a nasogastric catheter, a central venous pressure catheter and a foley catheter was placed into the patients. All the patients were given fluid-electrolyte resuscitation. In the preoperative period, the patients were simultaneously administered two antibiotics (intravenous ceftriaxone 1 g and metronidazole 500 mg). Antibiotic therapy was continued in the postoperative period and was stopped on the fifth day. Hemodynamically unstable patients were operated on under emergency conditions. Patients who were hemodynamically stable were assessed by physical examination, laboratory tests and imaging methods (radiography, ultrasonography, computed tomography), peritoneal lavage before proceeding with the surgery. One of these procedures for patients who were scheduled for surgery were performed primary repair+proximal diverting stoma (PDS), resection+anastomosis, primary closure or resection of injured bowel+PDS. Distal washout and presacral drainage were not performed for rectal injuries. Midline laparotomy was performed all patients.

Besides the demographic characteristics of the patients such as age and gender; the mechanism of the injury, the time between injury and surgery, accompanying body injuries (head and neck, face, chest, abdomen, extremities and external structures), vital signs at emergency admittance, GCS at admission, findings during the performed surgery and the treatment methods were also recorded. Follow up data after surgery, observed complications and the duration of time until discharge were evaluated. Trauma and/or operation related complications were defined as morbidity and deaths due to trauma and/or operation were defined as mortality.

With the obtained data, the AIS scores of each patient were calculated by using the 2008 revised AIS (AIS was calculated according to update 2008 dictionary in the www.aaam.org website). The ISS scores were calculated for each patient with the data from the three regions (regions: head & neck, face, chest, abdomen, extremity, external) with the highest scores The RTS were calculated for each patient by using the findings of respiratory rate at admittance to the emergency room, systolic blood pressure and GCS data. The TRISS were calculated for each patient by using the patient ISS, RTS, age and trauma mechanism

data. In order to calculate the ISS, RTS and the TRISS, the calculation tool available on the web site www.trauma.org were used.

All colonic injuries were divided into two categories as non-destructive (Flint scale grade 1–2) and destructive (Flint scale grade 3). The patients were divided into two groups, blunt injury group (BIG) and penetrating injury group (PIG), and a comparison was made between these two forms of trauma. The present study was approved by the Dicle University ethics committee and complies with the requirements of the Declaration of Helsinki.

Statistical analysis

Statistical analysis was performed by using the SPSS for Windows 11.5 (SPSS Inc. Chicago, IL, USA) program. Descriptive statistics were used for the evaluation of the data. The Kolmogorov-Smirnov test was used to determine the distribution of the data. The Chi-square test was used for the comparison of qualitative data between groups and the Mann–Whitney U test was used for the comparison of quantitative data. The data were evaluated in terms of mean standard deviation. The regression test was used to determine the factors effecting morbidity and mortality. A p value <0.05 was accepted as being statistically significant.

Results

Between January 2005 and December 2010, 3857 trauma patients were followed and treated by the general surgery department and the incidence of colorectal injury was detected to be 4 %. Colorectal injuries due to blunt trauma comprised 7.7 % of all colorectal injuries. The common causes of injury were gunshot wound ($n = 128$, 66 %), cuts and puncture wounds ($n = 51$, 26.3 %), traffic accidents ($n = 12$, 6.2 %) and falls from a height ($n = 3$, 1.5 %). The majority of the patients with colorectal injuries had Flint grade 1 injuries (53.1 %). Sixty two percent of the cases were managed by primary closure. The morbidity of the patients were 32 % and mortality was 12.4 %. The descriptive data of the study is presented in Figs. 1, 2 and 3.

A hundred and fifty one (77.8 %) patients had accompanying additional organ injuries. Fifty-eight (29.9 %) patients had two or more additional organ injuries. The most common organ injuries seen with colon injuries were small bowel injuries (Table 1).

Comparison of characteristics of BIG and PIG are presented in Table 2. When compared to the PIG, the rates of morbidity ($p = 0.02$), mortality ($p = 0.02$) and the rates of patients treated after 8 hours ($p = 0.008$) of the injury in the BIG were significantly higher. In the BIG, the mean RTS was significantly lower than in the PIG ($p = 0.037$) (Table 2).

Flint injury scale

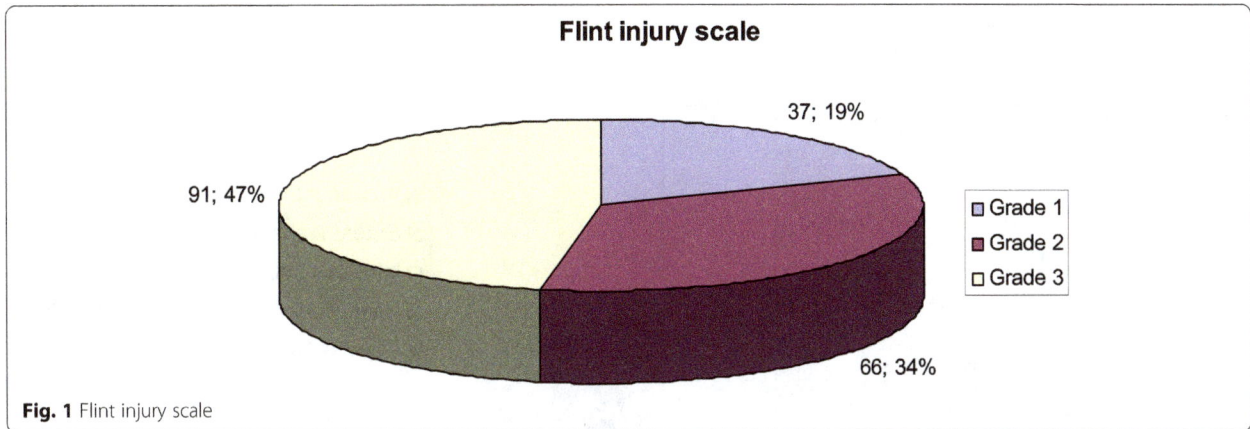

Fig. 1 Flint injury scale

The effects of gender ($p = 0.03$), the type of trauma ($p = 0.02$), the degree of colon injury ($p < 0.001$), the treatment methods ($p < 0.001$), the presence of additional organ injury ($p = 0.02$), the ISS ($p < 0.001$), RTS ($p < 0.001$), and the TRISS ($p < 0.001$) were found to be significant on mortality rates. The types of trauma ($p = 0.02$), the TRISS ($p = 0.008$), the ISS ($p < 0.001$), the RTS ($p = 0.03$), the treatment methods ($p = 0.001$), the TSI ($p < 0.001$) and the degree of colon injury ($p < 0.001$) were observed to have significant effects on morbidity (Table 3).

Regression analysis showed that Flint injury degree, TSI and treatment type had no significant effect on mortality. The ISS (OR 1.1; CI 95 % 1.01–1.2; $p = 0.02$), the RTS (OR 0.37; CI 95 % 0.21–0.67; $p = 0.001$) and the types of trauma (penetrating-blunt distinction) (OR 0.5; CI 95 % 0.01–0.39; $p = 0.004$) had significant effects on mortality. While the effects of TSI (OR 5.3; CI 95 % 1.5–18.8;

$p = 0.01$) and Flint injury degree (OR 3.2; CI 95 % 1.47–7.23; $p = 0.004$) were found to be significant for morbidity; there were no significant correlation observed between morbidity and the TRISS, RTS, ISS or the types of treatment (Table 4).

Discussion

It is difficult to determine the incidence of colorectal traumatic injury. In general war series, it has been reported to be as high as 5–10 %. Recently, in the Iraq war data that evaluated more than 3400 trauma patients, the incidence of colorectal injury was found to be 5.1 %. A recent study of colorectal injuries encountered in Afghanistan and Iraq reveals that 71 % of injuries occurred secondary to penetrating trauma, 23 % were secondary to blast, and 5 % occurred during blunt trauma. In civilian series it is observed to be 1–3 %. This rate is lower in blunt trauma

Treatment
PDS: Proximal diverting stoma

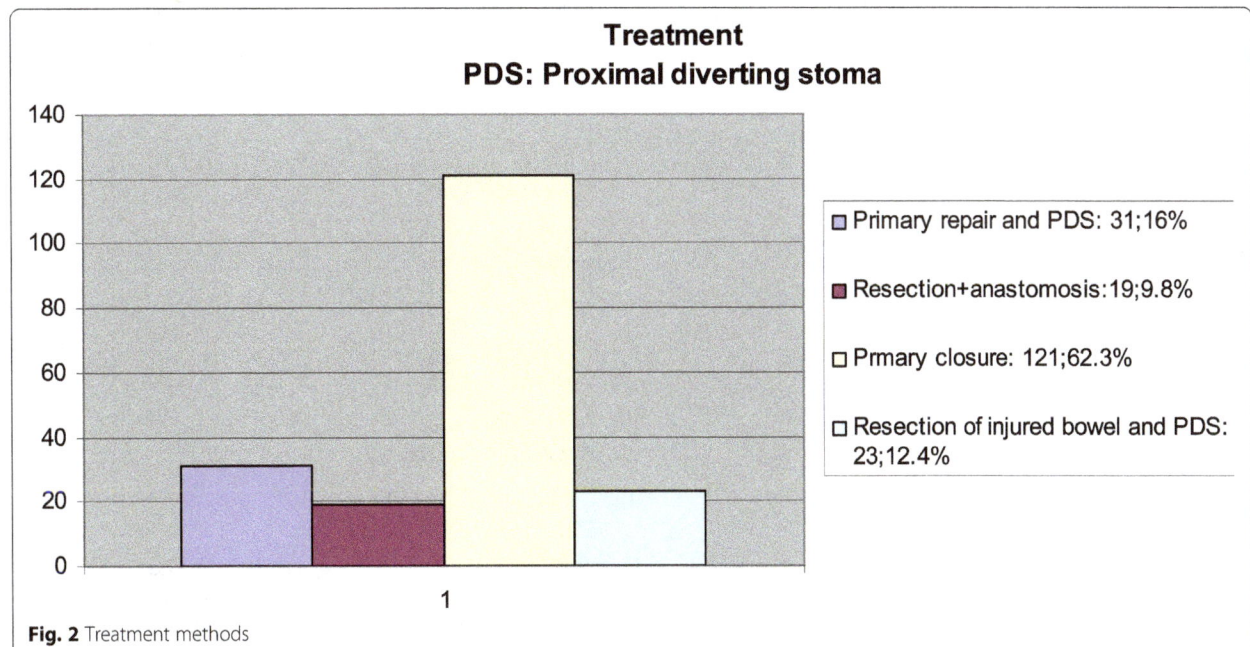

Fig. 2 Treatment methods

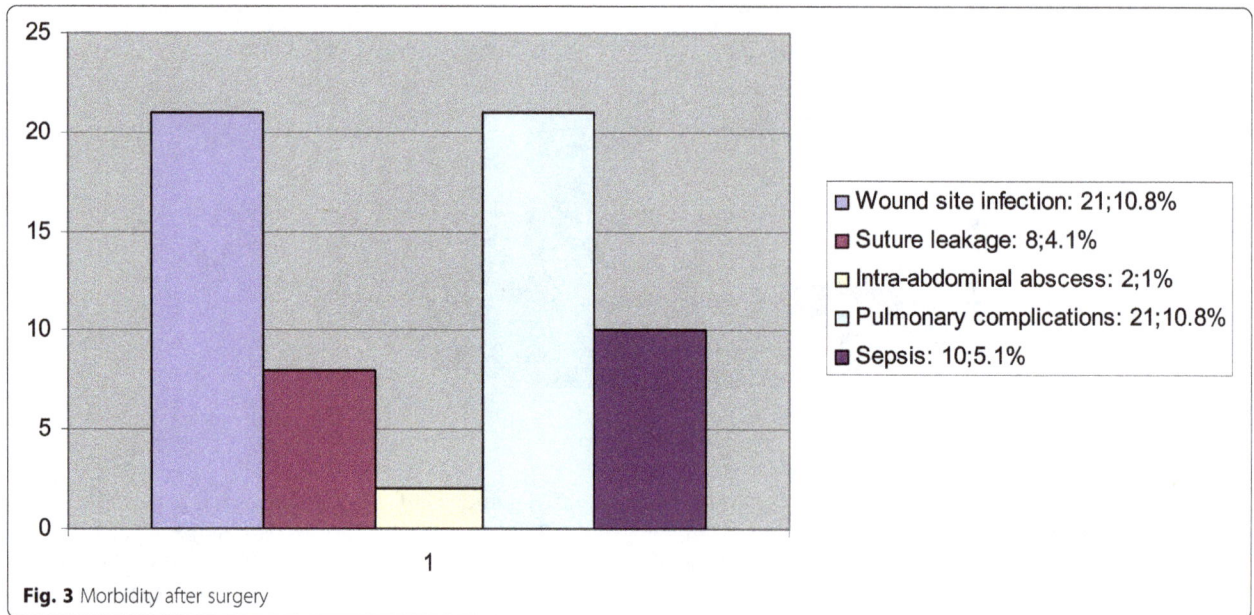

Fig. 3 Morbidity after surgery

Legend:
- □ Wound site infection: 21;10.8%
- ■ Suture leakage: 8;4.1%
- □ Intra-abdominal abscess: 2;1%
- □ Pulmonary complications: 21;10.8%
- ■ Sepsis: 10;5.1%

[4, 10–12]. During the peace time, 80–90 % of colon injuries are non-destructive colon injuries. In contrast, in war time, 72 % of colon injuries are destructive injuries [7]. In our study destructive injuries ratios were 46.9 %. These high rates of destructive and penetrating injuries may result from the low intensity war between an armed organisation and government forces in our region between 1985 and 2010, and resulting increase of other types of crimes due to social disorder.

Table 1 The other organs with injuries

Addition organ wounds	Number	Percent
Small bowel	101	52
Stomach	28	14,4
Kidney	22	11,3
Vascular	18	9,2
Diaphragm	17	8,7
Liver	16	8,2
Lung	14	7,2
Spleen	11	5,6
Bladder	8	4,1
Pancreas	3	1,5
Cardiac	3	1,5
Gall bladder	2	1
Ureter	2	1
Urethra	2	1
Oesophagus	1	0,5
Testicle	1	0,5
Multiple small bowel	41	21,1

Table 2 Comparison of characteristics of blunt injury group and penetrating injury group

	PIG ($n = 179$)	BIG ($n = 15$)	P value
Age (years), mean ± SD	28.9 ± 12.5	31.2 ± 11.2	0.3
Gender, males, n (%)	159 (88.8)	13 (86.6)	0.68
Treatment, n (%)			
Primary repair	132 (73.7)	8 (53.3)	0.13
Stoma procedure	47 (26.3)	7 (46.7)	0.13
Flint injury scale			
Grade 1 and 2	96 (53.6)	7 (46.7)	0.8
Grade 3	83 (46.4)	8 (53.3)	0.8
TSI, n(%)			
< 8 hours	165 (92.1)	10 (66.6)	0.008
> 8 hours	14 (7.9)	5 (33.4)	0.008
ISS, mean ± SD	29.7 ± 14.2	33.5 ± 11.8	0.08
RTS, mean ± SD	7.2 ± 1.3	7 ± 0.9	0.03
TRISS, mean ± SD	85 ± 26.1	88.2 ± 12.3	0.07
Hospitalization (days), mean ± SD	11.2 ± 9.3	9.8 ± 8.1	0.23
Morbidity, n (%)	53 (29.6)	9 (0.6)	0.02
Wound site infection	18 (10.1)	3 (20)	
Suture leakage	8 (4.5)	-	
Intraabdominal abscess	2 (1.1)	-	
Pulmonary complications	16 (8.9)	5 (33.3)	
Sepsis	9 (5)	1 (6.7)	
Mortality, n (%)	19 (10.6)	5 (33.4)	0.02

PIG penetrating injury group, *BIG* blunt injury group, *TSI*, trauma-surgery interval, *ISS* injury severity score, *RTS* revised trauma score, *TRISS* trauma-injury severity score

Table 3 Factors affecting morbidity and mortality following colorectal injury

	Morbidity			Mortality		
	Yes (n = 62)	No (n = 132)	P value	Yes (n = 24)	No (n = 170)	P value
Age, mean ± SD	28.3 ± 11.5	29.5 ± 12.7	0.54	30.5 ± 14.2	28.9 ± 12.1	0.57
Gender (male), n (%)	52 (83.8%)	120 (90.9%)	0.15	18 (75%)	154 (90.5%)	0.03
Treatment, n (%)						
Primary repair	35 (56.5%)	105 (79.5%)	0.001	8 (33.3%)	132 (77.6%)	<0.001
Stoma procedure	27 (43.5%)	27 (20.4%)		16 (66.7%)	38 (22.4%)	
Flint injury scale, n (%)						
Grade 1 and 2	17 (27.4%)	86 (65.2%)	<0.001	3 (12.5%)	100 (58.8%)	<0.001
Grade 3	45 (72.6%)	46 (34.8%)		21 (87.5%)	70 (41.2%)	
TSI, n (%)						
<8 hours	47 (75.8%)	128 (97%)	<0.001	19 (79.2%)	156 (91.8%)	0.07
>8 hours	15 (24.2%)	4 (3%)		5 (20.8%)	14 (8.2%)	
ISS	35.4 ± 14.5	27.5 ± 13.1	<0.001	51.7 ± 8.6	27 ± 11.8	< 0,001
RTS	6.86 ± 1.6	7.36 ± 1.1	0.03	4.84 ± 2	7.53 ± 0.73	< 0,001
TRISS	77.2 ± 31	88.9 ± 21.1	0.008	36.6 ± 28.9	92 ± 15.4	< 0,001
Additional organ injuries, n (%)						
None	11 (17.7%)	32 (24.2%)	0.07	1 (4.2%)	42 (24.7%)	0.02
1 organ	28 (45.2%)	65 (49.2%)		11 (45.8%)	82 (48.2%)	
2 or more organs	23 (37.1%)	35 (26.5%)		12 (50%)	46 (27.1%)	
Region, n (%)						0.8
Caecum	5 (8%)	7 (5.3%)	0.36	0	12 (7%)	
Right colon	8 (13%)	14 (10.6%)		4 (16.6%)	18 (10.6%)	
Transverse colon	18 (29%)	50 (37.9%)	0.36	9 (37.5%)	59 (34.7%)	
Left colon	12 (19.4%)	15 (11.3%)		4 (16.6%)	23 (13.5%)	
Sigmoid colon	9 (14.5%)	32 (24.2%)		5 (20.8%)	36 (21.2%)	
Intraperitoneal rectum	3 (4.8%)	5 (3.9%)		1 (4.2%)	7 (4.1%)	
Extraperitonral rectum	7 (11.3%)	9 (6.8%)		1 (4.2%)	15 (8.9%)	
Group, n (%)						
Penetrating	53 (85.5%)	126 (95.6%)	0.02	19 (79.2%)	160 (94.1%)	0.02
Blunt	9 (14.5%)	6 (4.5%)		5 (20.8%)	10 (5.9%)	

TSI trauma-surgery interval, *ISS* injury severity score, *RTS* revised trauma score, *TRISS* trauma-injury severity score

Table 4 Statistics of morbidity and mortality in multivariate analysis

Factors	P value	OR	CI % 95 range		P value*	OR*	CI % 95 range*	
Group	0.149	0.367	0.94	1433	0.004	0.500	0.006	0.390
Flint injury scale	0.004	3.261	1.471	7.228	0.346	0.300	0.250	3.668
Treatment	0.382	0.701	0.316	1.556	0.222	0.362	0.710	1.847
ISI	0.01	5.303	1.493	18.835	0.132	4.633	0.629	34.151
RTS	0.776	0.906	0.460	1.785	0.001	0.376	0.211	0.671
ISS	0.507	1.015	0.971	1.062	0.019	1.104	1.017	1.199
TRISS	0.834	1.005	0.960	1.052				

*Statistics of Mortality in Multivariate Analysis. *TSI* trauma-surgery interval, *ISS* injury severity score, *RTS* revised trauma score, *TRISS* trauma- injury severity score

In the study by Ng et al., that evaluated 1367 patients with blunt trauma, they found the incidence of colorectal injury to be 0.1 % [13]. Similarly, Carillo et al. found the incidence of colorectal injury to be 0.5 % following blunt trauma [14]. In a multicenter prospective study conducted with 297 patients in the years after 2000 by Demetriades et al., two-thirds of the destructive injuries requiring resection were treated with primary repair; colon related mortality was found to be significantly lower in the primary repair group (0 % and 4 %, $p = 0.012$) and no difference was observed in terms of colon related complications (22 % and 27 %, $p = 0.373$) [4]. In the study by Miller et al., while 153 patients (73 %) without destructive injuries had primary suturing performed, of the 56 patients with destructive injuries, 40 (19 %) had resection and anastomosis and 16 (7.6 %) had stomas [15]. In our study, 140 patients (71 %) had primary repair performed and 54 patients (29 %) had stomas. Morbidity was found to be significantly higher in the ostomy group than in the primary repair group (primary repair: 25 %, ostomy: 50 %, $p < 0.001$). While 70.4 % of the stoma performed patients had destructive injuries, 37.9 % of the primary repair performed patients had destructive injuries ($p < 0.001$). High morbidity in the stoma group by univariate analysis may be associated with high ratio of destructive injury patients. In civilian injuries, the incidence of anastomotic leakage following primary repair is between 1 and 15 % [16, 17]. In their evaluation of 2964 patients, Curran et al. reported this incidence as being 2.4 % [18]. Demetriades at al. in a multicenter prospective trial involving 19 trauma centers that included 297 patients with destructive colon injuries requiring resection, found that there were no difference between primary repair and stoma in term of anastomotic leakage [4]. Cleary et al., reported hemodynamic instability and shock as risk factors for anastomotic leakage and infective complications [19]. In our study, anastomotic leakage was 4.1 %. There was a significant relationship between anastomotic leakage ratio and more than 8 hours of TSI ($p < 0.001$) and the increase in the degree of injury ($p = 0.004$). We detected the anastomotic leakage ratio to be 3.6 % in the primary repair group and 5.6 % in the stoma group ($p < 0.05$). Although we did not reach a clear conclusion as to why more anastomotic leakage was observed in the stoma group, the significantly low levels of RTS observed in the stoma group might suggest that there was more hemodynamic instability in the stoma performed patient group (7.39 vs. 6.69 and $p < 0.05$).

Pinedo, Çöl and Gümüş et al. did not find any significant relationship between age and gender with morbidity in their studies [20–22]. In our study, there was no significant relationship between age and gender with morbidity.

In many studies, the most common organ injury accompanying colon injuries were reported as being small bowel injuries [21–25]. In the studies by Çöl et al., detected at least one accompanying organ injury in 70 % of the patients [21]. In the study by Adesanya et al., where they investigated penetrating colon injuries, the organ injuries most commonly accompanying colon injuries were found to be the small bowel (73.3 %), the liver (25 %) and the stomach (23.3 %) [25]. In our study, the ratio of accompanying organ injury was 77.8 % and the most common accompanying organ injured was the small bowel. In literature, although the second most common organ injuries accompanying colorectal injury after the small bowel were reported as being the spleen or liver [23, 25]. In our study, the spleen ranked fifth. We observed that stomach, kidney and vascular injuries more commonly accompanied colorectal injuries than spleen injuries. This difference can be explained by the fact that higher percentage (92.3 %) of the patients had penetrating injury and 56 % of the colorectal injuries were in the transverse and sigmoid colon. While there was an increase in mortality when colorectal injury was accompanied by two or more organ injuries, ($p = 0.021$), there was no significant increase in observed morbidity ($p = 0.07$). In our study, there was no significant correlation detected between wound localization and mortality or morbidity ($p > 0.05$).

In a study by Singh et al., where they compared the predictive capacity of scoring systems related to trauma; they observed that the RTS and TRISS were better than ISS in predicting the likelihood of survival. Again in the same study: The RTS ranged from 2.746 to 7.8408. There was a graded increase in mortality with decreasing RTS score. There was a graded increase in mortality with increasing ISS scores [6]. In our study univariate analysis, there were significant relationships observed between ISS increase and both RTS and TRISS decrease with increased morbidity and mortality. While in multivariate analysis there were no relationship between these scoring systems and morbidity. Therewere relationships between ISS, RTS and mortality in multivariate analysis. Increased ISS was associated with increased mortality and increased RTS was associated with decreased mortality. We suggest that this arises from the higher ratios of destructive injuries observed in our patients. The positive effect of a TSI < 8 hours on morbidity had been known since the study of Stone and Fabian, which was confirmed with later studies [2, 4, 22, 26]. In our study, 9.8 % of the patients were taken to surgery after 8 hours and 90.2 % were taken to surgery earlier than 8 hours. In patients taken to surgery after 8 hours, the high morbidity was significant ($p = 0.010$ and OR = 5.303 % CI 1.493–18.835).

When the mortalities occurring in the first 24 hours were excluded from the study, the TSI was observed to have significant effect on mortality ($p < 0.05$).

Conclusion

Objective criteria are needed for evaluation of trauma patients. Using these scoring systems should be used routinely for follow up and predicting morbidity and mortality. Rapid transfer to the hospital, early diagnosis and treatment of patients with possible traumatic colorectal injury will reduce morbidity and mortality rates. Predicting mortality by using scoring systems and a close follow up of the patients postoperatively may reduce morbidity and mortality rates. Our study shows that there are correlations between trauma scoring indexes and morbidity and mortality. This results imply that there is a need for randomized, prospective controlled studies for adopting these scoring indexes for a better patient treatment and care.

Competing interests

The authors declare that they have no competing interests.

Authors' contributions

NA analyzed the results and wrote the manuscript and participated in the study design. VA participated in the study design and assisted in the acquisition of data and provided intellectual contributions to the manuscript draft. İA participated in the study design and assisted in the acquisition of data and provided intellectual contributions to the manuscript draft. US participated in the study design and assisted in the acquisition of data and provided intellectual contributions to the manuscript draft. ŞK participated in the study design and assisted in the acquisition of data and provided intellectual contributions to the manuscript draft. BD participated in the study design and assisted in the acquisition of data and provided intellectual contributions to the manuscript draft. All authors read and approved the final manuscript.

Author details

[1]Diyarbakır Gazi Yaşargil Education and Research Hospital, Transplantation Center, Diyarbakır, Turkey. [2]Department of General Surgery, Diyarbakir Gazi Yaşargil Education and Research Hospital, Diyarbakır, Turkey. [3]Department of General Surgery, Akdeniz University Hospital, Antalya, Turkey. [4]Department of Cardiovascular Surgery, Diyarbakır Gazi Yaşargil Education and Research Hospital, Diyarbakır, Turkey. [5]Department of İnfectious Disease, Diyarbakır Gazi Yaşargil Education and Research Hospital, Diyarbakır, Turkey. [6]Atatürk State Hospital, Antalya, Turkey.

References

1. Brady RR, O'Neil S, Berry O, Kerssens JJ, Yalamarthi S, Parks RW. Traumatic injury to the colon and rectum in Scotland: demographics and outcome. Colorectal Dis. 2012;15(1):e 16–22.
2. Govender M, Madiba TE. Current management of large bowel injuries and factors influencing outcome. Injury. 2010;41(1):58–63.
3. JDuBose J. Colonic trauma: indications for diversion vs. repair. Gastrointest Surg. 2009;13(3):403–4.
4. Demetriades D, Murray JA, Chan L, Ordoñez C, Bowley D, Nagy KK, et al. Penetrating colon injuries requiring resection: diversion or primary anastomosis? An AAST prospective multicenter trial. J Trauma. 2001;50:765–75.
5. Aydin SA, Bulut M, Ozgüç H, Ercan I, Türkmen N, Eren B, et al. Should the new injury severity score replace the injury severity score in the trauma and injury severity score? Ulus Travma Acil Cerrahi Derg. 2008;14:308–12.
6. Singh J, Gupta G, Garg R, Gupta A. Evaluation of trauma and prediction of outcome using TRISS method. J Emerg Trauma Shock. 2011;4(4):448–9.
7. Sammour T, Kahokehr A, Caldwell S, Hill AG. Venous glucose and arterial lactate as biochemical predictors of mortality in clinically severely injured trauma patients—a comparison with ISS and TRISS. Injury. 2009;40:104–8.
8. Yağmur Y, Güloğlu C, Uğur M, Akkuş Z, Elik Y. Evaluation of patients with multiple injuries: comparison of injury severity score and revised trauma score. Ulus Travma Acil Cerrahi Derg. 1997;3:73–7.
9. Orhon R, Eren ŞH, Karadayı Ş, Korkmaz İ, Coşkun A, Eren M, et al. Comparison of trauma scores for predicting mortality and morbidity on trauma patients. Ulus Travma Acil Cerrahi Derg. 2014;20(4):258–64.
10. Steele SR, Wolcott KE, Mullenix PS, Martin MJ, Sebesta JA, Azarow KS, et al. Colon and rectal injuries during operation Iraqi Freedom: are there any changing trends in management or outcome? Dis Colon Rectum. 2007;50(6):870–7.
11. Johnson EK, Steele SR. Evidence-based management of colorectal trauma. J Gastrointest Surg. 2013;17(9):1712–9.
12. Cho SD, Kiraly LN, Flaherty SF, Herzig DO, Lu KC, Schreiber MA. Management of colonic injuries in the combat theater. Dis Colon Rectum. 2010;53(5):728–34.
13. Ng AK, Simons RK, Torreggiani WC, Ho SG, Kirkpatrick AW, Brown DR. Intra-abdominal free fluid without solid organ injury in blunt abdominal trauma. J Trauma. 2002;52(6):1134–40.
14. Carrillo EH, Somberg LB, Ceballos CE, Martini Jr MA, Ginzburg E, Sosa JL, et al. Blunt traumatic injuries to the colon and rectum. J Am Col Surg. 1996;183(6):548–52.
15. Miller PR, Fabian TC, Croce MA, Magnotti LJ, Elizabeth Pritchard F, Minard G, et al. İmproving outcomes following penetrating colon wounds: application of a clinical pathway. Ann Surg. 2002;235(6):775–81.
16. Stewart RM, Fabian TC, Croce MA, Pritchard FE, Minard G, Kudsk KA. Is resection with primary anastomosis following destructive colon wounds always safe? Am J Surg. 1994;168(4):316–9.
17. Sharpe JP, Magnotti LJ, Weinberg JA, Shahan CP, Cullinan DR, Marino KA, et al. Applicability of an established management algorithm for destructive colon injuries after abbreviated laparotomy: a 17-year experience. J Am Coll Surg. 2014;218(4):636–41.
18. Curran TJ, Borzotta AP. Complications of primary repair of colon injury: literature review of 2964 cases. Am J Surg. 1999;177(1):42–7.
19. Cleary RK, Pomerantz RA, Lampman RM. Colon and rectal injuries. Dis Colon Rectum. 2006;49(8):1203–22.
20. Pinedo-Onofre JA, Guevara-Torres L, Sanchez-Aquilar JM. Penetrating abdominal trauma. Cir Cir. 2006;74(6):431–42.
21. Col C, Dolapcı M, Yılmaz A. Procedures without colostomy in the surgical emergent treatment of colonic injuries. Ulus Travma Acil Cer Derg. 1997;3:42–7.
22. Gümüş M, Kapan M, Önder A, Böyuk A, Girgin S, Taçyıldız I. Factors affecting morbidity in penetrating rectal injuries: a civillian experience. Ulus Travma Acil Cer Derg. 2011;17(5):401–6.
23. Muffoletto JP, Tate JS. Colon trauma: primary repair evolving as the standart of care. J Nat Med Assoc. 1996;88(9):574–8.
24. Musa O, Ghildiyal JP, CPandey M. 6 Year prospective clinical trial of primary repair versus diversion colostomy in colonic injury cases. Indian J Surg. 2010;72(4):308–11.
25. Adesanya AA, Ekanem EE. A ten-year study of penetrating injuries of the colon. Dis Colon Rectum. 2004;47(12):2169–77.
26. Stone HH, Fabian TC. Management of perforating colon trauma: randomization between primary closure and exteriorization. Ann Surg. 1979;190(4):430–5.

11

Sigmoid volvulus and ileo-sigmoid knotting: a five-year experience at a tertiary care hospital

Phillipo L Chalya* and Joseph B Mabula

Abstract

Background: Sigmoid volvulus is a common cause of intestinal obstruction in developing countries where it affects relatively young people compared to developed countries. No prospective study has been done on this subject in Tanzania and Bugando Medical Centre in particular. This study describes in our region, the clinical presentation, management and outcome of sigmoid volvulus.

Methods: This was a descriptive prospective study of patients operated for sigmoid volvulus at Bugando Medical Centre from March 2009 to February 2014.

Results: A total of 146 patients (M: F = 5.1: 1) representing 14.2% of all cases of bowel obstruction were studied. The median age at presentation was 48 years. The disease significantly affected the older males compared with females (P = 0.012). The majority of the patients 102, (93.2%) presented acutely and had to undergo emergency surgical intervention, the rest were either sub-acute or chronic. Out of the 146 patients studied, 24 (16.4%) had ileo-sigmoid knotting. The majority of patients, 102(69.9%) were treated with resection and primary anastomosis, of which 63.0% were emergency cases. Colostomy was offered to 30.1% of cases. No patient had sigmoidoscopic derotation. Complications mainly surgical site infections were reported in 20.5% of cases. The overall median length of hospital stay was 14 days. Overall mortality rate was 17.1%. The main predictors of mortality were advanced age (>60 years), concomitant medical illness, late presentation (≥24 hours), presence of shock on admission and presence of gangrenous bowel (P < 0.001). The follow up of patients in this study was generally poor as more than half of patients were lost to follow up.

Conclusion: Sigmoid volvulus is not uncommon in our setting and commonly affects males than females. Most of the patients presented acutely, requiring immediate resuscitation and surgical approach. Findings from this study suggest that in viable bowel, sigmoid resection and primary anastomosis is feasible as it may not adversely affect outcome. Temporary colostomy should be considered if the bowel is gangrenous or perforated. Early diagnosis and timely definitive treatment are essential in order to decrease the morbidity and mortality associated with this disease.

Keywords: Sigmoid volvulus, Clinical presentation, Management, Outcome, Tanzania

Background

Sigmoid volvulus, first described by von Rokitansky in 1836 [1], is a condition in which the sigmoid colon wraps around itself and its own mesentery, causing a closed-loop obstruction which, if left untreated, often results in life-threatening complications, such as bowel ischemia, gangrene, and perforation [2,3]. It is an important cause of colonic obstruction worldwide [1-3]. In developed countries, sigmoid volvulus ranks the third among large intestine obstructions following cancer and diverticular diseases [4]. It represents 4% of all cases in developed countries and 50% in developing countries [5].

The etiology of sigmoid volvulus is multifactorial and controversial [4,6-9]. Those who possess a sigmoid colon with a long loop and narrow base of mesenteric attachment would be more prone to volvulus [8]. Anatomical predispositions, advanced age, a high-fibre diet, medications altering

* Correspondence: drphillipoleo@yahoo.com
Department of Surgery, Catholic University of Health and Allied Science-Bugando, Mwanza, Tanzania

intestinal motility, chronic constipation, previous abdominal surgery, neurological or psychiatric illness, pregnancy, high altitude and megacolon have all been reported in association with development of the condition [4,6-9].

Sigmoid Volvulus may present with acute sigmoid torsion, recurrent previous torsion or ileosigmoid knotting [10]. Sigmoid volvulus generally affects adults, with the highest incidence seen in the 4th-8th decades of life [5]. However, patients tend to be younger in developing countries as opposed to developed countries where the average age is 62 to 72 years [5,11]. The disease is more common in males and occurs in ratios ranging from 2:1 to 10:1 [1,5,11]. Classically, patients present with a triad of abdominal pain, constipation and abdominal distention [12]. Abdominal X-ray radiograph always revealed findings typical of volvulus in only 65.0% of cases [12,13]. Many other authors have reported similar symptoms and signs plus; vomiting, empty rectal ampulla, associated mental and other medical illnesses in sigmoid volvulus presentation [11-13].

The management of sigmoid volvulus posses a great challenge in resource limited societies as found in Africa [9,13,14]. Late presentation of the disease coupled with lack of advanced diagnostic (such as abdominal Computed Tomography (CT) scan and Magnetic Resonance Imaging (MRI) and therapeutic facilities for non-operative procedures are a common feature in resource-limited setting like Tanzania [13,14]. Early and correct diagnosis of this disease is essential for appropriate treatment aimed at correcting abnormal pathophysiological changes and restoring intestinal transit caused by the volvulus [2,14].

Despite significant progress in the treatment of this disease, no consensus has been reached [2,14]. Generally, the aim of treatment of sigmoid volvulus is to relieve the obstruction and decompress the twisted sigmoid colon [14]. Many authorities now agree that, in uncomplicated sigmoid volvulus (without perforation or gangrene) sigmoid resection with immediate primary anastomosis is a first choice single-stage operation as it does not increase morbidity or mortality rates [14,15]. On the other hand, if the sigmoid colon is gangrenous then Hartmann's procedure is recommended [13-16]. Some authors advocate nonoperative such as sigmoidoscopic decompression and derotation as the primary emergency treatment of choice in uncomplicated acute sigmoid volvulus followed by interval semi-elective resection and primary anastomosis several days after successful decompression and emergency surgery is reserved for gangrene or failed decompression [1,17,18]. Emergency surgery is the appropriate treatment for those who present with diffuse peritonitis, intestinal perforation or ischemic necrosis [18,19]. Nonoperative treatment is adopted if there is no evidence of these conditions. However, late presentation of the disease, lack of facilities for nonoperative treatment and associated high

rate of recurrence, nonoperative treatment may not be feasible in resource-limited setting.

Sigmoid volvulus is often associated with a high mortality because it affects elderly patients who may have severe co morbid conditions. Patients older than 70 years represent a high risk group if subjected to surgical intervention [19]. However, when volvulus necessitates emergency surgery, it also carries a substantial mortality even in relatively young patients [20]. The highest mortality usually occurs in cases of resection and primary anastomosis of gangrenous sigmoid colon [21].

There is a paucity of information regarding sigmoid volvulus in Tanzania and particularly the study area. This is partly due to a lack of published local data regarding this condition in this region. This study was designed to describe our experience on the management of sigmoid volvulus outlining the clinical presentation, treatment outcome of sigmoid volvulus in our local setting and to identify factors predicting the outcome.

Methods

Study design and setting

This was a descriptive prospective study of patients operated for sigmoid volvulus at Bugando Medical Centre from March 2009 to February 2014. Bugando Medical Centre is a tertiary care and teaching hospital for the Catholic University of Health and Allied Sciences-Bugando (CUHAS-Bugando) and has 1000 beds.

Study population

The study included patients who were operated for sigmoid volvulus at Bugando Medical Centre during the period of study. However, patients aged 10 years and below are usually admitted in the paediatric surgical wards and therefore were excluded from the study. Preoperative diagnosis of sigmoid volvulus was made clinically, radiologically and confirmed at laparotomy. Preoperatively, all the patients recruited into the study were resuscitated with intravenous fluids to correct fluid and electrolyte imbalance; nasogastric suction; urethral catheterization and broad-spectrum antibiotic coverage. Relevant preoperative investigations included packed cell volume, serum electrolytes, urea and creatinine, blood grouping and cross-matching. Radiological investigations including plan abdomen X-ray supine and erect views were done in all patients. Barium enema and Abdominal computed tomography (CT) was done in selected patients. No patients had sigmoidoscopy or Magnetic Resonance Imaging (MRI) investigations due to lack of these facilities' at our centre.

After resuscitation all patients under general anaesthesia were subjected to exploratory laparotomy through midline incision. They had pre-operative anaesthetic assessment using the American Society of Anaesthetists (ASA) classification [22] as shown in Table 1. To minimize variability

Table 1 American Society of Anaesthetists (ASA) classification

ASA class	Description
I	Healthy individual with no systemic disease
II	Mild systemic disease not limiting activity
III	Severe systemic disease that limits activity but is not incapacitating
IV	Incapacitating systemic disease which is constantly life threatening
V	Moribund, not expected to survive 24 hours with or without operation

in our study, the assignation of ASA class was performed by a consultant anesthetist adhering strictly to criteria above. Adequate hydration was indicated by an hourly urine output of 30 ml/hour. The operations were performed either by a consultant surgeon or a senior resident under the direct supervision of a consultant surgeon.

Intraoperatively, manual untwisting relieved the obstruction, and the distended hypertrophied sigmoid colon was decompressed by a tube passed through its wall, surrounded by seromuscular purse string of 2/0 vicryl and attached to a suction machine. The contents of the sigmoid colon, primarily gas and liquid feces, were evacuated as much as possible. A nasogastric tube was routinely used in all the cases to decompress the small bowel. The redundant sigmoid colon became evident, and the line of resection was decided. The descending colon and proximal rectum were mobilized, their vascularity was ensured and a resection and two-layered anastomosis with vicryl 2/0 and outer layer of interrupted silk 2/0. If the sigmoid colon was gangrenous, it was resected without untwisting and a Hartmann's procedure or double barreled colostomy fashioned. The patients underwent 1) emergency or elective sigmoid colon resection and primary anastomosis when the sigmoid colon was viable; 2) sigmoid colon resection and Hartmann's procedure or double barreled colostomy, when the colon was gangrenous. The peritoneal cavity was lavaged with warm normal saline and the abdomen closed by massclosure technique. A digital rectal dilatation was carried out as soon as the patient began to recover from anesthesia, to enhance drainage of mucoid colonic contents. Perioperative intravenous antibiotics were given to all the patients in combination with ampicillin 500 mg, gentamicin 80 mg and metronidazole 500 mg. Intravenous ampicillin was given 6 hourly, while gentamicin and metronidazole were given twice or every 8 hours respectively for a period of 72 hours. These were given for a further 48 hours for those with gangrenous bowel. Skin sutures were removed between 7 and 10 days and patients advised on follow-up. Data on each patient were entered into a pro forma prepared for the study. The study variables included socio-demographic (i.e. age and sex,

education, area of residence and occupation), associated pre-morbid illness, duration of symptoms, clinical presentation, radiological findings, timing of surgical procedure, ASA classification, operative findings and surgical procedure performed. The variables studied in the postoperative period were postoperative complications, hospital stay and mortality. Patients were followed up till discharge or death and thereafter for a period of six- twelve months.

Statistical data analysis

Statistical data analysis was done using SPSS software version 17.0 (SPSS, Inc, Chicago, IL). Data was summarized in form of proportions and frequent tables for categorical variables and mode and median for continuous variables. P-values were computed for categorical variables using Chi-square ($\chi2$) test and Fisher's exact test depending on the size of the data set. Independent student t-test was used for continuous variables. Multivariate logistic regression analysis was used to determine predictor variables that are associated with outcome. A p-value of less than 0.05 was considered to constitute a statistically significant difference.

Ethical consideration

Ethical approval to conduct the study was obtained from the Catholic University of Health and Allied Sciences/Bugando Medical Centre joint institutional ethic review committee before the commencement of the study. Patients who met the inclusion criteria were requested to sign a written informed consent before being enrolled into the study.

Results

Socio-demographic data

During the period of study, a total of 1028 adult patients were admitted to the adult general surgical wards of Bugando Medical Centre and underwent laparotomy for bowel obstruction. Out of these, the underlying cause of obstruction was sigmoid volvulus in 158 patients. Of these, 12 patients were excluded from the study due failure to meet the inclusion criteria. Thus, 146 patients representing 14.2% of all bowel obstruction cases (i.e. 146 out of 1028 patients) were enrolled into the study. The range of patients at presentation ranged from 18 to 82 years with a median age of 48 years (interquartile range, 46 to 52 years). The median age for males (54 years) at presentation was higher than that of their female counterparts (42 years) and this was statistically significant (P = 0.012). The peak age incidence was in the age group 51-60 years. Out of 146 patients, 122 (83.6%) were males and 24(16.4%) were females with a male to female ratio of 5.1: 1. Most of patients, 140 (82.2%) had either primary or no formal education and more than 80% of them were unemployed. The majority of patients, 112(76.7%) came from the rural areas located a considerable distance from the study area and more than three quarter of them had no identifiable health insurance.

Clinical presentation among patients with sigmoid volvulus

Majority of patients, 136 (93.2%) presented with acute bowel obstruction and the remaining 10 (6.8%) patients presented with sub-acute/chronic bowel obstruction. The duration of symptoms ranged from 1 to 16 days with a median duration of 6 days. Twelve (8.2%) patients presented within twenty-four hours of onset of symptoms, 14 (9.6%) between 24 and 48 hours, 22 (15.1%) between 48 and 72 hours and 98 (67.1%) over 72 hours afterwards. Gross abdominal distention in 140 (95.9%) patients, colicky abdominal pain in 134 (91.8%), constipation in 98 (67.1%), vomiting in 88 (60.3%) and fever in 46 (31.5%) patients were the main symptoms; while dehydration in 68 (46.6%) patients, abdominal tenderness in 60 (41.1%) and visible peristalsis in 62 (42.5%) patients were the main signs. The classic triad of abdominal pain, abdominal distention and constipation was reported in 136 (93.2%) patients. Forty-two (28.8%) of the patients were in shock (with a diastolic blood pressure of less than 90 mmHg) on admission. Twenty-six (17.8%) patients had history suggestive of previous episodes of which eleven (42.3%) had previously been admitted in peripheral hospitals with acute sigmoid volvulus and been managed with laparotomy and derotation without resection. Concomitant medical illness such as respiratory diseases (12), cardiovascular diseases (10), diabetes mellitus (8) and renal diseases (5) was reported 35 (24%) patients.

Diagnosis of sigmoid volvulus

Preoperative diagnosis of sigmoid volvulus was made clinically, radiologically and confirmed at laparotomy. All patients in this study had plain abdominal x-ray films available for review and demonstrated the classical plain abdominal x-ray features of sigmoid volvulus (grossly distended and twisted sigmoid loop filling the abdomen, with multiple air fluid levels and the 'omega' or 'coffee bean' sign) in 112 (76.7%) patients. Barium enema was done in 12 (8.2%) patients who had no evidence of peritonitis, bowel gangrene, or perforation and demonstrated the obstructive lumen. Abdominal computed tomography (CT) was performed in only 4 (2.7%) patients and demonstrated a twisted and dilated sigmoid colon with whirled sigmoid mesentery, in addition to twisted and dilated small intestinal segments. None of our patients had sigmoidoscopy done due to lack of this facility at our centre.

Pre-operative anaesthetic assessment

All patients were assessed pre-operatively using the American Society of Anesthetists (ASA) pre-operative grading (Table 1). According to ASA classification, 32 (21.9%) patients had ASA class I, 79 (54.1%) had ASA class II, 24 (16.4%) had ASA class III, 10 (6.8%) had ASA class IV and 1 (0.7%) patients had ASA class V. A high ASA score was found to be an independent predictor of gangrenous bowel (P = 0.000).

Treatment modalities

All the 146 patients underwent laparotomy. The majority of them, 136 (93.2%) were operated on emergency basis and required immediate resuscitation and relief of the sigmoid obstruction, while 10 (6.8%) patients had an elective surgery. Out of the 146 patients studied, 24 (16.4%) had ileo-sigmoid volvulus. Amongst the patients who had emergency operations, 112 (76.7%) had acute sigmoid volvulus and 24 (16.4%) had ileo-sigmoid volvulus, whereas 10 (6.8%) patients who presented with subacute or chronic sigmoid volvulus were operated on elective basis. Table 2 shows distribution of patients according to operative findings. The majority of patients, 102(69.9%) were treated with resection and primary anastomosis, of which 63.0% were emergency cases. Colostomy was offered to 30.1% of cases who had gangrenous and perforated bowel. All the patients who presented with sub-acute obstruction/chronic were treated with primary resection and anastomosis (Table 3). None of our patients in this study had sigmoidoscopic derotation due to lack of this facility at our centre. Delayed presentation (≥24 hours) (P = 0.011) and a high ASA score (P = 0.000) were found to be independent predictors of gangrenous bowel.

Treatment outcome

A total of 30 (20.5%) patients developed postoperative complications, of which surgical site infection was the

Table 2 Distribution of patients according to operative findings

Operative findings	Frequency	Percentages
Sigmoid colon (sigmoid volvulus)	**122**	**83.6**
• Viable	102	69.9
• Gangrenous/perforation	20	13.7
Ileo –sigmoid portion (ileo-sigmoid knotting)	**24**	**16.4**
• Viable ileum	1	0.7
• Gangrenous ileum	5	3.4
• Gangrenous both ileum and sigmoid	18	12.3
Peritonitis*	2	1.4
Adhesions*	6	4.1

*Occurred as operative findings in patients with either gangrenous or perforated bowel.

Table 3 Distribution of patients according surgical procedure performed

Diagnosis	Surgical procedure offered		Total
	Resection and primary anastomosis	Colostomy	
Acute sigmoid volvulus	92 (63.0)	20 (13.7)	112 (76.7)
Ileo-sigmoid knotting	0	24 (16.4)	24 (16.4)
Sub-acute/chronic sigmoid volvulus	10 (6.9)	0	10 (6.9)
Total	102 (69.9)	44 (30.1)	146 (100)

most common type accounting for 43.3% (Table 4). Complication rate was significantly higher in emergency operations than in elective operations (32.5% versus 11.9%) (P = 0.014) and in patients with gangrenous bowel undergoing bowel resection (42.3% v/s 13.2%) (P = 0.002). All complications resolved on conservative treatment alone except in three patients who required re-operation for wound dehiscence (2) and intraabdominal abscess (1) respectively.

The length of hospital stay (LOS) ranged from 1 to 34 days with a median of 14 days ((interquartile range, 12 to 16 days).The LOS for non-survivors ranged from 1 day to 11 days (median 4 days). The length of hospital stay was significantly longer in patients with advanced age, concomitant medical illness and presence of complications (P < 0.001).

In this study, 25 (17.1%) patients died in the hospital. Amongst the patients treated with primary resection and anastomosis, 17 (16.7% i.e 17/102) died while 8 (18.2% i.e. 8/44) of those who had colostomy died. This difference was not significant in multivariate logistic regression analysis (P = 0.289). According to multivariate logistic regression analysis, advanced age (>60 years) (OR = 2.5, 95% CI (1.2- 4.8), P = 0.012), concomitant medical illness (OR = 3.2, 95%CI (2.3-5.3), P = 0.003), late presentation (≥24 hours) (OR = 5.4, 95% CI (2.8- 6.9), P = 0.015), presence of shock on admission (OR = 3.2, 95%CI (2.2-8.5), P = 0.001) and presence of gangrenous bowel (OR = 3.2, 95%CI (1.1- 6.8), P = 0.000) were significantly associated with mortality.

Table 4 Postoperative complications (N = 30)

Postoperative complications	Frequency	Percentage
Surgical site infection	13	43.3
Chest infection	4	13.3
Wound dehiscence	2	6.6
Prolonged paralytic ileus	2	6.6
Urinary tract infection	2	6.6
Enterocutaneous fistulae	1	3.3
Intraabdominal abscess	1	3.3

Follow up of patients

Out of the 121 survivors, ninety seven (80.2%) were discharged well, eighteen (14.8%) were discharged home with colostomies and the remaining six (5.0%) patients were discharged against medical advice. No patient among survivors in this study had permanent disabilities. A total of 11 patients had their colostomies closed at the end of study period and the remaining 7 colostomies were not yet closed. The time interval from colostomy creation to colostomy closure ranged from 1 month to 5 months with a median of 4 months (+IQR of 3 to 6 months). Of the 121 survivors, fifty-eight (47.9%) patients were available for follow up at six to twelve months after discharge and the remaining 63 (52.1%) patients were lost to follow up.

Discussion

Since it was first described by von Rokitansky in 1836 [1], sigmoid volvulus remains a major cause of colonic intestinal obstruction, which results from twisting of the sigmoid colon on its own mesentery [2]. Globally, sigmoid volvulus shows geographic variation being higher in developing countries than in developed world [2,4,7]. It accounts for 2% to 5% of colonic obstructions in Western countries and 20% to 50% of obstructions in Eastern Countries including Africa [4,7]. In this study, sigmoid volvulus accounted for 14.2% of all diagnosed intestinal obstruction seen during the study period in our setting. This concurs with figures of 14.1% that was reported by Jumbi and Kuremu [23] in Kenya. There is no satisfactory explanation for the geographical distribution. It has been suggested that high fiber diet may contribute to the high incidence in Africa where the high fiber results in heavy loading of the sigmoid colon [24,25]. In East Africa, sigmoid volvulus is the second most common cause of intestinal obstruction after adhesions [23].

Sigmoid volvulus has been reported to occur in all age groups, from neonates to elderly [25]. Most often this condition is observed in adults, but the age at which it is most common also varies geographically. In developing countries, a man aged between 40 and 60 years is usually reported, whereas in developed countries, the mean age is between 60 and 70 years [5,11]. As reported in other African studies [11,13,14,23], the median age of 48 years in this study was younger than the age described in most developed countries; about 10 years difference has been reported in these studies [14,23]. We could not establish the reason for this age differences.

The male predominance demonstrated in this study was in keeping with previous observations reported in studies performed elsewhere [11,13,14,19,23]. There is a marked over-all preponderance of male patients with sigmoid volvulus, with a reported ratio of 2.5-9.1 [21,26]. It is suggested that the more spacious female pelvic area allowed a greater possibility of spontaneous reduction of a beginning volvulus [27]. Another predisposing factor is the mesocolon, which is longer in men but wider in women [8]. Heavy loading is more likely to cause sigmoid volvulus in the presence of a longer mesentery.

In keeping with other studies performed in developing countries [14,23], the majority of patients in this series came from the rural areas located a considerable distance from the study area and more than eighty percent had either primary or no formal education. Most of these patients were unemployed and had no identifiable health insurance. This observation has an implication on accessibility to healthcare facilities and awareness of the disease.

Clinically, sigmoid volvulus may present acutely as an emergency or subacutely especially when it is with associated recurrent symptoms of constipation and distention. As reported by other authors in developing countries [13-15], more than ninety percent of patients in this study presented with acute bowel obstruction. In developing countries like ours where over 60% of the populace cannot afford hospital treatment, patients seek hospitalization only when they had developed irreversible intestinal obstruction [13-15]. This observation is reflected in our study where more than ninety percent of patients presented late with acute intestinal obstruction and bowel perforations. The higher incidence rate of delayed presentation in developing countries like Tanzania is best explained by the challenges in health-related transportations, ignorance, poverty and lack of medical awareness [13-15,23]. This delayed presentation increases morbidity and mortality many-folds, as is evident from our results. We could not establish the reasons for the late presentation in this study.

The clinical presentation of sigmoid volvulus in our patients is not different from those in other studies [3-5,11,14,23], with abdominal pain, constipation and abdominal distention being common to all the patients. In this study, the classic triad of abdominal pain, abdominal distention and constipation was reported in 93.2% of the patients.

The diagnosis of acute sigmoid volvulus is established by clinical and radiological findings. In the majority of patients, a thorough physical examination and abdominal radiographs are adequate to achieve the diagnosis. Typical symptoms include sudden abdominal pain and distension followed by constipation. The most common signs are abdominal tenderness and asymmetrical abdominal distention. Other findings include abnormal bowel sounds, abdominal tympany, a palpable abdominal mass, empty rectum, and dehydration [28]. Plain radiographs are diagnostic in 57%-90% of patients [29,30]. The classical sign of acute sigmoid volvulus is the coffee bean sign. Abdominal Computed Tomography (CT) usually reveals a dilated colon with an air/fluid level and the "whirl sign", which

represents twisted colon and mesentery [31]. The classical plain abdominal x-ray features of sigmoid volvulus in this study were demonstrated in more than three quarters of patients. Abdominal CT scan was performed in only 2.7% of cases due to its high cost and irregular availability of this facility at our centre.

Previous studies performed in developing countries showed that ileo-sigmoid knotting accounts for 15-17% of the cases of sigmoid volvulus [11,14,23]. This concurs with our study in which ileo-sigmoid knotting was reported in 16.4% of the patients.

The ileo-sigmoid knot is a rare but serious abdominal emergency in which the ileum and sigmoid entangle each other to form a knot, which may lead to vascular compromise and gangrene of both the ileum and sigmoid colon. The condition is serious, generally progressing rapidly to gangrene of both ileum and sigmoid colon. However, the accurate preoperative diagnosis of ileo-sigmoid knotting is difficult, particularly when abdominal CT is not used. The disease is generally misdiagnosed as an obstructive or non-obstructive emergency in the preoperative period and the correct diagnosis is made upon laparotomy or, in some cases, autopsy [14,19,32]. This observation is reflected in our study in which all patients with ileo-sigmoid knotting presented acutely and all except one were found to have gangrenous bowel. Therefore, awareness of the condition is essential, for prompt diagnosis and optimal management.

The treatment of sigmoid volvulus remains controversial, and depends on the selected procedure and the most appropriate therapeutic approach in terms of the clinical status of the patient, the location of the problem, the suspicion or presence of peritonitis, bowel viability and the experience of the surgical team [33].

Initial nonoperative management, that is, sigmoidoscopic decompression as advocated by Bruudsgaard [34], followed by semi-elective sigmoidectomy and primary anastomosis has been widely accepted as standard management [11,35]. The nonresectional procedures such as sigmoidopexy and mesosigmoidoplasty have no need for bowel preparation and have lower morbidity and mortality rates but have high incidence of recurrence [35]. Where the decompression fails and there are signs of colonic gangrene, sigmoid resection and Hartmann's procedure or double barreled colostomy is done to avoid the high mortality associated with primary anastomosis in this situation [35,36]. Recently laparoscopic resection has been used in high-risk or elderly patients who may not tolerate conventional surgery [36]. A more critical appraisal is however needed for its general use. The treatment of choice at this time is resection with primary anastomosis in patients with viable sigmoid colons and Hartmann's procedure in those with gangrenous bowel [37]. Recurrence of sigmoid volvulus among patients treated with nonoperative approach is a common happening which ought to influence the choice of procedure to be performed. Most of our patients are poor and cannot afford to come back for interval sigmoid colectomy once the volvulus is reduced at sigmoidoscopy. It is for this reason that there is a tendency to perform resection and primary anastomosis. Irrespective of the presentation the major determining factor for primary resection and anastomosis is the presence or absence of complication such as gangrene or perforation. Many authors now prefer one stage primary resection and anastomosis procedure and colostomy if there are complications [10,16,18]. Colostomy is often advised in cases where the gut is gangrenous [13-16]. In the present study, the majority of patients (69.9%) were treated with resection and primary anastomosis, of which 63.0% were emergency cases. Colostomy was offered to 30.1% of cases who had gangrenous and perforated bowel. This treatment modality agrees with what was demonstrated by Okello et al [14] in Uganda. In this study, we found no significant difference between cases treated by primary anastomosis (one-stage resection) and those treated by two-staged resection (colostomy).This finding was consistent with that reported by Akcan et al [16] and Okello et al [14], that there is often no significant statistical difference whether a patient is treated with primary resection anastomosis or colostomy in terms of morbidity, complications and mortality. However, we found no prospective randomized studies done to compare the outcome in primary anastomosis and two-stage resections. Our study has confirmed that, in the hands of competent and experienced surgeons, resection and primary anastomosis in sigmoid volvulus patients with viable bowel, is safe and does not necessarily result in increased risk or a longer hospital stay. When the bowel is gangrenous, it is safer to resect and leave a temporary colostomy. In cases of ileo-sigmoid knotting, the secret behind a successful outcome lies in early diagnosis and prompt and appropriate treatment.

The presence of complications has an impact on the final outcome of patients presenting with bowel obstruction due to sigmoid volvulus. In keeping with other studies [11,14,23], surgical site infection was the most common postoperative complications in the present study. In our series, the complication rate was significantly higher in emergency operations than in elective operation and in patients with gangrenous bowel undergoing bowel resection.

The median duration of hospital stay in our study was 12 days, which is higher than that reported in other studies [14,23]. The length of hospital stay was significantly longer in patients with advanced age, concomitant medical illness and presence of complications. However, due to the poor socio-economic conditions in Tanzania, the duration of inpatient stay for our patients may be longer than expected.

Overall, the mortality of sigmoid volvulus in our setting was 17.1%, a figure that is slightly higher than 15.9% and 15.8% reported by Okello et al [14] and Oren et al [18]. Many other authors have reported mortality rates within the same range [10,11,23]. The high mortality rate in our study may be attributed to advanced age, presence of concomitant medical illness, late presentation (≥24 hours), presence of shock on admission and presence of gangrenous bowels. Addressing these factors responsible for high mortality in our patients is mandatory to be able to reduce mortality associated with this disease.

A total of 80.2% of our patients recovered well and were discharged. This figure is comparable with 84.1% reported by Okello et al [14] in Uganda. However, in this study the follow-up of patients was generally poor as more than half of patients (survivors) were lost to follow-up by the end of study period. Self discharge by patient against medical advice is a recognized problem in our setting. Similarly, poor follow up visits after discharge from hospitals remain a cause for concern. These issues are often the results of poverty, long distance from the hospitals and ignorance. Delayed presentation, discharge against medical advice and the large number of loss to follow up were the major limitations in this study. The fact that this study included only patients who were evaluated and treated at a single institution, findings from this study may not reflect the whole population in this region. Also, the prevalent of HIV infection (which was not assessed) in our setting is still high and this might have contributed to high mortality among our patients. However, despite this limitation, the study has provided local data that can help healthcare providers in the management of patients with sigmoid volvulus. The challenges identified in the management of sigmoid volvulus in our setting need to be addressed in order to deliver optimal care for these patients.

Conclusion

Sigmoid volvulus remains the commonest cause of colonic bowel obstruction at Bugando Medical Centre and contributes significantly to high morbidity and mortality. Most of the patients presented acutely, requiring immediate resuscitation and surgical approach. It is suggested that in viable bowel, sigmoid resection and primary anastomosis is feasible as it may not adversely affect outcome. Temporary colostomy should be considered if the bowel is gangrenous or perforated. Early diagnosis and timely definitive treatment are essential in order to decrease the morbidity and mortality associated with this disease.

Competing interests
The authors declare that they have no competing interests.

Authors' contributions

PLC participated in study design, literature search, data analysis, manuscript writing and editing. In addition PLC submitted the manuscript. JBM participated in data analysis, manuscript writing & editing. Both authors read and approved the final manuscript.

Acknowledgement

The authors are grateful to all who participated in the preparation of this manuscript. Special thanks go to our research assistants for their support during data collection and in the management of our patients.

References

1. Avots-Avotins KV, Waugh DE. Colon volvulus and the geriatric patient. Surg Clin North Am. 1982;62:248–60.

2. Katsikogiannis N, Machairiotis N, Zarogoulidis P, Sarika E, Stylianaki A, Zisoglou M, et al. Management of sigmoid volvulus avoiding sigmoid resection. Case Rep Gastroenterol. 2012;6:293–9.

3. Raveenthiran V. Observations on the pattern of vomiting and morbidity in patients with acute sigmoid volvulus. J Postgrad Med. 2004;50:27–9.

4. Lal SK, Morgenstern R, Vinjirayer EP, Matin A. Sigmoid volvulus an update. Gastrointest Endosc Clin N Am. 2006;16(1):175–87.

5. Onder A, Kapan M, Arikanoglu Z, Palanci Y, Gumus M, Aliosmanoglu I, et al. Sigmoid colon torsion: mortality and relevant risk factors. Eur Rev Med Pharmacol Sci. 2013;1:127–32.

6. Akinkuotu A, Samuel JC, Msiska N, Mvula C, Charles AG. The role of the anatomy of the sigmoid colon in developing sigmoid volvulus: a case-control study. Clin Anat. 2011;24:634–7.

7. Raveenthiran R, Madiba TE, Atamanalp SS, De U. Volvulus of the sigmoid colon. Colorectal Dis. 2010;12:1–17.

8. Bhatnagar BN, Sharma CL, Gupta SN, Mathur MM, Reddy DCS. Study on the anatomical dimensions of the human sigmoid colon. Clin Anat. 2004;17:236–43.

9. Madiba TE, MR H a, Sikhosana MH. Radiological anatomy of the sigmoid colon. Surg Radiol Anat. 2008;30:409–15.

10. Atamanalp SS, Yildirgan MI, Basoglu M, Kantarci M, Yilmaz I. Sigmoid colon volvulus in children: review of 19 cases. Pediatr Surg Int. 2004;20:492–5.

11. Sule AZ, Ajibade A. Adult large bowel obstruction: a review of clinical experience. Ann Afr Med. 2011;10:45–50.

12. Khan M, Ullah S, Jan MAU, Naseer A, Ahmed S, Rehman A. Primary anastomosis in the management of acute sigmoid volvulus with out colonic lavage. J Postgrad Med Inst. 2007;21:305–8.

13. Kotisso B, Bekele A. A three-year comprehensive retrospective analysis of Ilio-sigmoid knotting in Addis Ababa. Ethiop Med. 2006;44:377–83.

14. Okello TR, Ogwang DM, Kisa P, Komagum P. Sigmoid volvulus and ileosigmoid knotting at St. Mary's Hospital Lacor in Gulu, Uganda. East Cent Afr J Surg. 2009;14:58–64.

15. Sule AZ, Misauna M, Opaluwa AS, Ojo E, Obekpa PO. One stage procedure in the management of acute sigmoid volvulus without colonic lavage. Surgeon. 2007;5(5):268–70.

16. Akcan A, Akyildiz H, Artis T, Yilmaz N, Sozuer E. Feasibility of single-stage resection and primary anastomosis in patients with acute noncomplicated sigmoid volvulus. Am J Surg. 2007;193:421–6.

17. Atamanalp SS, Ören D, Aydınlı B, Öztürk G, Polat KY, Başoğlu M. Elective treatment of detorsioned sigmoid volvulus. Turk J Med Sci. 2008;38:227–34.

18. Oren D, Atamanalp SS, Aydinli B, Yildirgan MI, Başoğlu M, Polat KY. An algorithm for the management of sigmoid colon volvulus and the safety of primary resection: experience with 827 cases. Dis Colon Rectum. 2007;50:489–97.

19. Atamanalp SS. Sigmoid volvulus. EAJM. 2010;42:142–7.

20. Roseano M, Guarino G, Culviello A. Sigmoid volvulus: diagnostic and therapeutic features (considerations on 10 cases). Ann Ital Chir. 2001;72:79–84.

21. Bhuiyan MM, Machowski ZA, Linyama BS, Madiba MC. Management of sigmoid volvulus in Polokwane-Mankweng Hospital. Afr J Surg. 2005;43:17–9.

22. Wolters U, Wolf T, Stutzer H, Schroder T. ASA classification and perioperative variables as predictors of postoperative outcome. Br J Anaesth. 1996;77:217–22.

23. Jumbi G, Kuremu RT. Emergency resection of sigmoid volvulus. East Afr Med J. 2008;85:398–405.

24. Berry AR. Oxford Textbook of surgery. In: Volvulus of colon. 2nd ed. 2000. p. 1515–9.

25. Lou Z, Yu ED, Zhang W, Meng RG, Hao LQ, Fu CG. Appropriate treatment of acute sigmoid volvulus in the emergency setting. World J Gastroenterol. 2013;19:4979–83.

26. Khanna AK, Kumar P, Khanna R. Sigmoid volvulus: study from a north Indian hospital. Dis Colon Rectum. 1999;42:1081–4.

27. Bac B, Aldemir M, Tacyildiz I, Keles C. Predicting factors for mortality in sigmoid volvulus. Dicle Med J. 2004;31:9–15.

28. Atamanalp SS, Ozturk G. Sigmoid volvulus in the elderly: outcomes of a 43-year, 453-patient experience. Surg Today. 2011;41:514–9.

29. Osiro SB, Cunningham D, Shoja MM, Tubbs RS, Gielecki J, Loukas M. The twisted colon: a review of sigmoid volvulus. Am Surg. 2012;78:271–9.

30. Burrell HC, Baker DM, Wardrop P, Evans AJ. Significant plain film findings in sigmoid volvulus. Clin Radiol. 1994;49:317–9.

31. Hirao K, Kikawada M, Hanyu H, Iwamoto T. Sigmoid volvulus showing "a whirl sign" on CT. Intern Med. 2006;45:331–2.

32. Atamanalp SS, Oren D, Basoglu M, Yildirgan MI, Balik AA, Polat KY, et al. Ileosigmoidal knotting: outcome in 63 patients. Dis Colon Rectum. 2004;47:906–10.

33. Mulas C, Bruna M, García-Armengol J, Roig JV. Management of colonic volvulus. Experience in 75 patients. Rev Esp Enferm Dig. 2010;102:239–48.

34. Bruusgaard C. Volvulus of the sigmoid colon and its treatment. Surgery. 1947;22:466–78.

35. Nuhu A, Jah A. Acute sigmoid volvulus in a West African population. Ann Afr Med. 2010;9:86–90.

36. Liang JT, Lai HS, Lee PH. Elective laparoscopically assisted sigmoidectomy for the sigmoid volvulus. Surg Endosc. 2006;20:1772–3.

37. Madiba TE, Thomson SR. The management of sigmoid volvulus. J R Coll Surg Edinb. 2000;45:74–80.

12

Review of 58 patients with necrotizing fasciitis in the Netherlands

Sander F. L. van Stigt[1*], Janneke de Vries[2], Jilles B. Bijker[3], Roland M. H. G. Mollen[4], Edo J. Hekma[5], Susan M. Lemson[6] and Edward C. T. H. Tan[1]

Abstract

Background: Necrotizing fasciitis is a rare, life threatening soft tissue infection, primarily involving the fascia and subcutaneous tissue. In a large cohort of patients presenting with Necrotizing fasciitis in the Netherlands we analysed all available data to determine the causative pathogens and describe clinical management and outcome.

Methods: We conducted a retrospective, multicentre cohort study of patients with a necrotizing fasciitis between January 2003 and December 2013 in an university medical hospital and three teaching hospitals in the Netherlands. We only included patients who stayed at the Intensive Care Unit for at least one day.

Results: Fifty-eight patients were included. The mortality rate among those patients was 29.3 %. The central part of the body was affected in 28 patients (48.3 %) and in 21 patients (36.2 %) one of the extremities. Most common comorbidity was cardio vascular diseases in 39.7 %. Thirty-nine patients (67.2 %) were operated within 24 h after presentation. We found a type 1 necrotizing fasciitis in 35 patients (60.3 %) and a type 2 in 23 patients (39.7 %).

Conclusions: Our study, which is the largest study in Europe, reaffirmed that Necrotizing fasciitis is a life threatening disease with a high mortality. Early diagnosis and adequate treatment are necessary to improve the clinical outcome. Clinical awareness off necrotizing fasciitis remains pivotal.

Keywords: Necrotizing fasciitis, Outcome, Soft tissue infections, LRINEC score, The Netherlands, ICU

Background

Necrotizing fasciitis (NF) is a part of the Necrotizing Soft Tissue Infections. It's a rare, life threatening soft tissue infection, primarily involving the fascia and subcutaneous tissue. Although the symptoms were already described in the fifth century BC by Hippocrates [1, 2], even in modern medicine it still has a high mortality rate ranging from 6 to 76 % [1, 3–6]. The term necrotizing fasciitis was introduced by Wilson in 1952 [1, 7].

The rapidly progressive infection can affect any part of the body. The portal of entry usually is a minor injury of the affected site or a surgical wound. However, no definitive cause can be found in 20–50 % [8–10].

Medical conditions associated with necrotizing fasciitis are diabetes mellitus (31–44 %), obesity (28 %), smoking (27 %), alcoholabusus (17 %), cirrhosis (8–15 %),

malignancy (3 %), corticosteroid therapy (3 %) and chronic renal failure (3 %) [11, 12].

The incidence of NF is low with 0.4 cases per 100.000 in the United Kingdom [13].

Clinical symptoms consist of local symptoms like erythema, swelling, changes in skin colouring, intense pain, bullae and sometimes subcutaneous emphysema and general symptoms such as fever, nausea, vomiting and malaise [2, 8, 11].

Necrotizing fasciitis can be classified in four clinical forms, depending on the causative organisms [2]. In Type 1 at least one anaerobic species is isolated with one or more facultative anaerobic streptococci (other than group A) and members of the Enterobacteriaceae (e.g., *E.coli, Enterobacter, Klebsiella, Proteus*) [14]. Type 2 is generally monomicrobial and caused by hemolytic streptococcus group A, sometimes with co-infection of *Staphylococcus aureus*. Most articles show type 1 is more common, with a relative incidence up to 75 % [8, 9]. Some studies also describe type 3, caused by the marine *Vibrio spp*. The portal

* Correspondence: Sander.vanStigt@radboudumc.nl
[1]Department of Surgery, Traumasurgery Radboud University Medical Center, Geert Grooteplein-Zuid 10, 6525 GA Nijmegen, The Netherlands
Full list of author information is available at the end of the article

of entry for this type 3 NF is a puncture wound caused by fish or marine insects and is rarely observed in Europe [11]. Type 4 describes fungal cases of candida NF, which are very rare [2, 15].

The diagnosis of NF should be considered in patients with clinical symptoms as mentioned above, but can be very difficult. To clarify the diagnosis, Wong et all described the "Laboratory Risk Indicator for Necrotizing Fasciitis" (LRINEC) score, which is based on routinely performed laboratory tests [6] (Table 1). They found a score ≥6 had a positive predictive value of 92 % and a negative predictive value of 96 %. However, this test has not been validated in larger, prospective studies. Therefore, surgical exploration remains the gold standard to definitively establish the diagnosis of necrotizing fasciitis [8, 16]. Aggressive surgical debridement (<24 h) is associated with a lower mortality [17, 18].

Appropriate treatment of a patient with NF can only be achieved through close cooperation between the surgeon, intensivist and microbiologist.

The aim of our study was to analyse all available data of a large cohort of patients presenting with NF in four teaching hospitals in the Netherlands. Also, we determined the causative pathogens in our population, described clinical management and clinical outcome in this Dutch cohort and compared that with previous other studies.

Methods
Study design
The study was designed as a retrospective cohort study.

Table 1 The Laboratory Risk Indicator for Necrotizing Fasciitis (LRINEC score)

		Score
C-reactive protein (mg/l)	<150	0
	≥150	4
Leucocyte count (10⁹/l)	<15	0
	15–25	1
	>25	2
Haemoglobine (mmol/l)	>8.4	0
	6.8–8.4	1
	<6.8	2
Sodium (mmol/l)	≥135	0
	<135	2
Creatinine (μmol/l)	≤141	0
	>141	2
Glucose (mmol/l)	≤10	0
	>10	1
Total		13

Patients
All consecutive adult patients who were diagnosed with NF were eligible for inclusion at the Radboud University Medical Center Nijmegen (Radboudumc) (a 900 beds university hospital), the Gelderse Vallei Hospital Ede (GVH) (a 500 beds hospital), Rijnstate Hospital Arnhem (RH) (a 950 beds hospital) and Slingeland Hospital Doetinchem (SH) (a 340 beds hospital) between January 2003 and December 2013. These hospitals are located in the Central-Eastern part of the Netherlands, belonging to one surgical training region.

For inclusion, patients had to stay at the intensive care unit for at least one day. Patients were found by hospital data system, diagnostic codes and microbiological results.

Data collection
Diagnosis of necrotizing fasciitis was proven by histopathologic examination of tissue samples or surgical findings when no tissue sample was analyzed. This means the presence of an affected fascia, which was documented in the procedure note as a necrotizing fasciitis, was diagnostic. Vital parameters (e.g., temperature, blood pressure, heart rate), clinical symptoms of the affected body part and laboratory results at presentation, as well as all demographic data were collected from the patient charts. Results of blood and wound cultures, the number of surgical interventions, operative findings, length of stay at the intensive care unit (ICU), total duration of hospitalization and the mortality rate were documented. For all patients the LRINEC score was calculated from the laboratory findings.

We considered Type 2 FN as caused by a monoculture of hemolytic streptococcus group A (*Streptococcus pyogenes*), or in rare cases caused by *Staphylococcus aureus* or hemolytic streptococcus group C or G.

And in contrast Type 1 FN was seen as caused by different combinations of anaerobic bacteria, aerobic gram negative rods from the Enterobacteriaceae group and streptococci other than *Streptococcus pyogenes*.

Results
Initial assessment
A total of 58 patients were included (19 Radboudumc; 15 GVH, 16 RH, 8 SH). Thirty-four patients were male (58.6 %) and 24 were female (41.4 %). The median age was 62 years (range 21–81 years).

Localisation of the fasciitis was in the central part of the body in 28 patients (48.3 %) and in one of the extremities in 21 patients (36.2 %). In 8 patients (13.8 %) there was a combination of central part of the body with one of the extremities. In one patient the head was the affected.

The most common comorbidity was cardiovascular diseases (39.7 %). Other co-morbidities included were obesity

(25.9 %), diabetes mellitus (24.1 %) and malignancy (19.0 %). Thirteen patients (22.4 %) had no comorbidities.

Etiology of the necrotizing fasciitis was a minimal trauma in 16 patients (27.6 %) (median 4 days, range 1–30). Fourteen patients had undergone an operation a few days before they developed necrotizing fasciitis (median 3.3 days, range 1–60). Seven of them had undergone a sterile operation (e.g., inguinal hernia repair or lumpectomie), the other seven patients a contaminated operation (e.g., appendicitis or bowel resection) (Table 2). In 28 patients (48.3 %) there was no portal of entry or no known cause for the NF.

Nineteen patients (32.8 %) had a fever at time of presentation with a body temperature of >38.5 °C. Signs and symptoms at admission were swelling (54 cases, 93.1 %), erythema (52 cases, 89.7 %), tachycardia (33 cases, 57.9 %) and blisters (14 cases, 24.1 %). Other symptoms like crepitation or loss of sensibility were rare. Figure 1a shows a swelling and erythema matching a necrotizing fasciitis.

Forty-six patients had a LRINEC score ≥ 6 (79.3 %), 33 patients had a score ≥ 8 (56.9 %) and 8 patients had a score ≥ 10 (13.8 %). The mean LRINEC score was 7.4.

Microbiology

All 58 patients had positive cultures. We found a type 1 necrotizing fasciitis in 35 patients (60.3 %) and a type 2 in 23 patients (39.7 %). In 9 out of 35 patients (25.7 %) with a type 1 NF, we isolated a monoculture, mostly *E. coli*. In the other 26 patients (74.3 %), a total of 61 (mixed) pathogens were isolated (Table 3).

Treatment and follow up

All patients underwent one or more operations. Thirty-nine patients (67.2 %) were operated within 24 h and 16 patients (27.6 %) underwent their first operation after 24 h. In 3 patients the exact time of operation was not clear.

Forty-nine patients (84.5 %) underwent radical necrotectomy. In 6 cases (10.3 %) an amputation was necessary. In 3 patients the NF was so extensive, that because of poor prognosis, radical necrotectomy was not conducted.

The mean number of debridement procedures of the patients who survived was 2.8 (range 1–8). In 26 patients

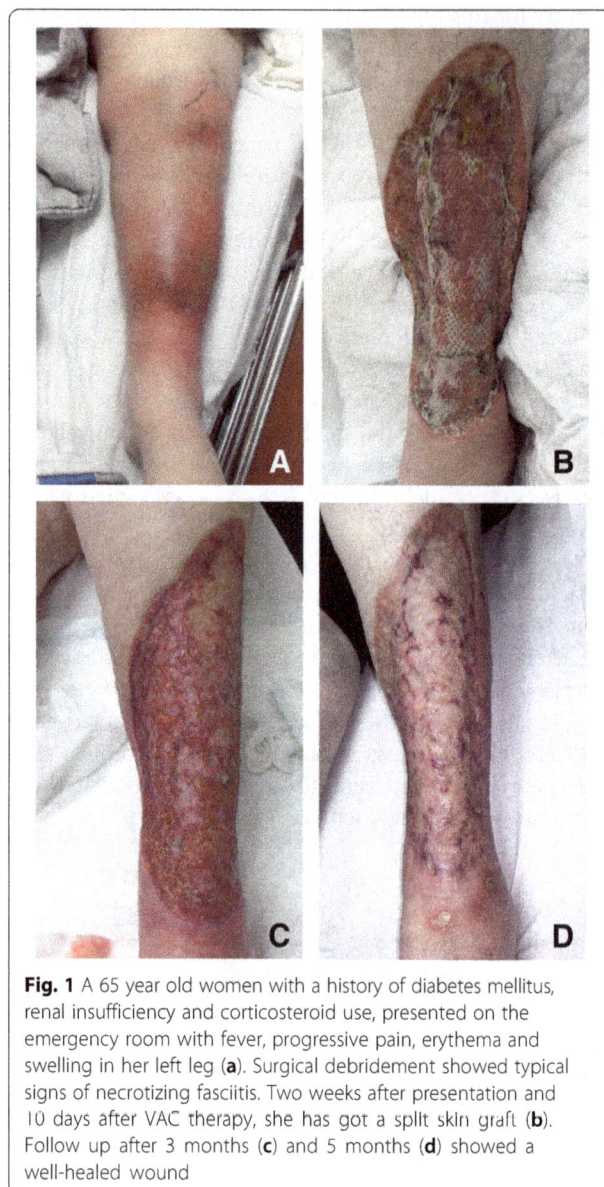

Fig. 1 A 65 year old women with a history of diabetes mellitus, renal insufficiency and corticosteroid use, presented on the emergency room with fever, progressive pain, erythema and swelling in her left leg (**a**). Surgical debridement showed typical signs of necrotizing fasciitis. Two weeks after presentation and 10 days after VAC therapy, she has got a split skin graft (**b**). Follow up after 3 months (**c**) and 5 months (**d**) showed a well-healed wound

Table 2 Operations prior to necrotizing fasciitis

Sterile	Number	Contaminated	Number
Inguinal hernia repair	2	Bowel resection	4
Renal transplantation	1	Hemorrhoidectomy	2
Laparoscopic cholecystectomy	1	Appendectomy	1
Adnex extirpation	1		
Lumpectomie	1		
Vasectomy	1		
Total	7		7

(44.8 %) we used vacuum assisted closure therapy, which in 12 patients was followed by definitive reconstruction by split skin grafts (Fig. 1b-d). Other patients received split skin grafts without VAC® (Vacuüm Assisted Closure) therapy, primary wound closure or reconstruction by the plastic surgeon.

The mortality was 17 out of 58 patients (29.3 %). The median age of the patients who died was 64 years (range 38–72 years). The median age of the survivors was 59 years (range 21–81 years). Nine patients died within 2 days because of multi organ failure or cessation of treatment due to poor prognosis. Two patients died in the first week after admission. Six patients died several weeks or months (range 15–73 days) after admission because of a new septic period, cardiac failure or general weakness.

Table 3 Cultures in necrotizing fasciitis type I, $n = 35$ patients

Micro organism	Monoculture	Present in mixed culture	Total
Escherichia coli	6	13	19
Klebsiella pneumoniae	1		1
Proteus mirabilis		3	3
Citrobacter freundii		1	1
Enterobacter cloacae		2	2
Serratia marcescens		1	1
Pseudomonas aeruginosa	1	1	2
Acinetobacter baumannii		1	1
Stenotrophomonas maltophilia		1	1
Aeromonas sobria		1	1
Bacillus species		1	1
Haemolytic streptococci, not group A		3	3
Enterococcus species		4	4
Streptococcus pneumoniae		1	1
Viridans streptococci		3	3
S.milleri group		6	6
Clostridium perfringens		2	2
Anaerobe gram negative rods, mainly B.fragilis	1	5	6
Anaerobic mixed culture		5	5
Mixed culture		7	7
Total cultures	9 (13 %)	61 (87 %)	70 (100 %)
Total patients	9 (26 %)	26 (74 %)	35 (100 %)

From 38 patients histological examinations were taken. In two cases an autopsy was performed. All patients showed typical signs of NF.

The mean duration of hospitalization of the patients who survived was 46 days (range 11–166). The mean stay on the intensive care unit was 11 days (range 1–42).

Discussion

Necrotizing fasciitis is a part of the Necrotizing Soft Tissue Infections (NSTI) and is a rare life threatening disease that still has a high mortality and morbidity. We included 58 patients with necrotizing fasciitis in four different hospitals. To our knowledge, this study is the first Dutch study and involves one of the largest European cohorts. Previous large studies have been conducted in Asia and Australia [5–7, 19, 20]. Because we exclusively wanted to include patients with the fulminant form of necrotizing fasciitis, patients with NF admitted for at least one day in the intensive care unit, were included.

Patients with a subacute fasciitis [21] or a doubtful diagnosis were excluded from our study.

Many patients presented with classical symptoms like erythema, swelling and tachycardia, had abnormal blood results and had a clear minimal trauma or a surgical wound as the portal of entry. Despite the classical presentation, up to 30 % was not operated on within 24 h after admission. This is consistent with the literature, which shows even higher numbers of delay of surgical treatment up to 40 % [7, 20]. Also, Goh et all describes 71.4 % misdiagnosis of NF as cellulitis or abscess in their systematic review [12]. This illustrates the diagnostic dilemma that is present in a large number of patients.

The LRINEC score can be a useful tool to help diagnose NF [6]. In the initial study, a score of 6 or above was shown to have a positive predictive value of 92 % and a negative predictive value of 96 % [6]. However, no prognostic studies for validating this score, and the cut-off value of ≥6, are available [22]. Twenty-one percent of our patients had a LRINEC score below 6. However, this was a selected group in which the diagnostic process had already been completed. The LRINEC score was used retrospectively and therefore did not aid in the diagnosis. If we want to use the LRINEC score in this way, an adequate validation is necessary.

The most common risk factor for NF in the literature is diabetes mellitus [5, 7, 11, 12, 23, 24], however, there are major differences between studies (Bucca at all 21 %, Wong at all 70.8 %) [6, 25]. In our study only 24.1 % of the patients had diabetes. The most common comorbidity we found was cardiovascular diseases in almost 40 % of the patients. Over 50 % of them had a serious cardiac event like infarction or arrhythmia. The other patients only had hypertension. The number of patients with no comorbidities (22.4 %) is comparable to other studies [5, 19].

Many of the larger studies on NF are published in South East Asia or Australia. These countries live in close relation to marine life. In addition to type 1 and type 2 NF, type 3 was described regularly. We had no patients in our study with NF type 3. Huang described 11.9 % wound cultures with *Vibrio spp*, it was the most common pathogen leading to bacteraemia (29.5 %) in their population [7]. This difference in pathogens may also have influenced the course of the disease and outcome of patients with NF. In our study we found 60.3 % of patients with type 1 NF and 39.7 % with type 2 NF. This is similar to other studies [3, 8, 9]. Studies with higher numbers of type 2 NF describe up to 63.3 % type 2. These studies used other criteria to distinguish between type 1 and 2, classifying all monomicrobial infections as type 2 [7, 24, 26].

The treatment of patients with NF is challenging and consists of adequate surgical debridement, supportive care by the intensivist and starting broad spectrum antimicrobials [25, 27]. The choice of antibiotics depends on the suspected causative microorganism(s), part of the body that is affected and clinical picture. Antibiotic therapy can be narrowed down as culture results are known. The most important factor is early surgical aggressive debridement, which is associated with a lower mortality when performed within 24 h [17, 18].

Mortality in our study population was 29 %, which is slightly higher than in other reports of patients with NF [5, 7, 10, 19, 20, 24, 25, 28]. This can be explained by the different inclusion criteria and possible different microorganism(s). Due to the inclusion criteria of at least 1 day ICU-stay we possibly included a more seriously ill population compared to other reports.

Recent years have shown an increase in the use of the vacuum assisted therapy [29]. We used the VAC® therapy in nearly half of our patients with good results.

Our study was limited by the retrospective character. Another limitation is, because of the rarity of NF, patients of four different hospitals are included. Different routines in the hospitals, although they belong to the same training regions, and the relative long period of inclusion can explain some missing data.

Conclusions

We present the first Dutch and the largest European study of patients with necrotizing fasciitis. Our study reaffirmed that NF is a life threatening disease with a high mortality. Early diagnosis and adequate treatment are necessary to improve the clinical outcome. Clinical awareness of necrotizing fasciitis remains pivotal.

Our recommendations for further research are a prospective study to validate the LRINEC score and to explore the correlation between the score and clinical outcome.

Abbreviations
GVH, Gelderse Vallei Hospital Ede; ICU, Intensive Care Unit; LRINEC, Laboratory Risk Indicator for Necrotizing Fasciitis; NF, Necrotizing Fasciitis (NF); NSTI, Necrotizing Soft Tissue Infections; Radboudumc, Radboud University Medical Center Nijmegen; RH, Rijnstate Hospital Arnhem; SH, Slingeland Hospital Doetinchem; VAC®, Vacuüm Assisted Closure.

Acknowledgements
No acknowledgements.

Funding
No fundings to declare.

Authors' contributions
SvS, performed the study, collected all data with help of the local surgeons, analysed the data and wrote the manuscript. JdV, microbiological support and supervision, critically revising the manuscript. JB, design of the manuscript, interpretation of data. RM, collected data GVH, critically revising the manuscript. EH, collected data RH, critically revising the manuscript. SL, collected data SH, critically revising the manuscript. ET, conceived the study, collected data RUMC, revising the manuscript critically, supervisor. All authors read and approved the final manuscript.

Competing interest
The authors declare that they have no competing interests.

Author details
[1]Department of Surgery, Traumasurgery Radboud University Medical Center, Geert Grooteplein-Zuid 10, 6525 GA Nijmegen, The Netherlands. [2]Department of Medical Microbiology, Radboud University Medical Center, Geert Grooteplein-Zuid 10, 6525 GA Nijmegen, The Netherlands. [3]Department of Anesthesiology, Gelderse Vallei Hospital, Willy Brandtlaan 10, 6716 RP Ede, The Netherlands. [4]Department of Surgery, Gelderse Vallei Hospital, Willy Brandtlaan 10, 6716 RP Ede, The Netherlands. [5]Department of Surgery, Rijnstate Hospital, Wagnerlaan 55, 6815 AD Arnhem, The Netherlands. [6]Department of Surgery, Slingeland Hospital, Kruisbergseweg 25, 7009 BL Doetinchem, The Netherlands.

References
1. Wong CH, Wang YS. The diagnosis of necrotizing fasciitis. Curr Opin Infect Dis. 2005;18:101–6.
2. Morgan MS. Diagnosis and management of necrotizing fasciitis: a multiparametric approach. J Hosp Infect. 2010;75:249–57.
3. McHenry CR, Piotrowski JJ, Petrinic D, Malangoni MA. Determinants of mortality for necrotising soft tissue infections. Ann Surg. 1995;221:558–65.
4. Tilkorn DJ, Citak M, Fehmer T, Ring A, Hauser J, Al Benna S, et al. Characteristics and differences in necrotizing fasciitis and gas forming myonecrosis: a series of 36 patients. Scand J Surg. 2012;101(1):51–5.
5. Su Y-C, Chen H-W, Hong Y-C, Chen C-Y, Hsiao C-T, Chen I-C. Laboratory risk indicator for necrotizing fasciitis score and the outcomes. ANZ J Surg. 2008;78:968–72.
6. Wong CH, Khin LW, Heng KS, Tan KC, Low CO. The LRINEC (Laboratory Risk Indicator for Necrotizing Fasciitis) score: a tool for distinguishing necrotizing fasciitis from other soft tissue infections. Crit Care Med. 2004;32(7):1535–41.
7. Huang K-F, Hung M-H, Lin Y-S, Lu C-L, Lui C, Chen C-C, Lee Y-H. Independent predictors of mortality for necrotizing fasciitis: a retrospective analysis in a single institution. J Trauma. 2011;71:467–73.
8. Sarani B, Strong M, Pascual J, Schwab CW. Necrotizing fasciitis: current concepts and review of the literature. J Am Coll Surg. 2009;208:279–88.
9. Wong CH, Chang HC, Pasupathy S, Khin LW, Tan JL, Low CO. Necrotizing fasciitis: clinical presentation, microbiology, and determinants of mortality. J Bone Joint Surg Am. 2003;85-A(8):1454–60.
10. Vayvada H, Demirdover C, Menderes A, Karaca C. Necrotising fasciitis in the central part of the body: diagnosis, management and review of the literature. Int Wound J. 2013;10(4):466–72.
11. Angoules AG, Kontakis G, Drakoulakis E, Vrentzos G, Granick MS, Giannoudis PV. Necrotising fasciitis of upper and lower limb: a systematic review. Injury. 2007;38(5):S19–26.
12. Goh T, Goh LG, Ang CH, Wong CH. Early diagnosis of necrotizing fasciitis. Br J Surg. 2014;101(1):119–25.
13. Ellis Simonsen SM, van Orman ER, Hatch BE, Jones SS, Gren LH, Hegmann KT, et al. Cellulitis incidence in a defined population. Epidemiol Infect. 2006;134:293–9.
14. Mandell GL, Bennett JE, Dolin R. Principles and practice of infectious diseases. 7th ed. Philadelphia: Churchill Livingstone; 2010. p. 1307–8. Part II.
15. Davoudian P, Flint NJ. Necrotizing fasciitis. Contin Educ Anaesth Crit Care Pain. 2012;12(5):245–50.
16. Stevens DL, Baddour LM, Sexton DJ, Edwards MS, Baron EL. Necrotizing soft tissue infections. Available online at: http://www.uptodate.com. Accessed 11 Dec 2014.
17. Cheung JP, Fung B, Tang WM, Ip WY. A review of necrotising fasciitis in the extremities. Hong Kong Med J. 2009;15(1):44–52.
18. Bilton BD, Zibari GB, McMillan RW, Aultman DF, Dunn G, McDonald JC. Aggressive surgical management of necrotizing fasciitis serves to decrease mortality: a retrospective study. Am Surg. 1998;64:397–400.
19. Das DK, Baker MG, Venugopal K. Risk factors, microbiological findings and outcomes of necrotizing fasciitis in New Zealand: a retrospective chart review. BMC Infect Dis. 2012;12:348.
20. Nisbet M, Ansell G, Lang S, Taylor S, Dzendrowskyj P, Holland D. Necrotizing fasciitis: review of 82 cases in South Auckland. Intern Med J. 2011;41(7):543–8.

21. Wong CH, Wang SW. What is a subacute necrotizing fasciitis?: A proposed clinical diagnostic criteria. J Infect. 2006;52(6):415–9.

22. Holland MJ. Application of the Laboratory Risk Indicator in Necrotizing Fasciitis (LRINEC) score to patients in a tropical tertiary referral centre. Anaesth Intensive Care. 2009;37:588–92.

23. Elliott DC, Kufera JA, Meyers RA. Necrotizing soft tissue infections. Risk factors for mortality and strategies for management. Ann Surg. 1996;244: 672–83.

24. Kalaivani V, Hiremath BV, Indumathi V. Necrotising soft tissue infection-risk factors for mortality. J Clin Diagn Res. 2013;7(8):1662–5.

25. Bucca K, Spencer R, Orford N, Cattigan C, Athan E, McDonald A. Early diagnosis and treatment of necrotizing fasciitis can improve survival: an observational intensive care unit cohort study. ANZ J Surg. 2013;83(5):365–70.

26. Ryssel H, Germann G, Kloeters O, Radu CA, Reichenberger M. Necrotizing fasciitis of the extremities: 34 cases at a single centre over the past 5 years. Arch Orthop Trauma Surg. 2010;130:1515–22.

27. Ustin JS, Malangoni MA. Necrotizing soft-tissue infections. Crit Care Med. 2011;39:2156–62.

28. Arifi HM, Duci SB, Zatriqi VK, Ahmeti HR, Ismajli VH, Gashi MM, et al. A retrospective study of 22 patients with necrotising fasciitis treated at the University Clinical Center of Kosovo (2005–2010). Int Wound J. 2013;10(4):461–5.

29. Misiakos EP, Bagias G, Patapis P, Sotiropoulos D, Kanavidis P, Machairas A. Current concepts in the management of necrotizing fasciitis. Front Surg. 2014;1:36.

13

Prediction of neurosurgical intervention after mild traumatic brain injury using the national trauma data bank

Timothy E. Sweeney[1*], Arghavan Salles[1], Odette A. Harris[2], David A. Spain[1] and Kristan L. Staudenmayer[1*]

Abstract

Introduction: Patients with mild traumatic brain injury (TBI) as defined by an admission Glasgow Coma Score (GCS) of 14–15 often do not require neurosurgical interventions, but which patients will go on to require neurosurgical care has been difficult to predict. We hypothesized that injury patterns would be associated with need for eventual neurosurgical intervention in mild TBI.

Methods: The National Trauma Databank (2007–2012) was queried for patients with blunt injury and a diagnosis of TBI with an emergency department GCS of 14–15. Patients were stratified by age and injury type. Multiple logistic regression for neurosurgical intervention was run with patient demographics, physiologic variables, and injury diagnoses as dependent variables.

Results: The study included 50,496 patients, with an overall 8.8 % rate of neurosurgical intervention. Neurosurgical intervention rates varied markedly according to injury type, and were only correlated with age for patients with epidural and subdural hemorrhage. In multiple logistic regression, TBI diagnoses were predictive of need for neurosurgical interventions; moreover, after controlling for injury type and severity score, age was not significantly associated with requiring neurosurgical intervention.

Conclusions: We found that in mild TBI, injury pattern is associated with eventual need for neurosurgical intervention. Patients with cerebral contusion or subarachnoid hemorrhage are much less likely to require neurosurgical intervention, and the effects of age are not significant after controlling for other patient factors. Prospective studies should validate this finding so that treatment guidelines can be updated to better allocate ICU resources.

Keywords: Traumatic brain injury, National trauma data bank, Neurosurgery

Background

Traumatic brain injury (TBI) accounts for >1.3 million Emergency Department (ED) visits and >750,000 hospitalizations each year [1]. A large number of TBI patients present with a Glasgow Coma Score (GCS) of 14–15 and do not ultimately require an intervention for their injuries. Which patients ultimately require intervention has been difficult to predict, and there are no clear consensus guidelines for treatment of this patient subset (in contrast to the extensive guidelines for severe TBI [2]).

For instance, the American College of Emergency Physicians' Mild TBI policy from 2008 offers recommendations on discharging patients without intracranial hemorrhage, but patients with GCS 14–15 and positive CT findings are not discussed [3]. Many hospital guidelines currently suggest that all patients with intracranial hemorrhage of any severity be observed in the intensive care unit (ICU) due to risk of decompensation and possible need for intervention. However, these recommendations are not evidence-based [4]. The lack of clear consensus for treatment of mild TBI leads to a wide variability in clinical practice, with initial ICU admission rates ranging from 50–97 % for patients with a GCS of 15 and traumatic intracranial hemorrhage [5].

* Correspondence: tes17@stanford.edu; kristans@stanford.edu
[1]Department of Surgery, Stanford University Medical Center, 300 Pasteur Drive, Stanford, CA 94305, USA
Full list of author information is available at the end of the article

Several prior studies have been published examining what factors contribute to decompensation in patients with mild TBI [5–9]. Factors that are typically part of the resulting models include older age, high-volume intracranial hemorrhage and/or midline shift, anticoagulant therapy, and worsening injury. However, these studies have mostly been from single-center or regional databases and thus may not be generalizable.

We hypothesized that injury type would be associated with deterioration for patients who present with isolated mild TBI. To explore this, we evaluated the need for a neurosurgical procedure in patients who presented with isolated mild TBI using the National Trauma Data Bank.

Methods

We used the National Trauma Data Bank (NTDB) from 2007 to 2012. The year 2012 is the most recent year for which data are available. Patients were included if they were adults (> = 18 years of age) with an International Classification of Diseases, Ninth Revision, Clinical Modification (ICD-9-CM) diagnosis of intracranial injury (851.0–854.9), were admitted to the hospital, and had an ED total GCS of 14–15. Skull fracture diagnoses (800–801.9, 803–804.9) were not included as the ICD-9-CM diagnosis codes do not distinguish which type of intracranial lesion is present. Also, open fractures present an indication for operative intervention making determination of intracranial injury progression difficult. Patients were also excluded if they had sustained a penetrating mechanism of injury or if they had an abbreviated injury scale (AIS) severity score of >1 in any body region other than the head. Patients with missing data on ED vital signs were excluded.

Head injuries were binned into six categories by ICD-9-CM code: isolated cerebral laceration or contusion (851.0–851.9), isolated subarachnoid hemorrhage (852.0–852.1), isolated subdural hemorrhage (852.2-852.3), isolated epidural hematoma (852.4–852.5), and unspecified (853–854.9). Patients with more than one of the above types of TBI were categorized only as 'multiple TBI injuries.'

Whether a neurosurgical intervention was performed was also determined. Neurosurgical intervention was defined as having either an operative neurosurgical procedure or placement of a neuromonitoring device (e.g., Camino bolt or endoventricular drainage catheter). Surgeries and placement of catheters were identified using ICD-9-CM procedure codes of 01–02.

Injury severity score (ISS) calculated from the AIS severity codes was evaluated in this model. ISS is calculated as the sum of the square of the top three AIS severity scores (by body region). Since here we only included patients whose non-head AIS severity scores were < =1, the maximum ISS any patient can receive is the square of the AIS head severity score plus two. We thus discretized ISS from

0–6, 7–11, 12–18, 19–27, and >27, with the assumption that increasing ISS is solely due to worsening severity of head injury.

In the NTDB, coagulopathy is defined as any condition that places the patient at risk for bleeding in which there is a problem with the body's blood clotting process (e.g., vitamin K deficiency, hemophilia, thrombocytopenia, chronic anticoagulation therapy with Coumadin, Plavix, or similar medications.) This does not include patients on chronic aspirin therapy. More granular information about exact anticoagulant drugs, dosages, etc., are not available. The presence of coagulopathy was thus coded as a binary variable.

Multiple logistic regression was used to predict the need for neurosurgical intervention. Dependent variables included in the analysis were age; presence of coagulopathy; ED vital signs; injury severity score (ISS) coded as described above; head injury type (coded in a binary form according to the categories defined above). The same model was also run as a mixed-effects model with different hospital facilities as the random-effects variable to control for center effect.

All statistical analyses were carried out in the R language for statistical computing version 3.0.1. Comparisons between two cases were done with two-sided Student's t-tests. Significance levels were set at $P < 0.01$ unless otherwise stated.

Results

The NTDB 2007–2012 dataset contained 1.3 million cases of traumatic brain injury. After applying inclusion and exclusion criteria, there were a total of 50,496 patients (Table 1). Isolated subdural hemorrhages (SDH) were the most common injury pattern (N = 18,784, 37 %), and subarachnoid hemorrhages were the second most common isolated injury (N = 13,191, 26 %) (Table 1). Most patients were treated at a Level I or II trauma center (N = 34,961, 69.2 %), and the majority of patients were admitted directly to the intensive care unit (N = 29,043, 58 %). The overall rate of neurosurgical intervention was 8.8 %.

Patients who underwent neurosurgical intervention were overall older (mean 65 vs 60 years, $P < 0.0001$), had higher ISS (mean 19.7 vs 13.1, $P < 0.0001$), and had a slightly lower ED GCS (14.7 vs. 14.8, $P < 0.0001$) compared to those who did not. Isolated epidural hemorrhages were most frequently associated with neurosurgical procedures (18 %), followed by isolated subdural hemorrhages (16 %) and multiple injury types (8 %) (Fig. 1). Isolated subarachnoid hemorrhages and contusions were infrequently associated with need for neurosurgical procedures (1.5 and 2.5 %, respectively).

We found that patients with SDH who underwent neurosurgical procedures were older than those who did not (70.2 vs 65.7 years, $P < 0.0001$), whereas patients with

Table 1 Patient demographics, injury patterns, and disposition. For discrete variables, percentages are calculated by dividing by total patients (not by the number of patients with the given variable)

	All patients		No neurosurgical intervention		Neurosurgical intervention	
	N or mean	% or SD	N or mean	% or SD	N or mean	% or SD
Total Included Patients	50,496	100 %	46,022	91.2 %	4,474	8.8 %
Demographics						
Male gender (N, %)	30386	60.2	27407	59.6	2979	66.6
Age (years) (mean, SD)	60.6	20.5	60.2	20.7	65.2***	18.3
Physiology						
ED GCS (mean, SD)	14.8	0.4	14.8	0.4	14.7***	0.4
ED SBP (mean, SD)	144.4	26.4	144.1	26.4	147.6***	26.6
ED Pulse (mean, SD)	85.3	18	85.6	18	81.7***	18
ED RR (mean, SD)	18.1	3.7	18.2	3.8	17.9***	3.4
Injury Characteristics						
ISS at discharge (mean, SD)	13.7	6.5	13.1	6.1	19.7***	6.7
Traumatic Brain Injury Patterns						
Isolated Contusion (N, %)	5636	11.2 %	5497	11.9 %	139	3.1 %
Isolated SAH (N, %)	13191	26.1 %	12994	28.2 %	197	4.4 %
Isolated SDH (N, %)	18784	37.2 %	15807	34.3 %	2977	66.5 %
Isolated EH (N, %)	901	1.8 %	742	1.6 %	159	3.6 %
Multiple Injury Types (N, %)	11984	23.7 %	10982	23.9 %	1002	22.4 %
Comorbidities						
Total comorbidities (mean, SD)	0.9	1.1	0.9	1.1	0.9	1.2
Presence of Coagulopathy (N, %)	2340	4.6 %	2061	4.5 %	279	6.2 %
ACS Trauma Center Level						
NA/ Unverified (N, %)	14713	29.1 %	13214	28.7 %	1499	33.5 %
Level IV (N, %)	20	0 %	19	0 %	1	0 %
Level III (N, %)	802	1.6 %	730	1.6 %	72	1.6 %
Level II (N, %)	13200	26.1 %	12110	26.3 %	1090	24.4 %
Level I (N, %)	21761	43.1 %	19949	43.3 %	1812	40.5 %
ED Disposition						
Observation unit (N, %)	827	1.6 %	818	1.8 %	9	0.2 %
Floor bed (N, %)	13329	26.4 %	12756	27.7 %	573	12.8 %
Telemetry/step-down unit (N, %)	5292	10.5 %	5122	11.1 %	170	3.8 %
Intensive Care Unit (ICU) (N, %)	29043	57.5 %	26580	57.8 %	2463	55.1 %
Operating Room (N, %)	2005	4 %	746	1.6 %	1259	28.1 %
Outcomes						
LOS (mean days, SD)	5.4	6.5	4.8	5.5	11.2***	11.2
Expired during Admission (N, %)	1594	3.2 %	1141	2.5 %	453	10.1 %

N Number, *SD* Standard Deviation, *ISS* Injury Severity Score, *ED* Emergency Department, *GCS* Glasgow Coma Score, *SBP* Systolic Blood Pressure, *RR* Respiratory Rate, *SAH* Subarachnoid Hemorrhage, *SDH* Subdural Hemorrhage, *ED* Epidural Hemorrhage, *LOS* Length of Stay

*** $P < 0.0001$; Student's *t*-test for differences of continuous measures between "No Neurosurgical Intervention" and "Neurosurgical Intervention" groups

EDH who underwent neurosurgical procedures were younger (37 vs 48 years, $P < 0.0001$) (Table 2). Age was not a significant factor for the other injury types. On breaking out interventions by age group, there was a positive correlation with age and neurosurgical intervention rates for the SDH cohort, but a negative correlation for the EDH cohort (Fig. 2).

The dataset was next randomly split into a 2/3 training set and a 1/3 test set. A multiple logistic regression model for predicting neurosurgical intervention was created from

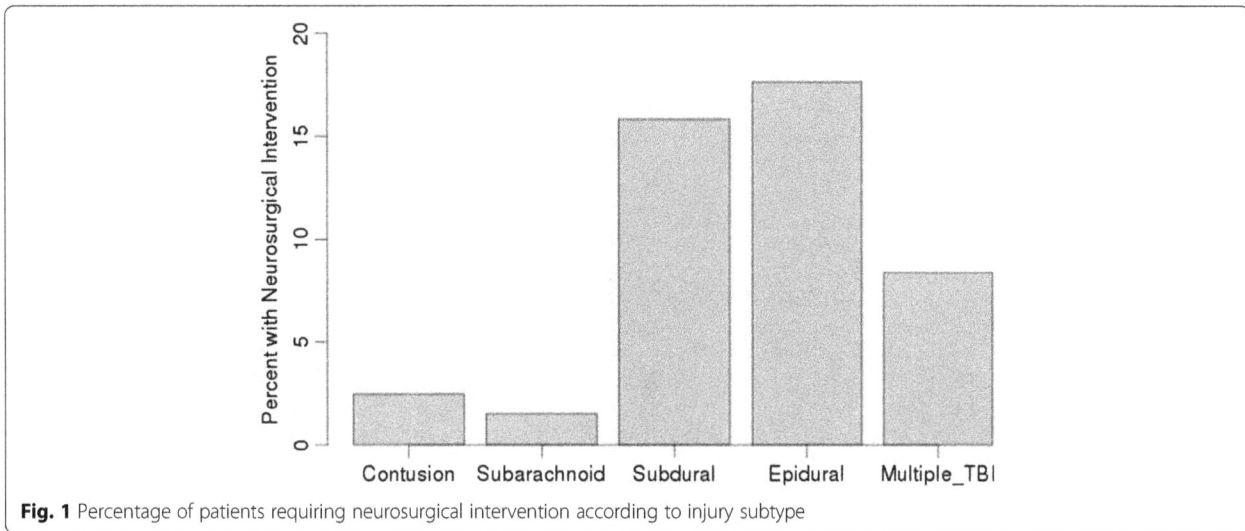

Fig. 1 Percentage of patients requiring neurosurgical intervention according to injury subtype

the training set (N = 33,327) (Table 3). After adjusting for injury severity, age, coagulopathy, and ED vital signs, injury pattern was strongly associated with need for neurosurgical intervention. Age was not significantly associated with need for neurosurgical intervention. The odds ratio for need for neurosurgical intervention for patients with an EDH vs. contusion was 6.4 (95 % CI 4.1–9.9). When applied to the held-out test set (N = 17,169), this model had good performance with an area under the receiver operator characteristics (ROC) curve for prediction of neurosurgery of 0.81 (Fig. 3a). It also showed excellent calibration (Hosmer-Lemeshow P = 0.8) (Fig. 3b). Interestingly, the calibration plot shows that our model's highest-risk decile has a modest expected (and observed) rate of neurosurgery of 38 %; the model is more effective at identifying very low-risk patients (lowest decile expected 0.5 % rate of neurosurgery). A mixed-effects model for which facility was used as a random effect was also performed; it showed no qualitative change in coefficients or significance (results not shown).

Table 2 Age and neurosurgical intervention for different injury patterns

Age (years)	No neurosurgical intervention	Neurosurgical intervention	P-value
	Mean ± SD	Mean ± SD	
Isolated Contusion	51.4 ± 21.8	48.5 ± 19.0	0.08
Isolated SAH	58.7 ± 20.1	56.1 ± 19.4	0.07
Isolated SDH	65.7 ± 19.1	70.2 ± 14.7	<0.0001
Isolated EH	48.0 ± 22.3	37.0 ± 17.2	<0.0001
Multiple Injury Types	59.4 ± 20.7	59.0 ± 20.0	0.56

P-values from Student's t-test for differences of continuous measures between "No Neurosurgical Intervention" and "Neurosurgical Intervention" groups
SD Standard Deviation, SAH Subarachnoid Hemorrhage, SDH Subdural Hemorrhage, ED Epidural Hemorrhage

Discussion

Traumatic brain injuries are an increasing source of emergency department visits and morbidity in the United States [10]. Mild traumatic brain injuries (those with a presentation GCS 14–15) with associated intracranial hemorrhage often present a clinical challenge, as acute decompensation in this cohort is rare but serious. As it has not been possible to predict which mild injuries will progress, many centers have policies of admitting all mild head injuries to a critical care or stepdown setting. This likely is beneficial for the small sub-group of patients who progress, but is associated with high costs and resource utilization.

Here we show that injury pattern may be important in determining which patients are at higher risk for ultimately requiring a neurosurgical intervention. Injury pattern is strongly associated with need for future neurosurgical procedures. In general, patients with SDH represent the largest number of interventions, and in this group older age is correlated with greater requirement for neurosurgical intervention. Previous reports have found that age is independently associated with higher associated rates of decompensation [7–9, 11], but this did not bear out when controlling for both injury type and physiologic variables. The finding that age is associated with need for intervention is likely due to the fact that patients with SDH are older, and there tend to be more of them than the other injury patterns (Table 2). These findings are consistent with the classic teaching of risk for SDH in elderly patients due age-related reductions in intracranial mass resulting in strain on bridging veins.

Epidural hemorrhages were far more infrequent (~2 %) than subdural hemorrhages but had the highest rates of neurosurgical intervention (21 %). Of those with epidural hemorrhages, younger patients had the highest rates of need for intervention. These findings are not particularly surprising given the fact that epidural hemorrhages often

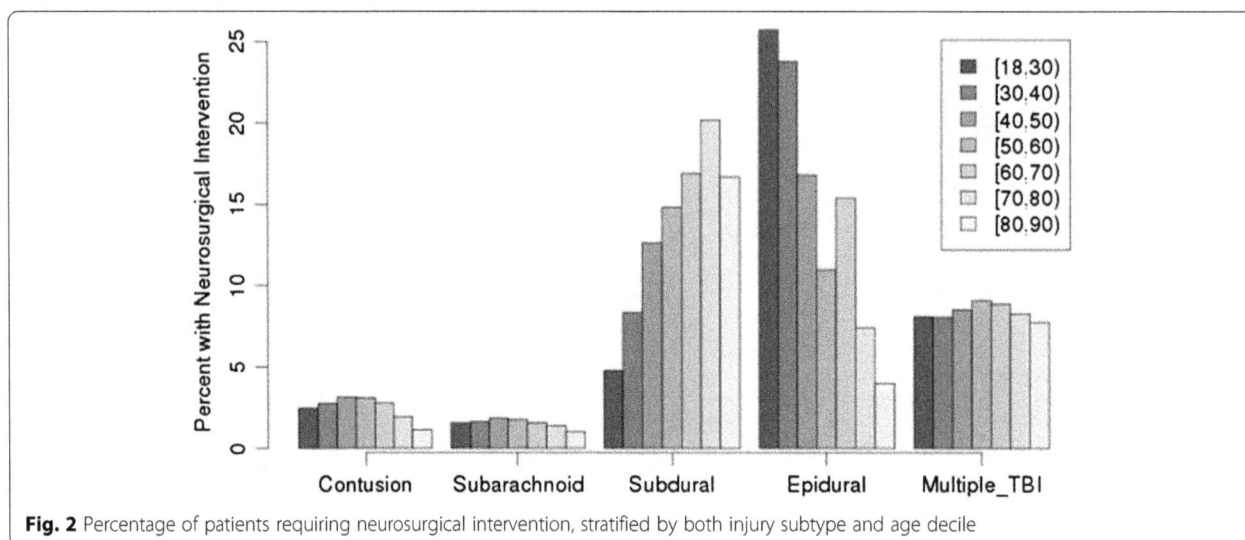

Fig. 2 Percentage of patients requiring neurosurgical intervention, stratified by both injury subtype and age decile

represent arterial bleeding and therefore have a higher risk of mass effect. The presence of multiple TBI patterns was also associated with higher rate of intervention. It may be that in these cases, higher force of impact resulted in multiple types of injuries and therefore these patients should be carefully monitored for worsening of their condition.

In contrast to SDH, SAH and contusions were much less often associated with the need for neurosurgical intervention. This is consistent with anecdotal reports of small

Table 3 Adjusted odds ratios for neurosurgical procedures. Multiple logistic regression run on 2/3 training set (n = 33,327)

	Odds ratio	(95 % CI)	P-value
(Intercept)	0.0893	(0.0099 – 0.78)	0.03
Age (years)	1.002	(0.999 – 1.01)	0.18
Anticoagulation Disorder	0.853	(0.66 – 1.09)	0.21
ED GCS	0.894	(0.781 – 1.03)	0.11
ED Systolic Blood Pressure	1.004	(1.002 – 1.01)	<0.001
ED Pulse	0.99	(0.986 – 0.993)	<0.0001
ED Respiratory Rate	0.962	(0.944 – 0.98)	<0.0001
ISS Category (vs. ISS 0–6)			
ISS 7-11	2.35	(1.44 – 4.09)	<0.01
ISS 12-18	3.37	(2.06 – 5.86)	<0.0001
ISS 19-27	18.9	(11.6 – 33)	<0.0001
ISS >27	7.01	(3.79 – 13.4)	<0.0001
Injury Category (vs. Contusion)			
Isolated SAH	0.95	(0.64 – 1.41)	0.79
Isolated SDH	4.9	(3.61 – 6.84)	<0.0001
Isolated EDH	6.42	(4.15 – 9.97)	<0.0001
Multiple Injury Types	2.34	(1.7 – 3.29)	<0.0001

CI Confidence Interval, *ISS* Injury Severity Score, *SD* Standard Deviation, *SAH* Subarachnoid Hemorrhage, *SDH* Subdural Hemorrhage, *ED* Epidural Hemorrhage

injuries with normal GCS not requiring advanced care. That said, while a 1–2 % rate of neurosurgical intervention may seem small, it still represents hundreds of patients who ultimately required advanced care. Patients with SAH and contusion were only part of the broader cohort with a very low predicted need for neurosurgical intervention. Further prospective studies will need to determine whether there are other characteristics or early signs that can predict which low-risk TBI patients with a GCS of 14–15 will deteriorate. If our findings are tested prospectively and characteristics that predict deterioration are validated, patients without these types of injuries may represent candidates for a non-monitored setting. This would have a large impact on resources and costs as together these injuries comprise 36 % of the TBI population in trauma centers in the United States.

The findings from this study are consistent with previous reports. There is evidence from single-center studies that type of head injury (e.g., subdural hemorrhage vs. epidural hematoma vs. contusion) might be associated with progression of injury [6, 12]. However, these are both single-center studies with small numbers. Other studies have tried to make prediction models of outcomes after minor head trauma [6, 7, 9, 13–17]. In particular, Nishijima et al. found that a rule with four parameters (abnormal mental status (GCS < 15), non-isolated head injury, age > 65 years, and swelling/shift on CT) was 98 % sensitive and 50 % specific for predicting need for any "critical care intervention." [11] However, the study included patients who had injuries other than TBI and the definition for "critical care intervention" included need for blood transfusion and central line placement. This does not help to answer the question of whether we can predict whether a mild isolated TBI will decompensate. In contrast, in our study we chose to evaluate isolated head

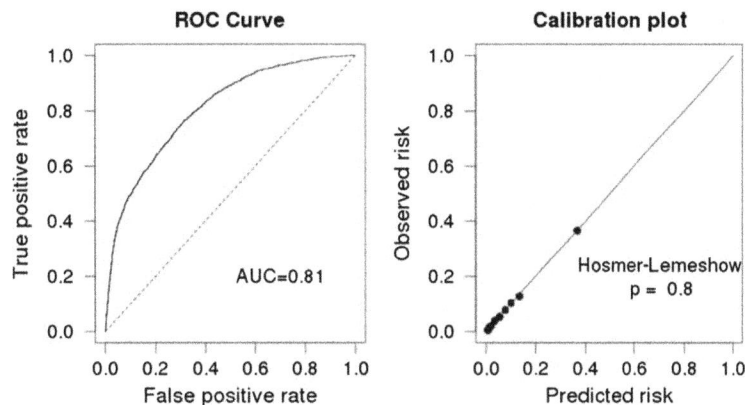

Fig. 3 Performance evaluation of the multiple logistic regression model on a held-out test set (n = 17,169). **a**. Receiver Operating Characteristic curve for the test set, area under the curve (AUC) = 0.81. **b**. Calibration plot; Hosmer-Lemeshow P = 0.8

trauma in order to prevent confounding that results from how non-TBI injuries may impact the course of a head injury.

Another factor thought to be associated with worsening of head injuries is pre-existing coagulopathy. In our multiple logistic regression model for predicting need for neurosurgical intervention, preexisting coagulopathy was not found to be a significant factor. This may be due to the fact that this variable may not be reliably recorded in trauma registries. Previous studies published from smaller, more granular trauma registries have shown that coagulopathy does predict decompensation [7, 8, 18].

This study has several limitations. First, this is a retrospective registry study that is subject to selection bias. In addition, we excluded all samples missing required data which relies on a missing-at-random assumption. Second, the NTDB does not capture neuro-critical care such as hyperosmolar therapy and hourly neurologic checks. Third, the NTDB does not capture information about the volume of intracranial hemorrhage, which may prove to be predictive. Finally, we did not model what happens in patients who sustain multi-system injury.

Despite these limitations, this study is the first to show an association between injury pattern and need for neurosurgical intervention in a national database. Overall, this study shows that in isolated blunt mild traumatic brain injury, SDH and EDH are associated with the highest rates of need for neurosurgical intervention, and that contusions and SAH are associated with low risks. Older age is associated with increasing rates of neurosurgical intervention after isolated SDH but is not a general predictor of need for neurosurgery in all types of injury. The accuracy of the model at predicting which patients are very unlikely to proceed to neurosurgical intervention suggests that these patients may not require higher levels of care (such as mandatory admission to an intensive care unit), albeit with a caveat that a 1-2 % rate of neurosurgical

intervention is not negligible. Improved prediction of the need for intervention can allow us to better match resource with patient need, saving lives and improving allocation of resources. Further prospective studies of outcomes after mild TBI should include injury type as a predictor so that these issues can be further elucidated.

Competing interests
OAH is a paid consultant for Emmanuel Law Corporation. The other authors have no disclosures.

Authors' contributions
Study conception and design: TES, AS, DAS, KLS. Data collection: TES, KLS. Data analysis and interpretation: TES, KLS, AS, OAH. Wrote manuscript: TES, KLS. Critical revision: TES, AS, OAH, DAS, KLS. All authors read and approved the final manuscript.

Acknowledgements
TES was supported by NLM training grant 2T15LM007033 and the Stanford Department of Surgery. We would like to thank Jay Bhattacharya and Eran BenDavid for helpful comments, and Lakshika Tennakoon for data preparation. The NTDB remains the full and exclusive copyrighted property of the American College of Surgeons. The American College of Surgeons is not responsible for any claims arising from works based on the original Data, Text, Tables, or Figures.

Author details
[1]Department of Surgery, Stanford University Medical Center, 300 Pasteur Drive, Stanford, CA 94305, USA. [2]Department of Neurosurgery, Stanford University Medical Center, 300 Pasteur Drive, Stanford, CA 94305, USA.

References
1. Coronado VG, Xu L, Basavaraju SV, McGuire LC, Wald MM, Faul MD, et al. Surveillance for traumatic brain injury-related deaths–United States, 1997–2007 MMWR. Surveill Summ. 2011;60:1–32.
2. Foundation BT, Surgeons AAoN, Surgeons CoN. Guidelines for the management of severe traumatic brain injury. J Neurotrauma 2007;24 Suppl 1:S1–106.
3. Jagoda AS, Bazarian JJ, Bruns JJ, Cantrill SV, Gean AD, Howard PK, et al. Clinical policy: neuroimaging and decisionmaking in adult mild traumatic brain injury in the acute setting. Ann Emerg Med. 2008;52:714–48.
4. Peloso PM, Carroll LJ, Cassidy JD, Borg J, von Holst H, Holm L, et al. Critical evaluation of the existing guidelines on mild traumatic brain injury. J Rehabil Med. 2004;43:106–12.

5. Nishijima DK, Haukoos JS, Newgard CD, Staudenmayer K, White N, Slattery D, et al. Variability of ICU use in adult patients with minor traumatic intracranial hemorrhage. Ann Emerg Med. 2013;61:509–17. e504.

6. Bee TK, Magnotti LJ, Croce MA, Maish GO, Minard G, Schroeppel TJ, et al. Necessity of repeat head CT and ICU monitoring in patients with minimal brain injury. J Trauma. 2009;66:1015–8.

7. Washington CW, Grubb RL. Are routine repeat imaging and intensive care unit admission necessary in mild traumatic brain injury? J Neurosurg. 2012;116:549–57.

8. Ratcliff JJ, Adeoye O, Lindsell CJ, Hart KW, Pancioli A, McMullan JT, et al. ED disposition of the Glasgow Coma Scale 13 to 15 traumatic brain injury patient: analysis of the Transforming Research and Clinical Knowledge in TBI study. Am J Emerg Med. 2014;32:844–50.

9. Nishijima DK, Sena M, Galante JM, Shahlaie K, London J, Melnikow J, et al. Derivation of a clinical decision instrument to identify adult patients with mild traumatic intracranial hemorrhage at low risk for requiring ICU admission. Ann Emerg Med. 2014;63(4):448–56.

10. Faul MXL, Wald MM, Coronado VG. Traumatic brain injury in the United States: emergency department visits, hospitalizations, and deaths. Atlanta (GA): Centers for Disease Control and Prevention, National Center for Injury Prevention and Control; 2010.

11. Nishijima DK, Shahlaie K, Echeverri A, Holmes JF. A clinical decision rule to predict adult patients with traumatic intracranial haemorrhage who do not require intensive care unit admission. Injury. 2012;43:1827–32.

12. Tong WS, Zheng P, Xu JF, Guo YJ, Zeng JS, Yang WJ, et al. Early CT signs of progressive hemorrhagic injury following acute traumatic brain injury. Neuroradiology. 2011;53:305–9.

13. Hukkelhoven CW, Steyerberg EW, Habbema JD, Maas AI. Admission of patients with severe and moderate traumatic brain injury to specialized ICU facilities: a search for triage criteria. Intensive Care Med. 2005;31:799–806.

14. Kuppermann N, Holmes JF, Dayan PS, Hoyle JD, Atabaki SM, Holubkov R, et al. Identification of children at very low risk of clinically-important brain injuries after head trauma: a prospective cohort study. Lancet. 2009;374:1160–70.

15. Steyerberg EW, Mushkudiani N, Perel P, Butcher I, Lu J, McHugh GS, et al. Predicting outcome after traumatic brain injury: development and international validation of prognostic scores based on admission characteristics. PLoS Med. 2008;5:e165. discussion e165.

16. Nishijima DK, Sena MJ. Holmes JF Identification of low-risk patients with traumatic brain injury and intracranial hemorrhage who do not need intensive care unit admission. J Trauma. 2011;70:E101–7.

17. Seddighi AS, Motiei-Langroudi R, Sadeghian H, Moudi M, Zali A, Asheghi E, et al. Factors predicting early deterioration in mild brain trauma: a prospective study. Brain Inj. 2013;27:1666–70.

18. Nishijima DK, Offerman SR, Ballard DW, Vinson DR, Chettipally UK, Rauchwerger AS, et al. Immediate and delayed traumatic intracranial hemorrhage in patients with head trauma and preinjury warfarin or clopidogrel use. Ann Emerg Med. 2012;59:460–8. e461-467.

14

A practical scoring system to predict mortality in patients with perforated peptic ulcer

Ebru Menekse[1*], Belma Kocer[2], Ramazan Topcu[3], Aydemir Olmez[4], Mesut Tez[1] and Cuneyt Kayaalp[5]

Abstract

Introduction: The mortality rate of perforated peptic ulcer is still high particularly for aged patients and all the existing scoring systems to predict mortality are complicated or based on history taking which is not always reliable for elderly patients. This study's aim was to develop an easy and applicable scoring system to predict mortality based on hospital admission data.

Methods: Total 227 patients operated for perforated peptic ulcer in two centers were included. All data that may be potential predictors with respect to hospital mortality were retrospectively analyzed.

Results: The mortality and morbidity rates were 10.1% and 24.2%, respectively. Multivariated analysis pointed out three parameters corresponding 1 point for each which were age >65 years, albumin ≤1,5 g/dl and BUN >45 mg/dl. Its prediction rate was high with 0,931 (95% CI, 0,890 to 0,961) value of AUC. The hospital mortality rates for none, one, two and three positive results were zero, 7.1%, 34.4% and 88.9%, respectively.

Conclusion: Because the new system consists only age and routinely measured two simple laboratory tests (albumin and BUN), its application is easy and prediction power is satisfactory. Verification of this new scoring system is required by large scale multicenter studies.

Keywords: Peptic ulcer, Perforation, Mortality, Scoring methods

Introduction

In treatment of peptic ulcer, incidence of elective surgery tended to decrease due to eradication of *Helicobacter pylori* during the recent three decades whereas incidence of emergency surgical interventions for complications of the disease did not decrease [1-3]. Moreover, population ageing and extensive use of non-steroid anti-inflammatory drugs increased the incidence of bleeding and perforation of peptic ulcer [1]. Only 5-10% of the patients with bleeding peptic ulcers require surgical intervention whereas almost all patients with perforated peptic ulcer (PPU) necessitate surgery [1]. The risk of mortality (6-30%) and morbidity (21-43%) at PPU unfortunately have not changed during the last decades [1,3-6]. Perforation was the cause of death in 70% of the patients with peptic ulcer and rate of mortality due to PPU is 10-fold higher than other acute abdominal factors such as acute appendicitis and acute cholecystitis [7].

Some scoring systems such as Boey, Peptic Ulcer Perforation Score (PULP) and ASA (American Society of Anesthesiologists) have been already developed for prediction of mortality at PPU [5,8,9]. PULP score appears to have the greatest predictability of mortality however it is impractical with its complexity [5]. Boey score is a more practical but its predictability value was found varying in several studies [5,10-12]. Both scoring systems require a well history taking to detect the duration of symptoms and co-morbidities [5,8]. However, those data cannot be taken reliably from some elderly patients. ASA as a scoring system is non-specific for PPU, its predictability is not superior than the others and its major drawback is its subjective assessment [5,10]. Detection of patients with high risk for mortality after PPU surgery can allow other treatment modalities except surgery or can necessitate some extra care protocols to decrease the mortality [6].

Our aim was to develop a new and easy applicable scoring system to predict mortality at PPU patients.

* Correspondence: drebrumenekse@gmail.com
[1]Department of General Surgery, Ankara Numune Training and Research Hospital, Ankara 06100, Turkey
Full list of author information is available at the end of the article

Patients and methods

The records of surgically treated PPU patients at Ankara Numune Training and Research Hospital and Inonu University Faculty of Medicine between dates 2009 and 2010 were reviewed as retrospectively. The computerized and documentary archives of patients in both of hospital were used in this study. The cases with malignant perforated tumors, marginal ulcer or incomplete data were excluded from the analysis.

The patients were diagnosed according to preoperative clinical features, routine laboratory tests, radiological findings and operative evidence. All the procedures were conducted via an open surgical approach.

The following data were collected: age, gender, white blood cell count (WBC), hemoglobin (Hb), urea, creatinine (Cre), albumin (Alb), systolic blood pressure (BP-S), diastolic blood pressure (BP-D), mean arterial pressure (MAP), pulse, perforation size, admission duration, ASA, Boey, PULP scores, duration of operation, medical illnesses, postoperative complications, reasons of mortality. Laboratory data's were used at the time of admission. The death that occurred within 30 days after surgical treatment or death at the same admission was defined as hospital mortality. The time interval longer than 24 hours between presumed perforation and surgery was accepted as a delayed admission. Factors associated with mortality and morbidity were analyzed using univariate and multivariate analysis. A clinical POMPP (Practical scoring system of mortality in patients with perforated peptic ulcer) score based on the final logistic regression model was constructed for mortality. Additionally, logistic regression analysis and receiver-operating characteristic (ROC) curve

analysis were used to calculate risk predictions for mortality in Boey, PULP and ASA scoring systems and their predictability on mortality was compared with the new scoring system. The definitions of the mentioned scoring systems are presented in the Table 1.

Perforation longer than 24 hours was differently defined by PULP and Boey scorings. This term was defined as time interval from perforation (onset of symptoms or aggravation of symptoms) until admission to hospital for PULP [5] whereas this term was defined as the time interval from perforation until surgery for Boey [13]. We also used the definition of Boey scoring system for perforation duration in all scorings. Therefore, total score of PULP may have resulted higher in our study than the original application.

Preoperative shock was defined as blood pressure < 100 mm Hg and heart rate >100 beats/ min for PULP whereas this term was described as only blood pressure < 100 mm Hg for Boey [5,13]. The parameter of preoperative shock was defined compatible with original form of each study in evaluation of these scoring systems in our study.

Statistical analysis

Shapiro-Wilk test was used for assessing normality. Continuous data are presented as mean ± SD while differences between groups were analyzed by means of Students t test. Categorical variables were analyzed with χ^2 tests. Logistic regression was used to identify variables associated with mortality. Variables with p ≤ 0.2 in the univariate analyses were included in multivariate analyses. Results of the multivariable analysis were shown as odds ratio (OR) and

Table 1 Comparison of scoring systems contents for mortality in patients with peptic ulcer perforation

Scoring systems	PULP - points		ASA - scores		BOEY - points		POMPP - points	
Substances	Age > 65	3	Normal health	1	Medical illness	1	Age > 65	1
	Comorbid active malign disease or AIDS	1	Mild systemic disease	2	Preoperative shock	1	BUN > 45 mg/dl	1
	Comorbid liver cirrhosis	2	Severe systemic disease	3	Duration of peptic ulcer perforation > 24 h	1	Albumin < 1.5 g/L	1
	Concomitant use of steroids	1	Severe systemic disease with a constant treat to life	4				
	Shock	1	Not expected survival for patients without surgery	5				
	Perforation time on admission >24	1						
	Serum creatinine >1.47 mg/dl	2						
	ASA 2	1						
	ASA 3	3						
	ASA 4	5						
	ASA 5	7						
High score		>6		>3		>1		>1
Total score		0-18		1-5		0-3		0-3

corresponding 95% confidence interval (CI). The analysis of the ROC curve used to define the optimal cut-off value for continuous variables in mortality. A clinical score based on the final logistic regression model was constructed; 1 point was given to indicate presence of each predictive factor.

Model discrimination was measured by the area under the receiver–operator characteristic (ROC) curve (AUC). The discrimination of a prognostic model is considered perfect, good, moderate and poor for AUC values of 1; >0,8; 0,6–0,8 and <0,6; respectively.

Results

We enrolled 325 patients underwent surgical treatment for PPU. A total of 98 patients were excluded because the fulfilled at least one of the exclusion criteria. The study population included remaining 227 patients with a mean age of 50.6 ± 19.6 (ranged16-95) years. Table 2 shows the clinical characteristics of PPU patients and comparison of these characteristics for mortality and morbidity according to univariate analysis. Hospital mortality was 10.1% (n: 23) in the patients while pneumonia, myocardial failure

combined with arrhythmia, septicemia and renal failure were found in 15, five, two and one patients, respectively. Morbidity rate was 24.2% (n: 55). The morbidities were pulmonary failure (n:24), wound infection (n:23), evisceration (n:10), renal failure (n:7), postoperative ileus (n:6), cardiac failure (n:5), suture leakage (n:3) and intraabdominal abscess (n:2)., respectively. Mean length of hospital stay was 7.9 ± 9.0 days (ranged 1–115).

The operative procedures included mainly simple closure (n: 218) or some definitive procedures (n:9) such as pyloroplasty or gastrectomy in cases of accompanying hemorrhage, large or multiple perforations.

Three variables were statistically significant in multivariate analysis: albumin level equal or less than 1.5 (OR = 0.0445), age over 65 (OR =1.1258), and BUN level higher than 45 (OR = 1.0353) (Table 3). A probability score was calculated by adding points given to these variables. Despite the differences in regression coefficients, 1 point was given for each of these risk factors to simplify procedure. The resulting predicting of mortality in perforated peptic ulcer (POMPP) score ranged between score 0 to 3.

Table 2 Clinical characteristics of patients in terms of mortality

Variable	Mortality	No Mortality	P	Morbidity	No morbidity	P
	n = 23	n = 204		n = 55	n = 172	
Age (years) (mean ± SD)	74.5 ± 12.1	47.9 ± 18.4	<0.0001	61.4 ± 18.1	47.2 ± 18.8	<0.0001
Sex; Male/Female (n,%)	18(9.1)/5(15.6)	180(90.9)/27(84.4)	NS†	43(21.7)/12(37.5)	155(78.3)/20(62.5)	0.047
White blood cell count (10/μL) (mean ± SD)	12.5 ± 7.8	13.7 ± 6.5	NS†	146.9 ± 86.7	132.0 ± 59.8	NS†
Hemoglobin (g/dl) (mean ± SD)	12.8 ± 2.8	15 ± 2.3	<0.0001	14.3 ± 3.2	14.9 ± 2.1	NS†
BUN (mg/dl) (mean ± SD)	123.5 ± 85.9	36.6 ± 20.9	<0.0001	70.5 ± 67.1	37.4 ± 26.2	<0.0001
Creatinine (mg/dl) (mean ± SD)	2.71 ± 2.07	1.15 ± 0.86	<0.0001	1.78 ± 1.32	1.20 ± 1.21	0.003
Albumin (g/L) (mean ± SD)	1.52 ± 0.51	2.57 ± 0.75	<0.0001	2.45 ± 0.69	3.12 ± 0.73	<0.0001
BP-S*(mm/Hg) (mean ± SD)	107 ± 28.4	125.9 ± 21.7	<0.0001	124.1 ± 28.6	123.9 ± 21.2	NS†
BP-D**(mm/Hg) (mean ± SD)	67.2 ± 19.4	76.7 ± 13.6	0.003	77.2 ± 16.9	75.3 ± 13.8	NS†
MAP***(mmHg) (mean ± SD)	80.4 ± 21.8	93.1 ± 15.03	<0.0001	92.8 ± 19.7	91.5 ± 14.9	NS†
Pulse (/ min) (mean ± SD)	113.2 ± 30.2	94.7 ± 14.3	<0.0001	104.6 ± 22.3	93.8 ± 14.7	<0.0001
Time from perforation to surgery (h) (n, %)						
<24 h	1 (1.2)	80 (98.8)	0.001	28 (17.4)	133 (82.6)	<0.0001
>24 h	22 (15.1)	124 (84.9)		27 (39.7)	41 (60.3)	
Perforation size (cm) (n, %)						
<0.5	15 (8.9)	153 (91.1)	0.02	4 (13.8)	25 (86.2)	0.001
0.5-1	1 (3.4)	28 (96.6)		36 (21.1)	135 (78.9)	
>1	7 (23.3)	23 (76.7)		15 (50)	15 (50)	
Operation time (min) (mean ± SD)	103.3 ± 42.4	81.6 ± 28.1	0.001	95.7 ± 46.8	80.3 ± 22.8	0.002
Other medical illnesses (n,%)						
Absent	4 (2.5)	155 (97.5)	<0.0001	22 (13.6)	140 (86.4)	<0.0001
Present	19 (27.5)	49 (72.1)		33 (48.5)	35 (51.5)	

*BP-S: Blood pressure-systolic, **BP-D: Blood pressure-diastolic, ***MAP: Median artery pressure, †NS: Non-significant.

Table 3 Independent predictor of mortality identified by multivariate logistic regression analysis

Predictors	P value	SE*	Odds ratio	95% CI
Albumin	0.0005	0.89	0.0445	0.0077 to 0.2577
BUN	0.0003	0.009	1.0353	1.0160 to 1.0550
Age	0.0013	0.03	1.1258	1.0474 – 1.2100

*Standard Error.

Three groups of patients were defined based on the POMPP score. In the first group, with a score 0, there was no mortality. The second group included patients with POMPP score 1, who had a 7.1% risk of mortality; this group comprised approximately 1.8% of the cohort. The third group, comprising approximately 4.8% of the patients, included those with a POMPP score of 2 whose risk of mortality 34.4% and last group with a POMPP score of 3 who had an 88.9% risk of mortality, this group comprised about 3.5% of the cohort (Table 4).

The area under the ROC curve (AUC) was 0.931 (95% CI, 0.89-0.96) (Figure 1). The AUC values of the other scoring systems evaluated in our study have been presented in Table 5. The specificity, sensitivity, negative likelihood and positive likelihood ratios for POMPP score exceeding 1 point were 89.2%; 82.6%; 0.19 and 7.66, respectively.

Discussion

We described a new and easily applicable scoring system to predict the postoperative mortality rate in patients with PPU. This scoring system simply based on only age and routinely measured two simple laboratory tests (albumin, BUN). Similarly to us, PULP or Boey scores were found that age over 65 or 60 was an independent risk factor for mortality [5,13]. Advanced age had been reported in several studies as an independent risk factor on mortality in PPU patients [4,14-18] and its importance is still remains [16,19].

Another parameter of POMPP scoring system was BUN level which is regulated as a result of several conditions such as protein catabolism, steroid intake and gastrointestinal bleeding. Regardless of renal functions, it is also accepted as a marker of a severity of disease

Table 4 Risk of mortality according to the POMPP score in patients with peptic ulcer perforation

POMPP Score	No Mortality n (%)	Mortality n (%)
0	130 (100)	0 (0)
1	52 (92.9)	4 (7.1)
2	21 (65.6)	11 (34.4)
3	1 (11.1)	8 (88.9)

[20]. In the study of Khuri et al., BUN > 40 mg/dl was found as a risk factor that increases 30-day mortality after non-cardiac operations [21]. In PULP and Jabolpur scoring systems, high level of serum creatinine was used in predicting risk for mortality [5,12]. In the study of Thorsen et al., serum creatinine level over 1.33 mg/dl was detected as an independent risk factor that indicates mortality risk in PPU [11]. Additionally, it was stated in this study that hypoalbuminemia and high creatinine levels may reflect some underlying pathologies and diseases such as presence of cancer, chronic severe disease and acute diseases that may cause dehydration or accompany with infection and sepsis [11]. We considered that high predictive power of low albumin and high BUN levels as well as advanced age in mortality is associated with the broad spectrum of underlying pathological events and diseases. Hypoalbuminemia alone had been shown as marker of increased risk of morbidity and mortality in PPU patients [22]. Thorsen et al. was found that hypoalbuminemia was a strong factor which might determine mortality solely (AUC: 0.78) [11]. Strong correlation between hypoalbuminemia and mortality in PPU patients is not surprising when reduction of albumin synthesis is considered in cases of dehydration, hepatic dysfunction, cancer, critical clinical course, systemic inflammatory response syndrome and sepsis [22,23].

PULP scoring system was constructed by testing a large patient population as the national data [5]. Even though, mortality predictive power of PULP scoring system was a little better than ours (PULP AUC: 0,955 vs. POMPP AUC: 9,931; p > 0,5), it is not easy to use the PULP in clinical practice. PULP is based on partially anamnesis and admission time was defined as the end of time interval which didn't reflect total duration of abdominal contamination. Additionally, three variables including missing data more than 20% were excluded from the PULP study and some more missing data below 20% were included in. Moller et al. was given AUC value of 0.83 for mortality prediction for PULP scoring system [5]. In a recent study by Thorsen et al. found the AUC value as 0.79 [11], whereas we have found it as 0.95. While calculating the PULP score in our study, we modified the defined time interval as from perforation onset to the surgery. For this reason, prediction of PULP in our analysis might be higher than the previously reported ones.

The other defined scoring system of Boey is more practical than the PULP. However, prediction values of Boey scoring system were quite varying in several studies as AUC values ranged between 0, 63 to 0, 86 [5,11,12,15,24]. In our analysis we found a better Boey value (AUC: 0.92) for prediction then the reported ones. On the other hand, Boey scoring system didn't involve advanced age which is generally an important parameter for mortality in PPU [8].

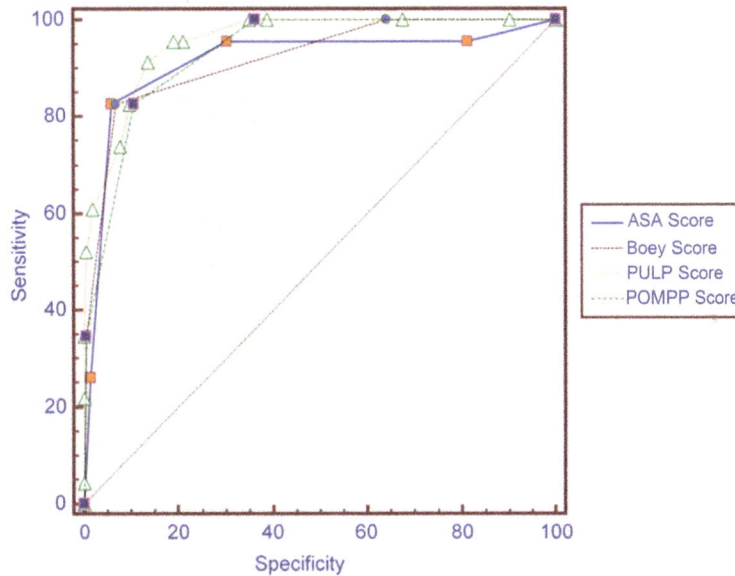

Figure 1 ROC curves analysis of POMPP, PULP, Boey and ASA scoring system.

Exclusion of advanced age might be caused by the fact that this scoring system was defined three decades before. Incidence of PPU complications increased in the population of advanced age due to prolonging mean lifetime in the present time and increased use of NSAIs in the advanced ages [25].

Several studies were analyzed the mortality prediction of ASA status in PPU patients and found AUC values between 0, 73 and 0, 91 [5,9,11,15]. ASA is not specific scoring system for neither PPU and it is mainly based on the co-morbid diseases and their severity [11,25,26]. Although co-morbidities are important risk factors for mortality, under diagnosed or unknown chronic diseases on emergency admission can result to underscoring of ASA. On the other hand, sepsis is as important as the additional medical diseases on the mortality of PPU [4,6,9]. Beside all that, the main problem of ASA scoring is that calculation is performed subjectively and differences between interpretations may be observed [10].

In fact, all of the scoring system models compared in our study had similar and well predictive power for

mortality in PPU patients. None of the previously described scoring systems were widely accepted in clinical practice yet. The reason can be their complexity, non-specificity or confused and subjective points in the mind of clinicians such as definitions of preoperative shock, perforation duration and severity of medical illnesses. We believe that three very clear parameters (age, albumin and BUN) can be easily adopted in the clinical practice to predict the surgical mortality of PPU patients. Respiratory support, circulatory stabilization, preoperative and postoperative care in ICU, frequent monitorization and perioperative care protocols can be added to the high risk patients with PPU [5,6]. It is demonstrated that if the high risk patients got extra perioperative care, the hospital mortality rate could be reduced from the standard care patients (17% and 27%, respectively, $p = 0.005$) [6]. Therefore, a simple and easy applicable system in predicting mortality for PPU patients may provide reduction in mortality rates.

As a limitation, our study population was only 227 but this number was noticeable when compared with other studies in the literature except cohort study of Moller [5,11,13,15]. Secondly, this was a retrospective analysis, and its prospective confirmation is evitable.

Table 5 The ROC curves results of different scoring system for mortality in peptic ulcer perforation

Scoring Systems	AUC	SE*	95% CI
ASA	0.914	0.0401	0.870 to 0.947
BOEY	0.920	0.0282	0.876 to 0.952
PULP	0.955	0.0164	0.919 to 0.978
POMPP	0.931	0.0195	0.890 to 0.961

*Standard Error.

Conclusion

POMPP is a very simple and appropriate scoring system for clinical practice that may allow surgeon to perform a rapid analysis and may help in predicting mortality rate in PPU with its construction based on objective data.

Competing interests

The authors declare that they have no competing interests.

Authors' contributions

Study conception or design: EM, BK. Data collection: AO, RT. Statistical analysis: MT, BK, EM, interpretation: EM, drafting or revision of the manuscript: BK, CK, MT, EM and critical reviewed and approval: EM, BK, RT, AO, MT, CK. All authors read and approved the final manuscript.

Author details

[1]Department of General Surgery, Ankara Numune Training and Research Hospital, Ankara 06100, Turkey. [2]Department of General Surgery, Faculty of Medicine, Sakarya University, Sakarya 54000, Turkey. [3]General Surgery Clinic, Turhal State Hospital, 60300 Tokat, Turkey. [4]Department of Surgery, Faculty of Medicine, Mersin University, 33343 Mersin, Turkey. [5]Department of Surgery, Faculty of Medicine, Inonu University, 44280 Malatya, Turkey.

References

1. Lee CW, Sarosi Jr GA. Emergency ulcer surgery. Surg Clin North Am. 2011;91:1001–13. doi:10.1016/j.suc.2011.06.008.
2. Sarosi Jr GA, Jaiswal KR, Nwariaku FE, Asolati M, Fleming JB, Anthony T. Surgical therapy of peptic ulcers in the 21st century: more common than you think. Am J Surg. 2005;190:775–9.
3. Lau JY, Sung J, Hill C, Henderson C, Howden CW, Metz DC. Systematic review of the epidemiology of complicated peptic ulcer disease: incidence, recurrence, risk factors and mortality. Digestion. 2011;84:102–13. doi:10.1159/000323958.
4. Kim JM, Jeong SH, Lee YJ, Park ST, Choi SK, Hong SC, et al. Analysis of risk factors for postoperative morbidity in perforated peptic ulcer. J Gastric Cancer. 2012;12:26–35. doi:10.5230/jgc.2012.12.1.26.
5. Møller MH, Engebjerg MC, Adamsen S, Bendix J, Thomsen RW. The Peptic Ulcer Perforation (PULP) score: a predictor of mortality following peptic ulcer perforation. A cohort study. Acta Anaesthesiol Scand. 2012;56:655–62. doi:10.1111/j.1399-6576.2011.02609.x.
6. Møller MH, Adamsen S, Thomsen RW, Møller AM. Peptic Ulcer Perforation (PULP) trial group. Multicentre trial of a perioperative protocol to reduce mortality in patients with peptic ulcer perforation. Br J Surg. 2011;98:802–10. doi:10.1002/bjs.7429.
7. Søreide K, Thorsen K, Søreide JA. Strategies to improve the outcome of emergency surgery for perforated peptic ulcer. Br J Surg. 2014;101:e51–64. doi:10.1002/bjs.9368.
8. Boey J, Choi SK, Poon A, Alagaratnam TT. Risk stratification in perforated duodenal ulcers. A prospective validation of predictive factors. Ann Surg. 1987;205:22–6.
9. Mäkelä JT, Kiviniemi H, Ohtonen P, Laitinen SO. Factors that predict morbidity and mortality in patients with perforated peptic ulcers. Eur J Surg. 2002;168:446–51.
10. Thorsen K, Søreide JA, Søreide K. Scoring systems for outcome prediction in patients with perforated peptic ulcer. Scand J Trauma Resusc Emerg Med. 2013;21:25. doi:10.1186/1757-7241-21-25.
11. Thorsen K, Søreide JA, Søreide K. What is the best predictor of mortality in perforated peptic ulcer disease? A population-based, multivariable regression analysis including three clinical scoring systems. J Gastrointest Surg. 2014;18:1261–8. doi:10.1007/s11605-014-2485-5.
12. Mishra A, Sharma D, Raina VK. A simplified prognostic scoring system for peptic ulcer perforation in developing countries. Indian J Gastroenterol. 2003;22:49–53.
13. Boey J, Wong J, Ong GB. A prospective study of operative risk factors in perforated duodenal ulcers. Ann Surg. 1982;195:265–9.
14. Kocer B, Surmeli S, Solak C, Unal B, Bozkurt B, Yildirim O, et al. Factors affecting mortality and morbidity in patients with peptic ulcer perforation. J Gastroenterol Hepatol. 2007;22:565–70.
15. Lohsiriwat V, Prapasrivorakul S, Lohsiriwat D. Perforated peptic ulcer: clinical presentation, surgical outcomes, and the accuracy of the Boey scoring system in predicting postoperative morbidity and mortality. World J Surg. 2009;33:80–5. doi:10.1007/s00268-008-9796-1.
16. Thorsen K, Søreide JA, Kvaløy JT, Glomsaker T, Søreide K. Epidemiology of perforated peptic ulcer: age- and gender-adjusted analysis of incidence and mortality. World J Gastroenterol. 2013;19:347–54. doi:10.3748/wjg.v19.i3.347.
17. Kujath P, Schwandner O, Bruch HP. Morbidity and mortality of perforated peptic gastroduodenal ulcer following emergency surgery. Langenbecks Arch Surg. 2002;387:298–302.
18. Hermansson M, Staël Von Holstein C, Zilling T. Peptic ulcer perforation before and after the introduction of H2-receptor blockers and proton pump inhibitors. Scand J Gastroenterol. 1997;32:523–9.
19. Di Saverio S, Bassi M, Smerieri N, Masetti M, Ferrara F, Fabbri C, et al. Diagnosis and treatment of perforated or bleeding peptic ulcers: 2013 WSES position paper. World J Emerg Surg. 2014;9:45. doi:10.1186/1749-7922-9-45.
20. Uchino S, Bellomo R, Goldsmith D. The meaning of the blood urea nitrogen/creatinine ratio in acute kidney injury. Clin Kidney J. 2012;5:187–91. doi:10.1093/ckj/sfs013.
21. Khuri SF, Daley J, Henderson W, Hur K, Demakis J, Aust JB, et al. The Department of Veterans Affairs' NSQIP: the first national, validated, outcome-based, risk-adjusted, and peer-controlled program for the measurement and enhancement of the quality of surgical care. National VA Surgical Quality Improvement Program. Ann Surg. 1998;228:491–507.
22. Møller MH, Adamsen S, Thomsen RW, Møller AM. Preoperative prognostic factors for mortality in peptic ulcer perforation: a systematic review. Scand J Gastroenterol. 2010;45:785–805. doi:10.3109/00365521003783320.
23. Ñamendys-Silva SA, González-Herrera MO, Texcocano-Becerra J, Herrera-Gómez A. Hypoalbuminemia in critically ill patients with cancer: incidence and mortality. Am J Hosp Palliat Care. 2011;28:253–7. doi:10.1177/1049909110384841.
24. Buck DL, Vester-Andersen M, Møller MH. Accuracy of clinical prediction rules in peptic ulcer perforation: an observational study. Scand J Gastroenterol. 2012;47:28–35. doi:10.3109/00365521.2011.639078.
25. Owens WD. American Society of Anesthesiologists Physical Status Classification System in not a risk classification system. Anesthesiology. 2001;94:378.
26. Daabiss M. American Society of Anaesthesiologists physical status classification. Indian J Anaesth. 2011;55:111–5. doi:10.4103/0019-5049.79879.

Diagnostic accuracy of oblique chest radiograph for occult pneumothorax: comparison with ultrasonography

Shokei Matsumoto[1*], Kazuhiko Sekine[2], Tomohiro Funabiki[1], Tomohiko Orita[1], Masayuki Shimizu[1], Kei Hayashida[1], Taku Kazamaki[1], Tatsuya Suzuki[3], Masanobu Kishikawa[4], Motoyasu Yamazaki[1] and Mitsuhide Kitano[1]

Abstract

Backgraound: An occult pneumothorax is a pneumothorax that is not seen on a supine chest X-ray but is detected by computed tomography scanning. However, critical patients are difficult to transport to the computed tomography suite. We previously reported a method to detect occult pneumothorax using oblique chest radiography (OXR). Several authors have also reported that ultrasonography is an effective technique for detecting occult pneumothorax. The aim of this study was to evaluate the usefulness of OXR in the diagnosis of the occult pneumothorax and to compare OXR with ultrasonography.

Methods: All consecutive blunt chest trauma patients with clinically suspected pneumothorax on arrival at the emergency department were prospectively included at our tertiary-care center. The patients underwent OXR and ultrasonography, and underwent computed tomography scans as the gold standard. Occult pneumothorax size on computed tomography was classified as minuscule, anterior, or anterolateral.

Results: One hundred and fifty-nine patients were enrolled. Of the 70 occult pneumothoraces found in the 318 thoraces, 19 were minuscule, 32 were anterior, and 19 were anterolateral. The sensitivity and specificity of OXR for detecting occult pneumothorax was 61.4 % and 99.2 %, respectively. The sensitivity and specificity of lung ultrasonography was 62.9 % and 98.8 %, respectively. Among 27 occult pneumothoraces that could not be detected by OXR, 16 were minuscule and 21 could be conservatively managed without thoracostomy.

Conclusion: OXR appears to be as good method as lung ultrasonography in the detection of large occult pneumothorax. In trauma patients who are difficult to transfer to computed tomography scan, OXR may be effective at detecting occult pneumothorax with a risk of progression.

Keywords: Oblique chest radiograph, Lung ultrasound, Occult pneumothorax, Diagnosis

Background

A traumatic pneumothorax is a common chest injury in which preventable trauma death can occur if appropriate treatment is delayed. The standard anteroposterior supine radiograph (APXR) is the recommended modality to evaluate trauma patients according to the Advanced Trauma Life Support Course guidelines [1]. However, the APXR fails to diagnose a significant proportion of

pneumothoraces in this situation. A pneumothorax identified on a computed tomography (CT) scan that was not seen on a preceding supine APXR is termed an "occult pneumothorax" (OPX) [2]. As CT scans are now frequently used to evaluate trauma patients as part of initial management, OPXs can be detected more easily. OPXs account for an astonishingly high 52 to 63 % of all traumatic pneumothoraces [3–5]. OPXs may become life threatening if tension develops, especially in patients receiving mechanical ventilation [6, 7]. Therefore, CT scans should be performed as soon as practicable. It is of note that CT scans are not always performed on patients

* Correspondence: m-shokei@feel.ocn.ne.jp
[1]Department of Trauma and Emergency Surgery, Saiseikai Yokohamashi Tobu Hospital, 3-6-1 Shimosueyoshi, Tsurumi-ku, Yokohama-shi, Kanagawa 230-0012, Japan
Full list of author information is available at the end of the article

in severe states of shocks and those in undeveloped countries.

Several studies have reported that lung ultrasonography (US) is an effective new and sensitive technique to evaluate chest trauma [3, 8–12]. However, lung US is operator dependent and operators need to learn the technique. We reported a method to detect OPX with oblique chest radiograph (OXR) without a CT scan or lung US [13] (Figs. 1 and 2). This method is simple, quick, and easily interpreted by anyone, including non-emergency, non-trauma physicians. However, the diagnostic accuracy of OXR for detecting OPX has not yet been evaluated. The aim of this study was to evaluate the usefulness of OXR in the diagnosis of OPX.

Patients & methods
Study design and clinical management
We conducted a prospective, noninferiority study at our emergency department in Saiseikai Yokohamashi Tobu Hospital, a tertiary-care center, from 1 January 2010 to 31 December 2014. All consecutive blunt trauma patients 18 years or older clinically suspected of OPX on arrival at the emergency department were included in this study. Clinical findings suggestive of OPX were at least one of the following conditions: (1) radiographic abnormality without overt pneumothorax finding on APXR (rib fracture, permeability decay of lung field) or (2) physical abnormalities (chest pain, bruise, subcutaneous emphysema). Exclusion criteria were overt pneumothorax, patients requiring immediate invasive interventions, transferred from another hospital, age younger than 18 years, refractory shock, cardiac arrest.

In accordance with ATLS guidelines, all patients had an examination and underwent APRX immediately upon admission. If the criteria were met, patients underwent OXR and lung US in the supine position in the emergency department, and underwent CT scans as soon as possible. OXR and lung US were performed on the bilateral-lung field as part of the routine method. In these patients, CT scans were considered the gold standard and were analyzed together with OXR and lung US. The decision to insert a chest tube for OPX was made on a case-by-case basis after a review of the images and clinical findings by attending physicians. There was no specific algorithm. This study was approved by our Institutional Scientific Board.

Diagnosis of pneumothorax by imaging test
All OXR was performed using mobile X-ray equipment (IME-200A, Toshiba, Tokyo, Japan) before lung US and CT scan were performed. A portable film cassette was set at 45 ° against a horizontal line in suspected hemithorax. The X-ray beams were sent vertically against the cassette over the pleural interface (Fig. 1). OXR criteria for a diagnosis of pneumothorax included a distinct visceral pleural line away from the chest wall. OXR was interpreted by an emergency radiologist (F.T.) without knowledge of other information and delineated the presence of pneumothorax.

All lung US examinations were performed by attending consultant emergency physicians (M.S., T.K., T.O. and S.M.) who were board-certified in Japanese Association for Acute Medicine and trained in lung US. Theydelineated the presence of pneumothorax at the time of examination, without prior knowledge of OXR findings. A lung US imaging unit (Viamo™, Toshiba, Tokyo, Japan) with a 3.5 MHz convex probe was used. Pleural interfaces were examined at the second to fourth intercostal spaces anteriorly and the sixth to eighth spaces in the midaxillary line. Lung US diagnosis of pneumothorax was based on the previously described scanning technique (disappearance of sliding signs and loss of comet-tail artifacts at the pleural interface) [9, 12, 14], and was not assessed with Doppler function.

All CT scans were performed with 64 multidetector CT scanners (Aquilion CT scanner, Toshiba, Tokyo, Japan). Immediately after emergency department resuscitation, thoracic CT scans were performed with contiguous 2 mm axial sections from the apicothorax to the symphysis pubis. The presence of pneumothorax on CT scans was judged by a supervised attending physician. Final dictated reports were reviewed by the first author (M.S.) and compared with other imaging tests. OPX size on CT was

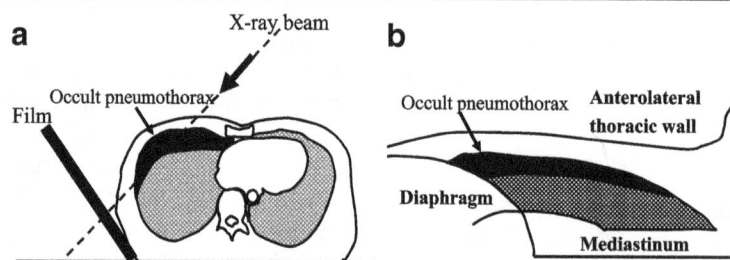

Fig. 1 a We previously reported a method to detect occult pneumothoraces by supine oblique chest radiography (OXR) without a CT scan. b X-ray beam is projected onto a film by this OXR method

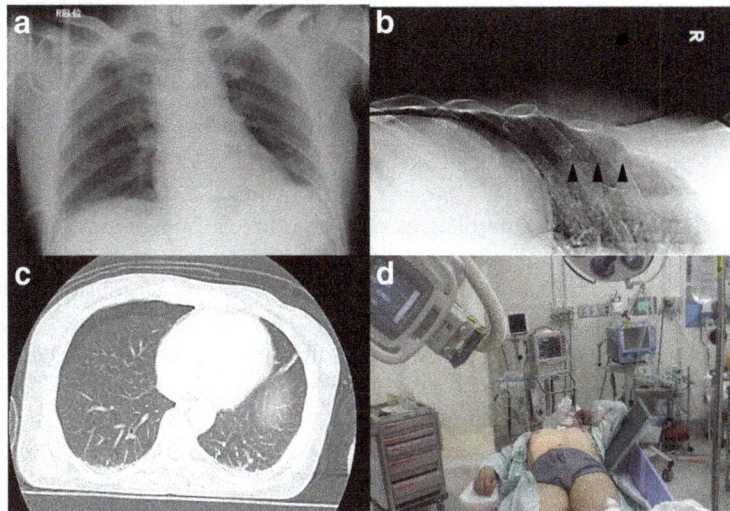

Fig. 2 A typical case of occult pneumothorax diagnosed by OXR. This 58-year-old woman was involved in a head-on car accident and arrived with dyspnea, right chest pain. **a** Anteroposterior supine radiograph shows no abnormality. **b** OXR on the right clearly reveals a distinct visceral pleural line (arrowheads). **c** CT scan proves the existence of an occult pneumothorax on the right side. **d** Supine oblique chest radiographs could be easily performed in a trauma resuscitation area

classified according to the previous report by Wolfman et al. as minuscule, anterior, or anterolateral [15] (Fig. 3).

Statistical analyses

All statistical analyses were performed using SPSS for Windows version 15.0 (SPSS Inc., Chicago, IL, USA). Analysis was made using the chi-squared test and Fisher's exact test as appropriate. The performance of lung US and OXR for the detection of pneumothorax was compared to CT scans as the gold standard. The diagnostic sensitivity, specificity, positive predictive value (PPV), negative predictive value (NPV), and accuracy for US and OXR were calculated using standard formulas. A value of $p < 0.05$ was considered statistically significant. The agreement between lung US and OXR was assessed using the k coefficient, which gauges whether the agreement is better than would occur by chance alone; a k value of 1 indicates perfect agreement.

Results

Patients suspected of occult pneumothorax

One hundred and fifty-nine patients were met the study criteria. During this study, a total of 3460 trauma patients attended the emergency department and 137 patients were diagnosed with traumatic pneumothorax. From this subset, 71 patients with traumatic pneumothorax were excluded owing to no suspicion of OPX by the attending physician, cardiopulmonary arrest or overt pneumothorax. The 159 patients underwent OXR, lung US, and CT and were included in the analysis. Of these patients, age 18 years to 99 years (median = 49.6 years), 110 (69.2 %) were men. These patients suffered from traffic accidents (71.5 %), falls (20 %), and others (8.5 %). There were 19 patients (11.9 %) who received mechanical ventilation. The average injury score was 14 ± 9.8.

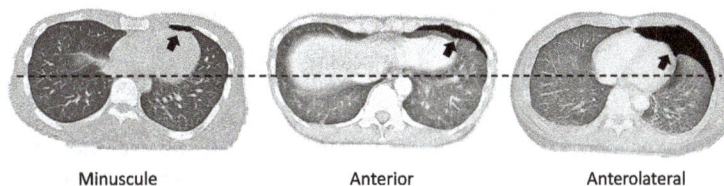

Minuscule   Anterior   Anterolateral

Fig. 3 Occult pneumothorax size on CT scan classification by Wolfman et al. [15]. Minuscule pneumothorax is defined as a thin collection of air up to 1 cm thick in the greatest slice and seen on no more than 4 cm length. Anterior pneumothorax is categorized as a collection of pleural air more than 1 cm thick, located anteriorly, not extending to the mid-coronal line, and which may be seen on 4 cm or more length. Anterolateral pneumothorax is defined as pleural air extending to the mid-coronal line at least

OPX diagnosed by CT gold standard and clinical management

According to the gold standard, OPX was present in 70 of these 318 thoraces (i.e., 159 patients enrolled × 2) (22.2 %). OPX involved the right side in 34 patients (52.5 %), the left side in 28 patients (42.6 %), and bilateral sides in 4 patients (4.9 %). Of the 70 OPXs, 19 were minuscule, 32 were anterior, and 19 were anterolateral. Of the 70 OPXs, 49 (70.0 %) were observed for stable cardiopulmonary condition. Sixteen OPXs underwent chest tube insertion at the time of initial care because of dyspnea, unstable condition, and disturbance of consciousness. In observed 54 OPXs, 16 (29.6 %) required a subsequent chest tube (11 of which were for progression of pneumothorax, 5 for progression of hemothorax). With a larger OPX size, the need for a chest tube increased significantly ($p < 0.001$). Viewed in terms of size (minuscule, anterior, and anterolateral) of OPX, the final chest tube insertion rate was 10.5 %, 40.6 %, and 89.5 %, respectively.

Comparative OPX and lung US performance

Table 1 shows the sensitivity, specificity, PPV, NPV, and accuracy for each diagnostic method. Both methods have high specificity for OPX diagnosis but low sensitivity. There was no significant difference between the accuracies of the two methods in terms of OPX diagnosis ($p = 0.88$). The agreement between the two methods for OPX diagnosis was 93.3 % ($k = 0.804$, $p < 0.001$). Of the 318 thoraces evaluated, OXR showed a true positive result for the detection of OPXs in 43 (12.8 %), a false positive in two (0.6 %), a true negative in 246 (73.2 %), and a false negative in 27 (11.9 %). Among 43 OPXs that could be detected by OXR, 26 (61.0 %) needed tube thoracostomy. Of these 27 false negative thoraces by OXR, 16 (69.6 %) were minuscule and 21 (77.8 %) could be conservatively managed without tube thoracostomy. In the remaining six patients, conservative management failed (three for progression of

hemothorax) and required a subsequent chest tube. Two false positive thorax by OXR was suspected to be due to the overlap of a large breast or skin (Fig. 4). The performance of lung US showed very similar findings to OXR. Lung US showed a true positive result for the detection of OPXs in 44 (13.8 %), a false positive in three (1 %), a true negative in 245 (77.0 %), and a false negative in 26 (8.2 %). These three false positive lung US patients had a history of tuberculous pleuritis.

Table 2 shows the sensitivity when viewed in terms of size of OPX for each diagnostic method. With a decrease in the size of the OPX, the sensitivity of both methods decreased significantly ($p < 0.001$). There was no significant difference in OPX size sensitivity between the two methods of OPX diagnosis.

Discussion

The currently reported incidence of OPX is between 2 and 8 % of all blunt trauma victims. The incidence of OPX among all traumatic pneumothoraces was between 52 and 72 % [3–5, 16–18]. Although pneumothorax has a high incidence in victims of major trauma, up to 76 % of all pneumothoraces may be occult to APXR interpreted by attending trauma teams in real time [19]. It was reported that most OPXs can be closely observed without a chest tube, even with positive pressure ventilation [20–22]. However, there are some OPXs that become worse as tension develops [15, 16, 23, 24]. Also, multiple traumas with high injury severity scores (ISSs) have been associated with failed observation [25, 26]. In this study, 15 of 66 patients with OPX were managed with immediate tube thoracostomy. Of the 51 patients who underwent observation, 16 (31.3 %) required subsequent chest tube insertion. Therefore, it is important that the early recognition of OPX can predict the development of tension, for which patients should be monitored and readied for chest tube insertion. CT scans detect OPX easily, but it is difficult for unstable patients to undergo a CT scan and most of these severe patients need positive pressure ventilation, which may pose a risk for progression. CT scans have the disadvantages of high cost and high doses of radiation. It is hoped that a simple method other than a CT scan or an US test for detecting OPX will attract attention.

To the best of our knowledge, this is the first study of supine OXR to detect OPX. In the primary care of trauma victims, patient movement is restricted by backboards. Upright chest radiography (CXR) is infrequently performed in the trauma bay, secondary to considerations for patient safety, especially regarding potential spine trauma and pelvic fracture. Because intrapleural air migrates into the anterior region of the pleural space (the most nondependent area) in the supine position [27], a small pneumothorax will not appear with APRX

Table 1 Performance of oblique chest radiography compared with lung ultrasonography in 158 patients with trauma

Parameter	Oblique x-ray	Lung US
Sensitivity (%)	61.4	62.9
	(0.56–0.64)	(0.57–0.66)
Specificity (%)	99.2	98.8
	(0.98–1.00)	(0.97–1.00)
Positive predictive value (%)	95.6	93.6
	(0.86–0.99)	(0.84–0.98)
Negative predictive value (%)	90.1	90.4
	(0.87–0.91)	(0.89–0.91)
Accuracy (%)	90.9	90.9
	(0.88–0.92)	(0.88–0.92)

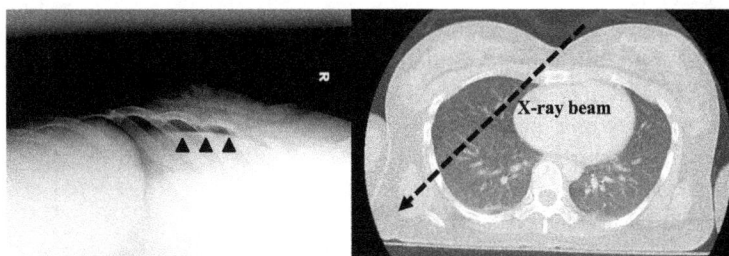

Fig. 4 False positive case of OXR. The overlap of a large breast causes a false positive. This look like a pleural visceral line on OXR (black arrowhead)

as the typical apicolateral pleural line is surrounded by intrapleural air. This means that the interface between the pneumothorax and the underlying lung is perpendicular, not parallel, to the incident x-ray beam, and cannot be easily seen. However, the x-ray beams produced by OXR could be parallel to the interface. The distribution of the intrapleural air is suitable for lung US test.

In this study, the x-ray beams of OXR were sent at 45 ° against the horizontal line. It is not certain that this angle is suitable. If the angle is close to horizontal, OXR may be able to detect smaller OPX. However, if the angle is extremely horizontal, the sternum or the other lung that overlaps an injured thorax may prevent the detection of OXR. As we considered smaller OPX to not be problematic and as the number was memorable, we defined the angle as 45 ° [13, 15].

In this study, both OXR and lung US were superior for detecting large OPXs. Other papers have reported the utility of lung US [3, 8–11]. The sensitivity in our study was lower than these previous papers. It is because there was difference in the indication criteria. Our study criteria excluded overt pneumothoraces unlike previous reports. We think that it is less important to reveal overt pneumothorax using lung US because it can be found clearly on APXR which is essential examination in primary care. Furthermore, these previous studies were performed in far fewer centers and raised the possibility of substantial bias for individual examiners. Also, these US examiners included emergency physicians, trauma surgeons, surgical residents, and radiologist. In this study, all

US examinations were performed by physicians who were trained in lung US, because not all staff were able to attain basic familiarity with lung US. Kirkpatrick and colleagues reported that US examination for detecting pneumothorax is relatively easy and the examination can be quickly learned [3]. However, there did not appear to be a learning curve over the duration of the study or differences in examiner accuracy. A good training system is essential for improving and maintaining the accuracy of US by emergency physicians and surgeons in clinical practice [28]. Although US is operator dependent, the practice and reading of OXR is simpler and easier.

In this study, the false positives of US for pneumothorax may stem from pleural adhesion with tuberculous pleuritis that were blocking lung sliding. A judgment of pneumothorax by US requires attention in Japan and developing countries where tuberculosis is more common compared to Western countries. Chest tube insertion for a patient with pleural adhesion is dangerous, especially using the Seldinger technique. Other causes of absent sliding signs include lung contusion, chronic obstructive pulmonary disease, a giant bulla, unilateral intubation, fibroid lung, and atelectasis lung [10, 14, 29, 30]. Subcutaneous emphysema is a finding suggestive of pneumothorax; however, it may produce comet-tail artifacts that have the potential of causing false negative. OXR had high specificity, however, there was two false positive case in this study. The positive finding of OXR is a collapsed lung surface (visceral pleural line) visible on X-rays. In the false positive case, a large breast was visualized by mimicking the visceral pleural line. When this false positive image of OXR was retrospectively evaluated, we could detect the presence of the lung marking distal to the false visceral pleural line. Therefore, it is important to evaluate not only the pleural visceral line but also the presence of lung marking. The majority of false negative cases of both US and OXR were minuscule pneumothorax. It is difficult to detect minuscule pneumothorax; however, this may be of low importance because most patients do not require thoracostomy.

It is important to indicate what type of patient OXR is suitable for. US is rapidly feasible following focused assessment with sonography for trauma (FAST). This is

Table 2 Sensitivity for detecting occult pneumothorax of oblique chest radiograph vs. lung ultrasonography viewed in terms of size of occult pneumothorax

	Occult pneumothorax size ($n = 70$)		
	Minuscule	Anterior	Anterolateral
	$n = 19$	$n = 32$	$n = 19$
Oblique X-ray sensitivity (%)	15.8	68.8	94.7
Lung US sensitivity (%)	10.5	75.0	94.7
p	0.63	0.59	1.0
Need for chest tube (%)	10.5	40.6	89.5

why lung US is called "Extended FAST" [3]. In this study, the majority of cases using both US and OXR could be performed within 3 min. OXR may be more laborious than US. Although OXR has a small radiological exposure compared to CT scans, patients using OXR are modestly irradiated. Therefore, it is better to limit use to patients at risk of OPX. Unfortunately, there are few useful clinical markers to predict OPX early in the resuscitation of trauma patients. Although the deep sulcus sign and the double diaphragm sign are APXR findings that suggest OPX, they lack credibility [18]. OXR may be useful to verify these subtle radiographic findings. Ball and colleagues reported that subcutaneous emphysema, pulmonary contusion, rib fractures, and female sex were independent predictors of OPX [31]. However, in a subsequent prospective study, they reported that only subcutaneous emphysema remained independently predictive of OPX [19]. There are many patients with OPX who do not have these findings. The incidence of OPX using this study's criteria is high (33.0 %), and they may be good criteria for OXR. Unfortunately, the incidence of OPX without this study criteria is unclear. As such, further studies are needed in order to determine the indication for OXR. In reality, there may be little chance to use OXR, because the majority of trauma centers in advanced countries have US and CT. We recommend the use of OXR when CT is unusable, for example, 1) in hospitals without CT or US devices, 2) in patients in which OPX is suspected by physiological and radiological findings, 3) in emergency operation rooms and intensive care units with hemodynamically unstable patients, 4) where there is no confidence in US findings, or 5) before air transport in large fires. Our study has several limitations. First, the number of patients with OPX was small and a selection bias may have occurred because our entry criteria insufficiently covered all cases of OPX in the emergency department Second, this study did not take into account the reproducibility or inter-reader agreement of diagnostic images. It appears that inter-reader variability exists for US aside from OXR. Third, the assessment of chest tube insertion was performed by the patient's attending physician. It is difficult to decide whether chest tube insertion is necessary or not. Additionally, attending physicians may consistently overrate the necessity of chest tube in cases of anterolateral OPX, because it is a notable finding.

Conclusion

OXR and lung US are good tools for the diagnosis of OPX. Furthermore, the detectability of OPX by OXR may eliminate the need for an immediate tube thoracostomy. OXR is simple and effective in trauma patients who are difficult to transfer to CT scan. Although there are several methods to detect OPX, each has its distinctive characteristics, advantages, and disadvantages. The methods that best meet the needs of the situation of trauma management should be chosen.

Abbreviations

APXR: Anteroposterior supine radiograph; CT: Computed tomography; OPX: Occult pneumothorax; US: Ultrasonography; OXR: Oblique chest radiograph; FAST: Focused assessment with sonography of trauma; NPV: Negative predictive value; PPV: Positive predictive value.

Competing interest

The authors declare no conflict of interest.

Author's contribution

OXR is the brainchild of Dr. Kishikawa. Sincere appreciation goes to Dr. Sekine, whose comments and suggestions were invaluable. I am also indebted to Dr. Kitano and Dr. Kishikawa for their useful comments and warm encouragement, Dr. Funabiki and Dr. Hayashida for providing advice about the analyzed data, and other authors for supporting the data collection. All authors read and approved the final manuscript.

Author details

[1]Department of Trauma and Emergency Surgery, Saiseikai Yokohamashi Tobu Hospital, 3-6-1 Shimosueyoshi, Tsurumi-ku, Yokohama-shi, Kanagawa 230-0012, Japan. [2]Department of Emergency Medicine, Saiseikai Central Hospital, 1-4-17 Mita, Minato, Tokyo 108-0073, Japan. [3]Department of Radiological Technology, Saiseikai Yokohamashi Tobu Hospital, 3-6-2 Shimosueyoshi, Tsurumi-ku,, Yokohama-shi 230-0011, Japan. [4]Division of Emergency Medicine, Fukuoka City Hospital, 13-1 Yoshizukahonmachi, Hakata-ku, Fukuoka 812-0046, Japan.

References

1. Surgeons ACo, editor. Advanced trauma life support course for doctors. Committee on Trauma. Instructors Course Manual.
2. Wall SD, Federle MP, Jeffrey RB, Brett CM. CT diagnosis of unsuspected pneumothorax after blunt abdominal trauma. AJR Am J Roentgenol. 1983;141(5):919–21.
3. Kirkpatrick AW, Sirois M, Laupland KB, Liu D, Rowan K, Ball CG, et al. Hand-held thoracic sonography for detecting post-traumatic pneumothoraces: the Extended Focused Assessment with Sonography for Trauma (EFAST). J Trauma. 2004;57(2):288–95.
4. Rhea JT, Novelline RA, Lawrason J, Sacknoff R, Oser A. The frequency and significance of thoracic injuries detected on abdominal CT scans of multiple trauma patients. J Trauma. 1989;29(4):502–5.
5. Neff MA, Monk Jr JS, Peters K, Nikhilesh A. Detection of occult pneumothoraces on abdominal computed tomographic scans in trauma patients. J Trauma. 2000;49(2):281–5.
6. Bridges KG, Welch G, Silver M, Schinco MA, Esposito B. CT detection of occult pneumothorax in multiple trauma patients. J Emerg Med. 1993;11(2):179–86.
7. In Blaosdell WF TD, editor. Trauma Management. New York: Thieme, Inc 1981
8. Dulchavsky SA, Schwarz KL, Kirkpatrick AW, Billica RD, Williams DR, Diebel LN, et al. Prospective evaluation of thoracic ultrasound in the detection of pneumothorax. J Trauma. 2001;50(2):201–5.
9. Kirkpatrick AW, Ng AK, Dulchavsky SA, Lyburn I, Harris A, Torregianni W, et al. Sonographic diagnosis of a pneumothorax inapparent on plain radiography: confirmation by computed tomography. J Trauma. 2001;50(4):750–2.
10. Brook OR, Beck-Razi N, Abadi S, Filatov J, Ilivitzki A, Litmanovich D, et al. Sonographic detection of pneumothorax by radiology residents as part of extended focused assessment with sonography for trauma. J Ultrasound Med. 2009;28(6):749–55.
11. Nagarsheth K, Kurek S. Ultrasound detection of pneumothorax compared with chest X-ray and computed tomography scan. Am Surg. 2011;77(4):480–4.
12. Soldati G, Testa A, Sher S, Pignataro G, La Sala M, Silveri NG. Occult traumatic pneumothorax: diagnostic accuracy of lung ultrasonography in the emergency department. Chest. 2008;133(1):204–11.

Diagnostic accuracy of oblique chest radiograph for occult pneumothorax: comparison...

113

13. Matsumoto S, Kishikawa M, Hayakawa K, Narumi A, Matsunami K, Kitano M. A method to detect occult pneumothorax with chest radiography. Ann Emerg Med. 2011;57(4):378–81.

14. Lichtenstein D, Meziere G, Biderman P, Gepner A. The comet-tail artifact: an ultrasound sign ruling out pneumothorax. Intensive Care Med. 1999;25(4):383–8.

15. Wolfman NT, Myers WS, Glauser SJ, Meredith JW, Chen MY. Validity of CT classification on management of occult pneumothorax: a prospective study. AJR Am J Roentgenol. 1998;171(5):1317–20.

16. Garramone Jr RR, Jacobs LM, Sahdev P. An objective method to measure and manage occult pneumothorax. Surg Gynecol Obstet. 1991;173(4):257–61.

17. Tocino IM, Miller MH, Frederick PR, Bahr AL, Thomas F. CT detection of occult pneumothorax in head trauma. AJR Am J Roentgenol. 1984;143(5):987–90.

18. Ball CG, Kirkpatrick AW, Fox DL, Laupland KB, Louis LJ, Andrews GD. Are occult pneumothoraces truly occult or simply missed? J Trauma. 2006;60(2):294–8. discussion 8–9.

19. Ball CG, Ranson K, Dente CJ, Feliciano DV, Laupland KB, Dyer D, et al. Clinical predictors of occult pneumothoraces in severely injured blunt polytrauma patients: A prospective observational study. Injury. 2009;40(1):44–7.

20. Brasel KJ, Stafford RE, Weigelt JA, Tenquist JE, Borgstrom DC. Treatment of occult pneumothoraces from blunt trauma. J Trauma. 1999;46(6):987–90. discussion 90–1.

21. Moore FO, Goslar PW, Coimbra R, Velmahos G, Brown CV, Coopwood Jr TB, et al. Blunt traumatic occult pneumothorax: is observation safe?–results of a prospective, AAST multicenter study. J Trauma. 2011;70(5):1019–23. discussion 23–5.

22. Mowery NT, Gunter OL, Collier BR, Diaz Jr JJ, Haut E, Hildreth A, et al. Practice management guidelines for management of hemothorax and occult pneumothorax. J Trauma. 2011;70(2):510–8.

23. Enderson BL, Abdalla R, Frame SB, Casey MT, Gould H, Maull KI. Tube thoracostomy for occult pneumothorax: a prospective randomized study of its use. J Trauma. 1993;35(5):726–9. discussion 9–30.

24. Collins JC, Levine G, Waxman K. Occult traumatic pneumothorax: immediate tube thoracostomy versus expectant management. Am Surg. 1992;58(12):743–6.

25. Hill SL, Edmisten T, Holtzman G, Wright A. The occult pneumothorax: an increasing diagnostic entity in trauma. Am Surg. 1999;65(3):254–8.

26. Barrios C, Tran T, Malinoski D, Lekawa M, Dolich M, Lush S, et al. Successful management of occult pneumothorax without tube thoracostomy despite positive pressure ventilation. Am Surg. 2008;74(10):958–61.

27. Ball CG, Kirkpatrick AW, Laupland KB, Fox DL, Litvinchuk S, Dyer DM, et al. Factors related to the failure of radiographic recognition of occult posttraumatic pneumothoraces. Am J Surg. 2005;189(5):541–6. discussion 6.

28. Emergency ultrasound guidelines. Ann Emerg Med. 2009 Apr;53(4):550–70.

29. Rowan KR, Kirkpatrick AW, Liu D, Forkheim KE, Mayo JR, Nicolaou S. Traumatic pneumothorax detection with thoracic US: correlation with chest radiography and CT–initial experience. Radiology. 2002;225(1):210–4.

30. Lichtenstein DA, Lascols N, Prin S, Meziere G. The "lung pulse": an early ultrasound sign of complete atelectasis. Intensive Care Med. 2003;29(12):2187–92.

31. Ball CG, Kirkpatrick AW, Laupland KB, Fox DI, Nicolaou S, Anderson IB, et al. Incidence, risk factors, and outcomes for occult pneumothoraces in victims of major trauma. J Trauma. 2005;59(4):917–24. discussion 24–5.

16

Prevention of lung-to-lung aspiration during emergency thoracic surgery

Jin-Young Hwang[1], Jiseok Baik[2], Sahngun Francis Nahm[3], Dongjin Kim[4], Young-Tae Jeon[3], Jinhee Kim[3], Seongjoo Park[3] and Sunghee Han[3*]

Abstract

Background: Lung separation is essential for an emergency thoracic surgery for massive hemoptysis. When using a double lumen tube (DLT), a commonly adopted lung separation device during thoracic surgery, a water-tight seal of endobronchial cuff is crucial to prevent lung-to-lung aspiration of blood. In this study, we investigated the fluid sealing characteristics of the endobronchial cuff of a DLT and examined the effect of gel lubrication on the fluid leakage beyond the endobronchial cuff of DLT.

Methods: An artificial tracheobronchial tree was intubated with a DLT. In the first phase of the study, the intra-cuff pressure of endobronchial cuff of DLT was set to 25, 50, or 100 cmH$_2$O (n = 7, each), and the non-dependent bronchus was filled with 5 ml of water. Fluid leakage to the dependent bronchus beyond the endobronchial cuff was collected for 6 h. The time until leakage was first detected and the time until 100% leakage occurred were measured. In the second phase, the endobronchial cuff was coated with either saline (group C, n = 10) or lubricant gel (group GEL, n = 10), and the same parameters were measured.

Results: In the first phase of the study, the times to first leakage and 100% leakage at an intra-cuff pressure of 25 cmH$_2$O were 21.0 (7.0 - 59.0) sec and 3.0 (2.0 - 4.0) min, respectively. Higher intra-cuff (50 and 100 cmH$_2$O) resulted in longer time for the first leakage and 100% leakage, but the duration was not long enough for clinical purpose. In the second phase, all the DLTs in group C showed 100% fluid leakage during the 6-hour period. In contrast, in group GEL, fluid leakage beyond the endobronchial cuff was detected only in 50% of the DLTs and none of the DLT showed 100% fluid leakage during the study. Among the DLTs which exhibited fluid leakage, the time to first leakage was 252.0 (171.0-305.0) min and the leakage volume at the end of the study period was 0.3[0.0-1.8]ml.

Conclusions: Endobronchial cuff of DLT cannot prevent fluid leakage beyond the endobronchial cuff, but lubricant gel coating on the endobronchial cuff can effectively reduce the lung-to-lung aspiration.

Keyword: Double lumen tube, Hemoptysis, Aspiration, Lung separation, Thoracic surgery, Endobronchial cuff

Introduction

Massive hemoptysis, traumatic or non-traumatic, is potentially lethal and has a high mortality rate [1,2]. Emergency surgery is an important treatment option [2-4] and sparing the non-bleeding lung from blood spill is critical in the perioperative period [1,5]. Patients undergoing thoracic surgery for hemoptysis are frequently placed in a lateral decubitus position to facilitate the surgical approach. In this position, the healthy lung is placed below the operative lung. Thus, preventing the gravity-driven drainage of blood from the operative lung into the healthy lung on the dependent side is an important clinical issue.

The double lumen tube (DLT) is the most commonly used lung isolation device during thoracic surgery [6]. When using the DLT, preventing leakage from one lung to the other depends on the sealing properties of the endobronchial cuff. It has been reported that endotracheal

* Correspondence: noninvasive@hanmail.net
[3]Department of Anesthesiology and Pain Medicine, Seoul National University Bundang Hospital, Seoul National University, College of Medicine, 300 Gumidong Bundanggu, Seongnamsi, Kyoneggido 463-707, South Korea
Full list of author information is available at the end of the article

cuff of the modern single lumen endotracheal tubes (SLT) cannot reliably prevent fluid leakage [7-9]. The endobronchial cuff of the DLT has high-volume low-pressure (HVLP) characteristics, similar to those of endotracheal cuff of SLT [10-12]. As yet, the fluid sealing characteristics of endobronchial cuff of DLT in the lateral decubitus position have not been investigated in detail. In the first phase of our study, we investigated the sealing characteristics of endobronchial cuff of DLT in a lateral decubitus position using an artificial tracheobronchial tree.

For SLT, several methods have been suggested to improve the sealing characteristics of the endotracheal cuff. Of interest, the application of lubrication gel to the SLT endotracheal cuff has been shown to effectively reduce fluid leakage [13,14]. Thus, in the second phase of the study, we hypothesized that lubrication gel coating on the DLT endobronchial cuff could reduce fluid leakage past the cuff to reduce lung-to-lung spillage. The sealing characteristics of either lubrication gel-coated or saline-coated endobronchial cuffs were compared with respect to the volume and timing of fluid leakage past the cuff.

Methods

Based on the previous reports [15], we simulated an artificial tracheobronchial tree with a 17-mm trachea that branched into 13-mm left and 16-mm right bronchi, and the study was conducted in two phases.

The first phase examined the fluid sealing characteristics of the DLT endobronchial cuff in the lateral decubitus position. The artificial tracheobronchial tree was intubated with a 35 Fr DLT (Broncho-cath^{TM}, Mallinckrodt, Ireland). It was positioned horizontally, with one bronchus in the dependent position and the other bronchus in the non-dependent position. The intra-cuff pressure was set at 25, 50, or 100 cmH2O (groups 25, 50 and 100, respectively) using a cuff inflator (Cuff Pressure Manometer^{TM}, Microcuff GmbH,Weinheim, Germany). After the cuff inflation, 5 ml of colored water were poured into the non-dependent side of the artificial bronchus to simulate blood or pus in the operative lung. Fluid leakage past the endobronchial cuff into the dependent bronchus was monitored. The leaked water was collected in a container placed below the open end of the dependent bronchus. The time until leakage was first detected and the time until 100% leakage occurred were measured. The time to 100% leakage was defined as the time point when 4.8 ml of fluid were collected in the container, because our pilot study revealed that 0.1- 0.2 ml of fluid was retained within the artificial tracheobronchial tree even when the cuff was completely deflated. The volume of fluid collected in the container was monitored for 6 h, and recorded by the minute during the first 15 min, at 30 min, and once per hour thereafter. Seven 35Fr DLTs were tested for each group.

In the second phase of the study, the effect of lubricating gel on the sealing characteristics of the cuff was investigated. The endobronchial cuff was lubricated with either saline or gel. In the saline-control group (group C; n = 10), the tube was dipped into bottle of saline before intubation. In the gel-lubrication group (group GEL; n = 10), 3 ml of water-soluble gel (K-Y Jelly^{TM}, Johnson & Johnson, Korea) were applied onto a 10 × 10-cm four-ply gauze pad, and the pad was used to coat the cuff with gel. The artificial tracheobronchial tree was intubated with the DLT and positioned horizontally. The endobronchial cuff was inflated to pressure of 25 cmH2O and the volume of fluid leaking past the endobronchial cuff was measured for 6 h as in the first part of the study. The parameters measured in the first part of the study were also measured.

Statistics

For the data from the first phase of the study, between-group comparisons were made using the Kruskal-Wallis test, with the Mann–Whitney U test as appropriate. The data from the second phase were compared using the Mann–Whitney U test. Value of P or the Bonferroni corrected P (P value multiplied by the number of comparisons) less than 0.05 were considered to indicate statistical significance. Data are presented as medians (interquatile).

Results

During the first phase of the study, the time until the first fluid leakage and the time until 100% leakage at each of the three intra-cuff pressures are presented in Table 1. The time to first leakage differed significantly among the groups. In pairwise comparisons, group 100 differed from groups 25 and 50, but no significant difference in time to first leakage was found between groups 25 and 50. The time to 100% leakage also differed significantly among the three groups. Compared with groups 25 and 50, group 100 exhibited a significantly longer time to 100% leakage. Groups 25 and 50 did not differ significantly with regard to time to 100% leakage. The volume of fluid that leaked over time at each intra-cuff pressure is presented in Figure 1. The volume of fluid that leaked differed significantly among the three groups from 1 min and 1 h. For the first hour, group 100 exhibited a significantly lower volume of leakage compared with groups 25 and 50, while groups 25 and 50 exhibited same amount of fluid leakage. By 2 h, 100% fluid leakage had occurred in all three groups, and there was no difference among them.

In the second phase of the study, the endobronchial cuff lubricated with gel had a significantly longer ($P = 0.001$) time to first leakage when compared with the saline control. The first fluid leakage was detected within 1 min [19.0 (9.8-34.3) s] in the group C. Among the 10 DLTs in the gel-coated group, only five showed fluid leakage during the 6-h study period, with a time to first fluid leakage

Table 1 Time to first leakage and to 100% leakage of double-lumen tubes at each intra-cuff pressure

Group	Time to first leakage (s)*	Corrected P-value*	Time to 100% leakage (min)[†]	Corrected P-value
25	21.0 (7.0-59.0)	0.495[a]	3.0 (2.0-4.0)	0.786[a]
50	48.0 (32.0-78.0)	0.002[b]	6.0 (4.0-12.0)	0.002[b]
100	191 (125.0-260.0)	0.002[c]	85.0 (70.0-130.0)	0.002[c]

Data are presented as median (interquartile).
Group 25: Intra-cuff pressure of 25 cm H$_2$O; group 50: Intra-cuff pressure of 50 cm H$_2$O; group 100: Intra-cuff pressure of 100 cm H$_2$O.
*P = 0.001 among all three groups.
[†]P < 0.001 among all three groups.
[a]Group 25 vs. group 50.
[b]Group 50 vs. group 100.
[c]Group 25 vs. group 100.

of 252.0 (171.0-305.0) min. The time to 100% leakage in the group C was 3.0 (2.0-4.0) min, whereas none of the DLTs in group GEL exhibited 100% leakage during the study period. The median fluid leakage in the group GEL at the end of the study period was only 0.3 (0.0-1.8) ml. Figure 2 illustrates the significantly greater volume of fluid leakage in the group C compared with the group GEL at each time point during the study.

Discussion

Our study showed that the DLT endobronchial cuff could not provide a water-tight seal against lung-to-lung fluid leakage in a lateral decubitus position but gel lubrication of the cuff effectively improved the sealing characteristics.

The modern polyvinylchloride–endotracheal cuff has HVLP characteristics [10]. An intra-cuff pressure of around of 25 cmH$_2$O is recommended for HVLP cuff to avoid mucosal damage [16,17]. However, it has been well documented that this pressure cannot prevent fluid leakage around the HVLP endotracheal cuff [8,18]. The endobronchial cuff of DLT also has HVLP characteristics

similar to those of the SLT endotracheal cuff [11,12], and our results show that in a lateral decubitus position, the DLT endobronchial cuff cannot provide a water tight seal under the recommended intra-cuff pressure of 25 cm H$_2$O as that of endotracheal cuff of SLT. For the endotracheal cuff of the SLT, some studies have reported that higher intra-cuff pressures of 50–60 cmH$_2$O can stop or reduce fluid leakage [7,9], whereas other groups have reported that an increase in intra-cuff pressure to 50 cmH$_2$O is unable to prevent leakage [8]. During the present study, we examined the effect of pressure escalating on sealing characteristics of the endobronchial cuff of DLT by applying intra-cuff pressures of 25, 50, and 100 cmH$_2$O to the endobronchial cuff. Compared with 25 and 50 cmH$_2$O, an intra-cuff pressure of 100 cmH$_2$O showed significantly longer times to both first leakage and 100% leakage. However, even at a pressure of 100 cm H$_2$O, the times to first fluid leakage (median; 191 sec) and 100% leakage (median; 85 min) do not seem to be long enough for complicated thoracic surgery for hemoptysis which poses a high risk for lung-to-lung aspiration. In addition, the intra-cuff pressure of 100 cm

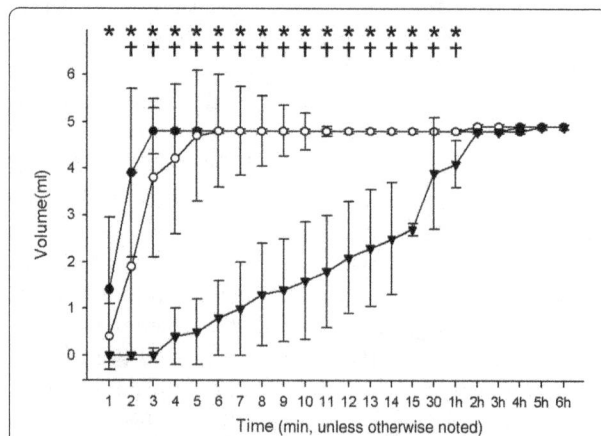

Figure 1 Changes in fluid leakage volume over time at each intra-cuff pressure. Data points are medians. Error bars represent interquartile ranges. Group 25: Intra-cuff pressure of 25 cm H$_2$O (●); group 50: Intra-cuff pressure of 50 cm H$_2$O (○); group 100: Intra-cuff pressure of 100 cm H$_2$O (▼). * P < 0.008 among all three groups. † Corrected P < 0.020, group 100 vs. group 25 and group 100 vs. Group 50.

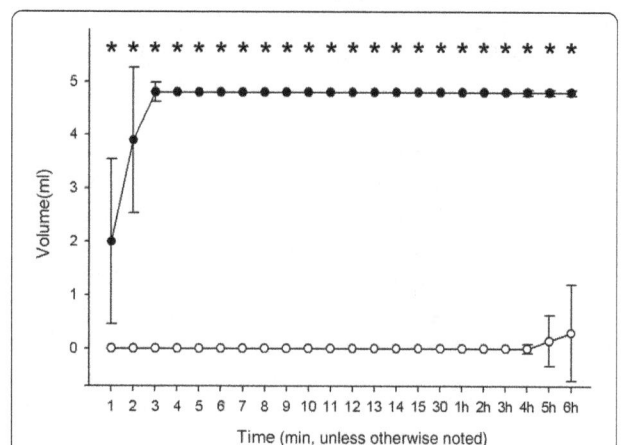

Figure 2 Changes in fluid leakage volume over time based on gel lubrication of cuff. Data points are medians. Error bars represent interquartile ranges. Saline group: endotracheal cuff was coated with saline (●); Gel group: endogracheal cuff was coated with lubrication gel (○).* P < 0.001 between the groups.

H_2O possesses a risk of airway injury [11,16,17]. Thus, despite the statistically beneficial results at 100 cm H_2O, the clinical benefit of increasing the endobronchial cuff pressure above 25 cm H_2O is doubtful.

Gel lubrication of the SLT cuff has been reported to prevent fluid leakage and reduce the risk for pulmonary aspiration [13]. The fluid leakage past the HLVP cuff occurs because the diameter of the high-volume cuff exceeds the diameter of the tracheal lumen. Upon inflation, numerous longitudinal folds are formed on the surface of the cuff and they permit fluid leakage around the cuff [7-9]. By using lubricant gel, these folds can be effectively sealed and fluid leakage past the HVLP cuff can be prohibited [13]. In agreement with previous study regarding endotracheal cuffs, the use of gel lubricants effectively reduced fluid leakage past the endobronchial cuff in this study. Gel lubricant has been widely applied to airway management in clinical practice such as facilitating endotracheal intubation [19,20], flexible bronchoscopy insertion [21], laryngeal mask airway insertion [22], and endotracheal stylet use [23]. In this respect, gel lubrication of the endobronchial cuff could be safely applied in clinical practice to reduce lung-to-lung contamination via a DLT in patients undergoing emergency thoracic surgery for hemoptysis.

Conclusions

To sum up, the endobronchial cuff of a DLT cannot provide an adequately water-tight seal against lung-to-lung contamination even with higher intra-cuff pressure than the recommended range, and gel lubrication of the endobronchial cuff effectively improves its sealing characteristics under a recommended intra-cuff pressure. We recommend consideration of the application of gel lubrication on the endobronchial cuff of DLT to reduce lung-to-lung aspiration during emergency thoracic surgery for hemoptysis.

Competing interests
The authors declare that they have no competing interests.

Authors' contributions
J-YH: concept and design, acquisition of data, drafting the manuscript. JB; concept and design, acquisition of data, drafting the manuscript. SF Nahm: analysis and interpretation of data, revise the manuscript critically. DK: concept and design, acquisition of data, revise the manuscript critically. Y-TJ: concept and design, interpretation of data, revise the manuscript critically. JK: concept and design, interpretation of data, revise the manuscript critically. SP: acquisition of data, drafting the manuscript. SH: concept and design, analysis and interpretation of data, revise the manuscript critically. All authors read and approved the final manuscript.

Authors' information
Jiseok Baik; M.D., Assistant professor. Jin-Young Hwang : M.D., Ph D., Assistant professor. Sahngun Francis Nahm: M.D., Ph D., Assistant professor. Dongjin Kim: M.D., Ph D., Clinical assistant professor. Young-Tae Jeon : M.D., Ph D., Associated professor. Jinhee Kim: M.D., Ph D., Professor. Seongjoo Park: M.D., Ph D., Clinical assistant professor. Sunghee Han: M.D., Ph D., Professor.

Author details
[1]Department of Anesthesiology and Pain Medicine, Borame Medical Center, Seoul National University, College of Medicine, Boramae-ro 5-gil, Dongjak-gu, Seoul, Kyoneggido 156-707, South Korea. [2]Department of Anesthesiology and Pain Medicine, Pusan National University Hospital, Biomedical Research Institute, Pusan National University, School of Medicine, 179 Gudeok-ro, Seo-Gu, Busan 602-739, South Korea. [3]Department of Anesthesiology and Pain Medicine, Seoul National University Bundang Hospital, Seoul National University, College of Medicine, 300 Gumidong Bundanggu, Seongnamsi, Kyoneggido 463-707, South Korea. [4]Department of Thoracic Surgery, Sejong General Hospital, 489-28 Hohyun-Ro, Sosa-Gu, Bucheon-Si, Kyoneggido 422-711, South Korea.

References
1. Jean-Baptiste E. Clinical assessment and management of massive hemoptysis. Crit Care Med. 2000;28(5):1642–7.
2. Karmy-Jones R, Jurkovich GJ, Shatz DV, Brundage S, Wall Jr MJ, Engelhardt S, et al. Management of traumatic lung injury: a Western Trauma Association Multicenter review. J Trauma. 2001;51(6):1049–53.
3. Shigemura N, Wan IY, Yu SC, Wong RH, Hsin MK, Thung HK, et al. Multidisciplinary management of life-threatening massive hemoptysis: a 10-year experience. Ann Thorac Surg. 2009;87(3):849–53.
4. Metin M, Sayar A, Turna A, Solak O, Erkan L, Dincer SI, et al. Emergency surgery for massive haemoptysis. Acta Chir Belg. 2005;105(6):639–43.
5. Winter SMID. Massive hemoptysis: pathogenesis and management. J Intensive Care Med. 1988;3(3):171–88.
6. Slinger PD, Campos JH. Anesthesia for thoracic surgery. In: Miller RD, editor. Miller's Anesthesia. 8th ed. New York: Elsevier; 2009. p. 1942–2006.
7. Pavlin EG, VanNimwegan D, Hornbein TF. Failure of a high-compliance low-pressure cuff to prevent aspiration. Anesthesiology. 1975;42(2):216–9.
8. Seegobin RD, van Hasselt GL. Aspiration beyond endotracheal cuffs. Can Anaesth Soc J. 1986;33(3 Pt 1):273–9.
9. Young PJ, Rollinson M, Downward G, Henderson S. Leakage of fluid past the tracheal tube cuff in a benchtop model. Br J Anaesth. 1997;78(5):557–62.
10. Bernhard WN, Yost L, Joynes D, Cothalis S, Turndorf H. Intracuff pressures in endotracheal and tracheostomy tubes. Related cuff physical characteristics. Chest. 1985;87(6):720–5.
11. Brodsky JB, Adkins MO, Gaba DM. Bronchial cuff pressures of double-lumen tubes. Anesth Analg. 1989;69(5):608–10.
12. Hannallah MS, Benumof JL, Bachenheimer LC, Mundt DJ. The resting volume and compliance characteristics of the bronchial cuff of left polyvinyl chloride double-lumen endobronchial tubes. Anesth Analg. 1993;77(6):1222–6.
13. Blunt MC, Young PJ, Patil A, Haddock A. Gel lubrication of the tracheal tube cuff reduces pulmonary aspiration. Anesthesiology. 2001;95(2):377–81.
14. Dave MH, Koepfer N, Madjdpour C, Frotzler A, Weiss M. Tracheal fluid leakage in benchtop trials: comparison of static versus dynamic ventilation model with and without lubrication. J Anesth. 2010;24(2):247–52.
15. Chow MY, Liam BL, Thng CH, Chong BK. Predicting the size of a double-lumen endobronchial tube using computed tomographic scan measurements of the left main bronchus diameter. Anesth Analg. 1999;88(2):302–5.
16. Seegobin RD, van Hasselt GL. Endotracheal cuff pressure and tracheal mucosal blood flow: endoscopic study of effects of four large volume cuffs. Br Med J (Clin Res Ed). 1984;288(6422):965–8.
17. Mehta S. Safe lateral wall cuff pressure to prevent aspiration. Ann R Coll Surg Engl. 1984;66(6):426–7.
18. Pitts R, Fisher D, Sulemanji D, Kratohvil J, Jiang Y, Kacmarek R. Variables affecting leakage past endotracheal tube cuffs: a bench study. Intensive Care Med. 2010;36(12):2066–73.
19. Stride PC. Postoperative sore throat: topical hydrocortisone. Anaesthesia. 1990;45(11):968–71.
20. Estebe JP, Delahaye S, Le Corre P, Dollo G, Le Naoures A, Chevanne F, et al. Alkalinization of intra-cuff lidocaine and use of gel lubrication protect against tracheal tube-induced emergence phenomena. Br J Anaesth. 2004;92(3):361–6.
21. British Thoracic Society Bronchoscopy Guidelines Committee aSoSoCCoBTS. British Thoracic Society guidelines on diagnostic flexible bronchoscopy. Thorax. 2001;56 Suppl 1:i1–21.

17

Pattern and predictors of mortality in necrotizing fasciitis patients in a single tertiary hospital

Gaby Jabbour[1], Ayman El-Menyar[2,3]* (iD), Ruben Peralta[4], Nissar Shaikh[5], Husham Abdelrahman[4], Insolvisagan Natesa Mudali[5], Mohamed Ellabib[4] and Hassan Al-Thani[4]

Abstract

Background: Necrotizing fasciitis (NF) is a fatal aggressive infectious disease. We aimed to assess the major contributing factors of mortality in NF patients.

Methods: A retrospective study was conducted at a single surgical intensive care unit between 2000 and 2013. Patients were categorized into 2 groups based on their in-hospital outcome (survivors versus non-survivors).

Results: During a14-year period, 331 NF patients were admitted with a mean age of 50.8 ± 15.4 years and 74 % of them were males Non-survivors (26 %) were 14.5 years older ($p = 0.001$) and had lower frequency of pain ($p = 0.01$) and fever ($p = 0.001$) than survivors (74 %) at hospital presentation. Diabetes mellitus, hypertension, and coronary artery disease were more prevalent among non-survivors ($p = 0.001$). The 2 groups were comparable for the site of infection; except for sacral region that was more involved in non-survivors ($p = 0.005$). On admission, non-survivors had lower hemoglobin levels ($p = 0.001$), platelet count ($p = 0.02$), blood glucose levels ($p = 0.07$) and had higher serum creatinine ($p = 0.001$). Non-survivors had greater median LRINEC (Laboratory Risk Indicator for NECrotizing fasciitis score) and Sequential Organ Failure Assessment (SOFA) scores ($p = 0.001$). Polybacterial and monobacterial gram negative infections were more evident in non-survivors group. Monobacterial pseudomonas ($p = 0.01$) and proteus infections ($p = 0.005$) were reported more among non-survivors. The overall mortality was 26 % and the major causes of death were bacteremia, septic shock and multiorgan failure. Multivariate analysis showed that age and SOFA score were independent predictors of mortality in the entire study population.

Conclusion: The mortality rate is quite high as one quarter of NF patients died during hospitalization. The present study highlights the clinical and laboratory characteristics and predictors of mortality in NF patients.

Keywords: Necrotizing fasciitis, Predisposing factors, Presentation, Management, Mortality

Background

Necrotizing fasciitis (NF) is a rare infectious disease which is rapidly progressive and potentially fatal in nature [1]. Despite the advanced medical treatment, the rate of mortality remains as high as 24-34 %; posing a challenge for the diagnosis and management [2]. The mortality in NF patients primarily depends upon the time of the medical and surgical interventions and extent of spread of infection to the primary site (subcutaneous tissue, fasciae, skin or muscles) [3]. NF patients with streptococcal infection are associated with increased risk of complications and mortality (up to 80 %) [4]. There are various predisposing factors for NF such as advanced age, diabetes mellitus, peripheral vascular disease, obesity, chronic renal failure and trauma [5]. Therefore, early recognition of these predisposing factors might help in the early definitive management [6]. Moreover, early surgical debridement is a known contributor to improve outcomes in NF patients [5].

To date, the most appropriate tool for diagnosis and discrimination of NF is the LRINEC (Laboratory Risk

* Correspondence: aymanco65@yahoo.com
[2]Clinical Research, Trauma Surgery, Hamad General Hospital, Doha, Qatar
[3]Clinical Medicine, Weill Cornell Medical School, Doha, Qatar
Full list of author information is available at the end of the article

Indicator for NECrotizing fasciitis score) scoring system proposed by Wong et al. [7]. It is based on laboratory parameters that are readily available for scoring in most institutions to predict survival and discriminate necrotizing from non-necrotizing infections. In addition, various predictors of mortality based on predisposing factors have been reported by different investigators. Previous studies have identified advanced age (>60 years), aeromonas and vibrio infection, liver cirrhosis, cancer, hypotension, band polymorphonuclear neutrophils (PMN) >10 %, and serum creatinine >2 mg/dL to be independent predictors of mortality in NF cases [8, 9]. Despite the fact that mortality depends upon the time of diagnosis, and management, the predisposing factors also play an important role in the outcome. The present study aims to determine the various predisposing and prognostic factors associated with mortality in NF patients.

Methods

All consecutive patients admitted to the surgical intensive care at Hamad General Hospital (HGH) with a diagnosis of necrotizing fasciitis were retrospectively included in this analysis between January 2000 and December 2013. Patients were categorized into 2 groups according to their hospital mortality (survivors versus non-survivors). The present study included patients for which the operative notes and or histopathological findings indicate NF. Data included age, sex, presentation and duration of symptoms, predisposing factors, risk factors, causative microbiological organisms, on-admission laboratory parameters, the Sequential Organ Failure Assessment (SOFA) and LRINEC score, number of operative debridement, length of intensive care and hospital stay, recurrence and in-hospital mortality. The anatomic site of infection was classified as extremity (upper and lower limbs), abdominal/groin, chest/breast, neck/facial, sacral and perineum. Exclusion criteria included patients not admitted in the ICU (uncomplicated mild forms of NF and were managed in the regular ward), patients with cellulitis or superficial infection not requiring aggressive debridement or antibiotics), and non-surgical patients.

The ratio of partial pressure of arterial oxygen and fraction of inspired oxygen (PaO2/FiO2), platelets count, bilirubin level, Glasgow coma score, mean arterial pressure (MAP), vasopressor use, creatinine level and urine output were used to calculate SOFA score [10]. The laboratory parameters such as C-reactive protein (CRP), WBC, hemoglobin, sodium level, creatinine concentration and glucose level were used to calculate the LRINEC score [7]. The various recorded parameters were analyzed according to the final outcome. This study was approved by the medical research center at HMC, Qatar with IRB#14066/14.

Statistical analysis

Data were presented as proportions, median (range) or mean (± standard deviation), as appropriate. Baseline demographic characteristics, laboratory findings, clinical presentation, bacteriology and predisposing factors were compared between non-survivors and survivors. Analyses were conducted using Student-t test for continuous variables and Pearson chi-square (χ^2) test for categorical variables; Fisher's exact test was used, if the expected cell frequencies were below 5. A 2-tailed $p < 0.05$ was considered significant. Multivariate logistic regression analysis was performed to look for the predictors of mortality in the overall NF cohort along with the odd ratio and 95 % confidence interval. Data analysis was carried out using the Statistical Package for Social Sciences version 18 (SPSS Inc, Chicago, Illinois).

Results

During the 14-year study period, a total of 331 admissions were recorded for NF; 74 % were males and the mean age was 50.8 ± 15.4 years. Among them, 246 were survivors (74.3 %) and 85 (25.7 %) were non-survivors. Non-survivors were 14.5 years older (61.6 ± 14.3 vs. 47 ± 14 years, $p = 0.001$) than survivors and the two groups were comparable for gender. Moreover, higher proportion of Qatari nationals (50.6 % vs. 27.2 %; $p = 0.001$) died due to NF as compared to non-Qatari (Arabs) (Table 1).

Clinical findings

On admission, the most common symptoms were local swelling (78 %), pain/tenderness (68 %) and fever (67 %). At presentation, non-survivors had significantly lower frequency of pain (57 % vs. 72 %; $p = 0.01$) and fever (48 % vs. 73 %; $p = 0.001$) than survivors. The frequency of diabetes mellitus (64 % vs. 47 %; $p = 0.007$), hypertension (53 % vs. 29 %; $p = 0.001$), renal impairment (30 % vs. 10 %; $p = 0.001$), coronary artery disease (25 % vs. 11 %; $p = 0.001$) and cerebrovascular accidents (8 % vs. 1 %; $p = 0.001$) were significantly higher among non-survivors as compared to survivor group. However, traumatic injuries (18 % vs. 8 %; $p = 0.04$) were observed more among survivors than non-survivors.

Site of infection

The most frequent site of infection was lower limb/thigh (53 %) followed by perineum (25 %), abdominal/groin region (11.5 %) and neck/facial region (6.3 %). Although, the 2 groups were comparable for the site of infection; sacral region had significantly higher frequency in non-survivors (4.7 % vs. 0.4 %; $p = 0.005$) than survivors.

Table 1 Comparison of necrotizing fasciitis by outcome (survivors versus non-survivors)

	All patients (n = 331)	Survivors (n = 246)	Non- survivors (n = 85)	P *
Males	246 (74.3 %)	75 %	73 %	0.73
Age in years[a]	50.8 ± 15.4	47 ± 14	61.6 ± 14.3	0.001
Nationality				
Qatari	110 (33.2 %)	27.2 %	50.6 %	0.001
Non-Qatari (Arabs)	73 (22.1 %)	20.3 %	27.1 %	
Others	148 (44.7)	52.4 %	22.4 %	
Symptoms				
Swelling	237 (78 %)	76.4 %	82.3 %	0.28
Pain/tenderness	208 (68.4 %)	72.4 %	57 %	0.01
Fever	203 (67 %)	73.3 %	48 %	0.001
Laboratory findings				
Hemoglobin (g/dl)[a]	11 ± 2.7	11.4 ± 2.7	10.1 ± 2.6	0.001
WBC(/µl)[a]	16.2 ± 8.6	16.4 ± 8.6	15.2 ± 8.6	0.28
Platelet count (/µl)[b]	269 ± 201	273 ± 141	230 ± 158	0.02
Sodium (mmol/l)[a]	133.5 ± 5.6	133.4 ± 5.4	133.9 ± 6	0.43
Serum Creatinine (µmol/l)[b]	97 (26–1263)	91 (26–1189)	135 (26–1263)	0.001
Serum Bilirubin(µmol/l)[b]	14.2 (3–381)	14 (3–233)	15 (4–381)	0.35
Serum Glucose[a]	12.0 ± 7.8	12.5 ± 8.4	10.7 ± 5.4	0.07
C-reactive protein[a]	221 ± 120	214 ± 120	232 ± 120	0.35
Procalcitonin (<24 h)[b,c]	10.5 (0.07-303)	3.3 (0.07-303)	9.8 (0.1-182)	0.28
Scoring				
SOFA[b]	9 (2–21)	9 (2–19)	12 (7–21)	0.001
LRINEC[b]	6 (1–13)	5 (1–13)	7 (2–13)	0.001
Site				
Lower limb/Thigh	175 (53 %)	53.3 %	51.8 %	0.81
Perineum	81 (25 %)	23.6 %	27 %	0.52
Abdominal/Groin	38 (11.5)	10.6 %	14 %	0.37
Upper Limb	13 (3.9 %)	4.1 %	3.5 %	0.82
Neck/Facial	21 (6.3 %)	7.3 %	3.5 %	0.21
Chest/Breast	8 (2.4 %)	2.8 %	1.2 %	0.38
Sacral	5 (1.5 %)	0.4 %	4.7 %	0.005
Gluteus	3 (0.9 %)	1.2 %	0 %	0.30
Histopathological confirmation	192 (58 %)	61 %	49.4 %	0.06
Morbidity				
Diabetes Mellitus	167 (52 %)	47 %	64 %	0.007
Renal impairment	49 (15.2 %)	10 %	30 %	0.001
Coronary Artery disease	46 (14.2 %)	11 %	25 %	0.001
Trauma	43 (15.5 %)	18.2 %	8 %	0.04
Number of debridement[b]	2 (1–8)	2 (1–7)	2 (1–8)	0.22
Combined antibiotics(>2)	94(33.6 %)	49.3 %	28.2 %	0.001
Septic shock	76 (27.8 %)	19 %	51.4 %	0.001
ICU stay in days[b]	5.5 (1–75)	5 (1–43)	9 (1–75)	0.002
Hospital stay in days[b]	16 (2–295)	15 (2–295)	20.5(2–273)	0.02

* = survivors vs. non-survivors, [a] = values in (mean ± SD), [b] = values in median and (range), c=<0.5ng/l low risk and >2.0 ng/l high risk sepsis

Laboratory findings

The initial blood investigations such as hemoglobin, leukocyte count, serum sodium, bilirubin and C-reactive protein were comparable among survivors and non-survivors. However, non-survivors had lower levels of hemoglobin (10.1 ± 2.6 vs. 11.4 ± 2.7; p = 0.001), platelet count (230 ± 158 vs. 273 ± 141; p = 0.02), blood glucose levels (10.7 ± 5.4 vs. 12.5 ± 8.4; p = 0.07) and had higher serum creatinine [135 (26–1263) vs. 91 (26–1189); p = 0.001] as compared to survivors. The median procalcitonin levels were non-significantly higher in non-survivors [9.8 (0.1-182) vs. 3.3 (0.07-303); p = 0.28] than that of survivors. In addition, non-survivors had significantly higher median LRINEC [7 (2–13) vs. 5 (1–13); p = 0.001] and SOFA scores [12 (7–21) vs. 9 (2–19); p = 0.001] in comparison to the survivors group. Also, non-survivors were less likely to receive combination of antibiotics (>2 antibiotics) than survivors (28.2 % vs. 49.3 %; p = 0.001).

Microbiological findings

Table 2 represents the involvement of microorganisms in the pathogenesis of NF. Monobacterial gram positive (42 %) were the most frequent organisms identified followed by polybacterial (34 %) and monobacterial gram negative (12.5 %). Among gram positive bacteria,

Table 2 Micro-organisms involved in necrotizing fasciitis

	Overall	Survivors	Non-survivors	P value
Positive wound culture	204 (77 %)	80.4 %	67.6 %	0.03
Positive blood and tissue culture	56 (21 %)	18 %	29.6 %	0.04
Polybacterial infection	90 (34 %)	32.5 %	38.0 %	0.002 for all
Monobacterial Gram positive	111 (42 %)	47.9 %	25.4 %	
Monobacterial Gram negative	33 (12.5 %)	11.3 %	15.5 %	
Fungal	30 (10.2 %)	6.9 %	19.2 %	
Gram positive				
Streptococcus	114 (38 %)	42 %	29 %	0.05
Staphylococcus	109 (37 %)	39 %	29 %	0.11
Enterococcus	14 (5 %)	4.5 %	5.3 %	0.78
Clostridium	3 (1 %)	1.4 %	0 %	0.30
Gram negative				
Bacteroides	61 (22 %)	20 %	22.4 %	0.64
E. Coli	34 (11 %)	10 %	16 %	0.16
Pseudomonas	23 (8 %)	5.4 %	14.5 %	0.01
Klebsiella	23 (8 %)	6 %	12 %	0.12
Aeromonas	4 (1.3 %)	0.9 %	2.6 %	0.26
Proteus	5 (1.7 %)	0.5 %	5.3 %	0.005
Morganella	2 (0.7 %)	0.5 %	1.3 %	0.42

streptococcus (38 %) and staphylococcus (37 %) were the most commonly identified organisms. Bacteriodes (22 %) and E-Coli (11 %) were the predominant gram negative microorganisms. Fungal infection was observed in 30 (10.2 %) cases. Among them 22 (73.3 %) cases were positive for tissue culture, 7 (23.3 %) were positive for tissue as well as blood culture and one (3.4 %) case was positive for blood culture alone. The frequency of poly-bacterial (38 % vs. 32.5 %, p = 0.002) and monobacterial gram negative infections (15.5 % vs. 11.3 %, p = 0.002) were more evident in non-survivors; while monobacterial gram positive organisms were commonly identified among survivors (47.9 % vs. 25.4 %; p = 0.002) compared to non-survivors.

Pseudomonas (14.5 % vs. 5.4 %; p = 0.01) and Proteus infections (5.3 % vs. 0.5 %; p = 0.005) were the most commonly associated microorganisms among non-survivors.

Management and outcomes

The median number of surgical debridements performed was 2 (ranged 1–8) and the hospital length of stay was 16 (2–295) days. The number of debridements was comparable in the 2 groups. The median ICU stay [9 (1–75) vs. 5 days (1–43); p = 0.002], overall hospital stay [20.5 (2–273) vs. 15 (2–295) days; p = 0.02] and the frequency of septic shock (48 % vs. 20 %; p = 0.001) were significantly higher in non-survivors than the survivor group. Recurrent admissions for NF were required for 13 (4 %) patients; of whom 11 patients were admitted twice and two patients required three admissions. A total of 85 patients died in the present study with an overall mortality rate of 26 %. Table 3 shows the major causes of mortality which mainly involved septic shock alone and a combination of bacteremia and multiorgan failure.

Table 4 shows multivariate analysis for the major predictors of mortality. SOFA scoring followed by age were the independent predictors of mortality in the present study cohort. The proportion of mortality based on the bacteriology results is given in Table 5.

None of the co-morbidities showed significant association with types of microorganisms and combination of antibiotics used except coronary heart disease (CHD). Significantly higher frequency of CHD patients were prescribed more than two antibiotic combinations (p = 0.009). Table 6 compares the co-morbidities with microbiological data and antibiotics used.

Discussion

The association of high morbidity and mortality in necrotizing fasciitis (NF) patients urges the need for early diagnosis and identification of potential risk factors of worse outcomes. The present study is interestingly large series of NF cases from a Middle Eastern small

Table 3 Major causes of mortality ($n = 85$) in necrotizing fasciitis patients

Variable	Number
- Septic shock	22
- Bacteremia & multiorgan failure	25
- End stage renal disease and sepsis	2
- sepsis and Cardiopulmonary arrest	3
- Disseminated intravascular coagulation and sepsis	1
- Pulmonary embolism and sepsis	1
- Acute respiratory distress syndrome	2
- Stomach cancer and sepsis	1
- Encephalopathy and sepsis	1
- Volume overload/HF and sepsis	1
- Necrotizing pancreatitis + multiorgan failure	1
- Hypoxic brain injury and sepsis	1
- Myocardial infarction and sepsis	1
Septic myocarditis	1
Cardiac arrest	3
Cardiogenic shock	2
Myocardial infarction	1
Pneumonia	2
Acute myeloid leukemia and sepsis	1
Acute pulmonary edema	1
Missing/not defined	12

Table 5 Mortality based on the bacteriology results

	Number of cases	Mortality
Polybacterial infection	90	27 (38 %)
Gram Positive alone	111	18 (25.4 %)
Gram negative alone	33	11 (15.5 %)
Fungal[a]	30	15 (21.1 %)
Total[b]	265	71

[a]overlap with Gram stain bacteria, [b]Confirmed results

of pain, tender local swelling, and fever [13, 14]. Consistent with earlier reports, this triad was more frequently observed among survivors in the current series. Moreover, out of proportion pain on physical examination and unresolved cellulitis are major diagnostic clues for NF, however, these clinical features often appear later in the disease course [9]. Therefore, delayed diagnosis is usually associated with high mortality (up to 25 %) among young adults which could even reach 44 % in elderly population [9, 15]. The number of in-hospital deaths in the present study is 26 % which is consistent with earlier studies.

The current literature suggests that NF could occur at any age but is mostly reported within the age range of 32 to 57 years [16, 17]. In the present study, the mean age was 51 years and the non-survivors were 14.5 years older than the survivors at the time of presentation. The reason of the frequently observed association of NF with advanced age could be explained in part by the pre-existing co-morbidities and immunosuppression. In this context, Golger et al. [18] reported advanced age, streptococcal toxic shock syndrome and immunocompromised status to be independent predictors of mortality in NF patients.

The frequently associated co-morbidities in NF are diabetes mellitus, malignancy, chronic cardiac disease, peripheral vascular disease, chronic renal disease, and immune-suppression [19]. Other predisposing factors include traumatic injuries, smoking, history of muscular injection and paraplegia. Diabetes mellitus, hypertension, and renal impairment were the most frequent co-morbidities associated with mortality in the current series. Diabetes mellitus remains the main co-morbidity in NF patients which is associated with prolonged hospitalization and increased mortality [13, 20]. In this study, patients with a history of diabetes mellitus showed considerably rapid progress of the severity of NF and mortality. This finding could be attributed in part to the hyperglycemic status that compromises the immunity status and fosters bacterial growth. However, the initial readings of serum sugar in the study cohort were non-significantly lower in non-survivors. Unfortunately, the current database did not include HbA1c to explain in-part this finding. The other common comorbidity in the

population country that assesses various contributing factors to mortality. NF is a fulminant life-threatening infection of the musculoskeletal soft tissues characterized with rapid progression that typically requires urgent surgical interventions [11, 12]. The classic and frequent manifestations associated with NF usually include a triad

Table 4 Multivariate analysis for predictors of mortality

	P value	Odd ratio	95 % confidence interval	
Gender	0.928	0.952	0.328	2.762
Age	0.001	1.06	1.03	1.11
Serum hemoglobin	0.416	1.088	0.888	1.333
Serum sodium	0.442	0.965	0.883	1.056
Serum glucose	0.887	0.995	0.926	1.069
Serum creatinine	0.557	0.999	0.997	1.002
SOFA score	0.020	1.23	1.03	1.49
Lower Limb NF	0.979	1.017	0.278	3.719
Perineum NF	0.891	1.096	0.296	4.059
Abdominal NF	0.671	1.496	0.234	9.574
Prior coronary artery disease	0.917	1.060	0.355	3.162
Monobacterial Gram positive	0.086	0.435	0.168	1.124

NF necrotizing fasciitis

Table 6 Comparison of co-morbidities with microbiological data and antibiotics

	Diabetes mellitus ($n = 167$)	Renal impairment ($n = 49$)	Coronary artery disease ($n = 46$)	Trauma ($n = 43$)
Polybacterial infection	51 (30.5 %)	14 (28.6 %)	10 (21.7 %)	18 (41.9 %)
Monobacterial Gram positive	54 (32.3 %)	12 (24.5 %)	11 (23.9 %)	16 (37.2 %)
Monobacterial Gram negative	19 (11.4 %)	7 (14.3 %)	6 (13.0 %)	0 (0.0 %)
Fungal	21 (12.6 %)	9 (18.4 %)	7 (15.2 %)	2 (4.6 %)
Antibiotic combination used (>2)	47 (28.1 %)	18 (36.7 %)	21 (45.6 %)[a]	13 (30.2 %)

[a] statistically significant

present study was hypertension, which might cause disruption of the microvascular supply and reduction of tissue oxygenation and antimicrobial delivery. The frequency of hypertension was significantly higher in the non-survivors group. Consistently, Huang et al. [8] demonstrated a high association of hypertension among NF non-survivors. Earlier studies have also outlined the increased risk of NF in the presence of the above-mentioned pathologies [21, 22]. Furthermore, elderly patients with such co-morbidities who are suspected to have NF should be evaluated thoroughly to rule out NF, even in the absence of the usual hard manifestations.

Although, NF might affect any part of the body, earlier studies have reported frequent involvement of the extremities, perineum, head & neck and truncal regions [23]. In the current series, the most frequent sites of infection included lower limbs, perineum, abdominal/groin and neck/facial regions. The site of infection and its expansion also affect mortality. It has been suggested that affection of the head and neck region is associated with higher mortality as accounted for the proximity with various vital anatomical structures [24]. Mao et al. [25] analyzed the craniocervical NF cases with and without thoracic extension and observed a poor survival with thoracic extension as compared to non-thoracic extension. An earlier study reported a lower rate of mortality in extremity infection in comparison to abdominal and perineal infections [26]. Urschel [27] suggested that NF infection extending proximally to pelvis or trunk might have worse prognosis. Therefore, early and aggressive treatment aimed at restriction of the infection with repeated surgical debridement could be useful in achieving better survival rates.

Unfortunately, the first stage of NF disease is frequently masked by non-specific manifestations, which prevents effective and timely specific therapy [28]. Therefore, early identification and diagnosis is mandatory and should not rely only on the clinical signs alone [6]. Consequently, prognostic indicators such as laboratory markers and specific patient characteristics obtained from the medical history would assist in the early diagnosis, risk stratification and decision making [29]. Earlier studies identified some laboratory findings such as anemia, elevated creatinine, and increased white cell count to be non-specifically

associated with NF which might affect prognosis. In the present series, non-survivors had significantly lower levels of hemoglobin and platelet count and had higher serum creatinine as compared to survivors. Similarly, an earlier study observed that non-survivors had significantly lower levels of hemoglobin and platelet and presented with higher levels of serum glucose and creatinine than the survivors [8]. An earlier study reported that aeromonas infection, advanced age, band PMNs >10 %, serum creatinine (>2.0 mg/dL), and an activated prothrombin time (>60 s) were found to be the independent predictors of mortality in NF patients [8]. In the present study the major predictors of mortality were age and SOFA scoring. SOFA score is a useful tool to assess the severity of NF based on the involvement of major organ systems. In the present series, non-survivors had significantly higher median SOFA scores which are in accordance with the current literature. The initial increase in SOFA score during the first two days of ICU admission successfully predicts high rates of mortality (50-95 %) [30]. This finding could be used as an alarming indictor and encourages physicians to refer those patients as early as possible to the tertiary care centers for the appropriate intensive care. Therefore, the use of validated prognostic factors in daily clinical practice, especially for initial diagnosis in emergency departments, would help physicians for timely management and obtaining better outcomes.

It has been suggested that bacteremia is one of the frequent complications of NF which has been associated with higher risk of mortality [31]. In the current study, 21 % of the patients had positive blood and tissue cultures and subsequently had higher mortality rate in comparison to those who had negative blood culture. Similarly, Huang et al. [8] observed four-fold increased rate of mortality in patients with positive blood cultures than those who had negative cultures.

Consistent with previous reports [13], gram positive microorganisms, mainly streptococcus and staphylococcus organism, were frequently identified in the present study cohort. On the other side, bacteriodes and E-coli were the predominant gram negative organisms. In the present study, monobacterial infections with pseudomonas and proteus were the most commonly associated microorganisms among non-survivors. However, earlier

Table 7 Summary of published studies of mortality in necrotizing fasciitis/NSTI patients worldwide

Authors	Year/country	Study type/duration	Mortality	Predictors of mortality
Dahm P et al. [40]	2000/USA	Retrospective/1984 to 1998	Overall mortality rate was 20 % (10/50)	The extent of the infection ($P = 0.0234$) was the only significant, independent predictor of outcome
Chin-Ho Wong et al. [29]	2003/Singapore	Retrospective/1997 to 2002	Total $n = 89$	A delay in surgery of > 24 h was correlated with increased mortality ($p < 0.05$; RR = 9.4)
Daniel A. Anaya et al. [32]	2005/USA	Retrospective/1996 to 2001	The overall mortality rate was 16.9 % (total $n = 166$)	Independent predictors of mortality included WBC > 30 000 × 103/μL, creatinine level > 2 mg/dL (176.8 μmol/L), and heart disease at hospital admission
Kwan MK et al. [41]	2006/Malaysia	Retrospective/1998 to 2002	Overall mortality rate was 36 % (total $n = 36$)	A poor WBC response, high serum urea and creatinine, and low haemoglobin level were the predictors for mortality
Golger A et al. [18]	2007/Canada	Retrospective/1994 to 2001	Ninety-nine patients satisfied the inclusion criteria. Overall mortality was 20 %	Advanced age (OR, 1.04; 95 % CI, 1.01 to 1.08; $p = 0.012$), streptococcal toxic shock syndrome (OR, 10.54; 95 % CI, 2.80 to 39.44; $p < 0.001$), and immunocompromised status (OR, 3.97; 95 % CI, 1.04 to 15.19; $p = 0.044$) were independent predictors of mortality
Mulla ZD et al. [42]	2007/USA	Case series/2001	The crude hospital mortality rate was 11.1 % (total $n = 216$)	Patients aged > or =44 years at the time of admission were 5 times as likely to die in the hospital than patients who were aged < or =43 years (adjusted RR 5.08, $P = 0.03$)
Hsiao CT et al. [9]	2008/Taiwan	Retrospective/2002 to 2005	[a]24/128 (19 %)	Aeromonas infection, Vibrio infection, cancer, hypotension, and band form WBC > 10 % were independent positive predictors of mortality ($P < 0.05$). Presence of hemorrhagic bullae was a negative predictor of mortality ($P < 0.05$)
Bair MJ et al. [43]	2009/Taiwan	Retrospective/1995 to 2006	The overall mortality was 17.0 %. total $n = 85$	Predictors of mortality included advanced age, class C liver cirrhosis, ascites, higher serum creatinine, and lower hemoglobin and platelet levels
Kuo Chou TN et al. [44]	2010/Taiwan	Retrospective/2000 to 2007	24/119 (20 %)	The presence of hemorrhagic bullous skin lesions/necrotizing fasciitis, primary septicemia, a greater severity of illness, absence of leukocytosis, and hypoalbuminemia were the significant risk factors for mortality
Kao LS et al. [45]	2011/USA	Retrospective/2004 to 2007	Mortality rates varied between 6 hospitals from 9 % to 25 % ($n = 296$)	Patient age and severity of disease (reflected by shock requiring vasopressors and renal failure postoperatively) were the main predictors of mortality
Huang KF et al. [8]	2011/Taiwan	Retrospective/2003 to 2009	Overall mortality was 12.1 % ($n = 57/472$) and the 30 day mortality was 11.0 % ($n = 52/472$)	Eight independent predictors of mortality : liver cirrhosis, soft tissue air, Aeromonas infection, age > 60 years, band polymorphonuclear neutrophils >10 %, activated partial thromboplastin time >60 s, bacteremia, and serum creatinine >2 mg/dL
Yeung YK et al. [46]	2011/Hong Kong	Retrospective	Overall mortality was 28 % (total $n = 29$)	Renal and liver failure, thrombocytopenia, initial proximal involvement, and hypotension on admission were predictors of mortality in UL NF. The ALERTS (Abnormal Liver function, Extent of infection, Renal impairment, Thrombocytopenia, and Shock) score with a cutoff of 3 appeared to predict mortality.
Nisbet M et al. [47]	2011/New Zealand	Retrospective/2000 to 2006	Twenty-five (30 %) patients died, 17 (68 %) within 72 h of admission. Total $n = 82$	Independent predictors of mortality include congestive heart failure ($P = 0.033$) and a history of gout ($P = 0.037$)
Krieg et al. [48]	2014/Germany	Retrospective/1996 to 2011	[a]24/64(32.8 %)	Independent predictors of mortality were skin necrosis on the initial clinical examination (OR = 15.48; 95 % CI = 2.02–118.91) and acute renal failure (OR = 118.91; 95 % CI 7.66–5135.79)

Table 7 Summary of published studies of mortality in necrotizing fasciitis/NSTI patients worldwide *(Continued)*

Lee YC et al. [49]	2014/Taiwan	Retrospective/1996 to 2011	18/100 (18 %)	Unknown injury events, presence of multiple skin lesions, leukocytes < 10,000 cells/mm^3, platelets < 100,000/mm^3, serum creatinine ≥1.3 mg/dL, serum albumin < 2.5 mg/dL, and delayed treatment beyond 3 days post-injury were associated with significantly higher mortality. Treatment delayed beyond 3 days is an independent factor indicating a poor prognosis (OR 10.75, 95 % CI 1.02-113.39, *p* = 0.048)
Khamnuan P et al. [50]	2015/Thailand	Retrospective/2009 to 2012	*n* = 290/1504 (19.3 %)	Female gender; age >60; chronic heart disease, cirrhosis, skin necrosis, pulse rate >130/min, systolic BP <90 mmHg, and serum creatinine ≥1.6 mg/dL
Khamnuan P et al. [51]	2015/Thailand	Retrospective observational cohort study/2009 to 2012	165 (69.6) in patients with severe sepsis (*n* = 237) 66 (5.5) without severe sepsis (*n* = 1,215) *P* <0.001	Female sex, diabetes mellitus, chronic heart disease, hemorrhagic bleb, skin necrosis, and serum protein <6 g/dL
Arif et al. [52]	2016/USA	Retrospective/2003 to 2013	9871 NF-related deaths 4 · 8 deaths/ 1000000 person-yr	Diabetes mellitus, obesity, and renal failure were significantly associated with NF-related death. However, age, sex, and race were independently associated with the rate of NF-related deaths
Hadeed GJ et al. [35]	2016/USA	Retrospective/2003 to 2008	11/87 (12.5 %)	Clinically significant difference based on the timing of surgical intervention (< or > 6 h) (17.5 % in late vs. 7.5 % in early intervention group), however no statistical significance

[a] = Deaths/total NF cases

studies reported clostridial [32], beta-streptococci [33], aeromonas and vibrio [9] infections to be associated with poor outcomes.

Prompt and aggressive debridement is important for the management of NF. The debridement aims to remove all necrotic tissue until the local infectious process is treated. There is a positive correlation between the survival rate and early diagnosis with appropriate surgical debridement in NF patients [34]. In the present study, the median number of debridement procedures performed per patient was two interventions, and these were comparable for both non-survivors as well as survivors. Data suggested that early surgical intervention is crucial in reducing morbidity and mortality in NF patients [35]. However, there is still a lack of clear definition on 'How early should we be'. Kobayashi et al. showed significantly lower mortality in the early intervention group (within 12 h after diagnosis) [36]. Delay of surgical treatment of >12 h was associated with an increased number of surgical debridement, septic shock and acute renal failure [36]. Hadeed et al. [35] reported outcomes of earlier surgical treatment (within the first 6 h) and found that although there was no statistically significantly difference in mortality between the study groups, higher mortality among late intervention group was clinically significant. Moreover, the outcomes in terms of the duration of hospital and intensive care unit stay were in favor of early intervention [35].

The appropriate and early antibiotic use and intensive care measures significantly appear to affect patients' outcomes. In the past decades, patients with NF have higher mortality rates (up to 70 %), however, currently with improved surgical and intensive care treatment, mortality rates have declined to less than 30 % [37, 38]. Not only delayed diagnosis and surgical intervention influences in-hospital mortality, but also, the development of secondary complications has unfavorable impact [39]. The major complications that significantly related to mortality in the present series were bacteremia, septic shock and multiorgan failure. Therefore, appropriate prevention and management of such complications are vital for improving the outcome in these vulnerable patients [39].

Table 7 summarizes the published studies of mortality in NF and NSTI worldwide between 2000 and 2016. There is no consensus for specific predictors of mortality between these 20 studies including the current study. The design and objectives of studies as well as the availability of clinical and laboratory data are the main reason of the diversity of predictors of mortality among these studies. The present study has several limitations. It is retrospective in nature. It lacks information regarding the exact time of commencing antibiotics, delay in diagnosis, the timing of surgical debridement and the type of surgery performed post diagnosis. Also, the sensitivity and minimum inhibitory concentration of the bacteria and percentage of multi drug resistant strains is not available . Data describing the empiric antibiotic treatment in the emergency room is also not available for analysis. Moreover, procalcitonin has been introduced recently at HGH; therefore not all the NF in the past underwent procalcitonin assessment at admission. Further prospective studies are required to determine the time interval between the diagnosis and treatment which could possibly influence the mortality among NF patients.

Conclusion

The mortality rate is quite high as one quarter of NF patients died in the hospital. The present study highlights the clinical characteristics and predictors of mortality in NF patients. It is important to have a high index of suspicion at initial presentation. Use of prognostic tools in the daily clinical practice will help physicians for the proper on-time management. The present study provides useful information on the severity and outcome of NF patients that will inform institutional guidelines for the on-time treatment of NF.

Abbreviations

CRP, C-reactive protein; LRINEC, laboratory risk indicator for necrotizing fasciitis score; MAP, mean arterial pressure; NF, necrotizing fasciitis; NSAID, non-steroidal anti-inflammatory drug; SOFA, sequential organ failure assessment.

Acknowledgement

We thank all the surgical intensive care unit staff, Hamad General Hospital, Doha, Qatar. All the authors have read and approved the manuscript, and all have no financial issue to disclose.

Funding

This research did not receive any specific grant from any funding agency in the public, commercial or not-for-profit sector.

Authors' contributions

GJ: acquisition of data, writing manuscript and review of manuscript; AE: conception and design of the study, interpretation of data, writing manuscript and critical review of manuscript; RP: study design, helped to draft manuscript and review of manuscript; NS: acquisition of data, writing manuscript and critical review of manuscript; HA: study design, acquisition of data and critical review of manuscript; INM: acquisition of data, writing manuscript and review of manuscript; ME: acquisition of data, writing manuscript and critical review of manuscript; HA: conception and design of the study, writing manuscript and critical review of manuscript. All authors read and approved the final manuscript.

Competing interests

The authors declare that they have no competing interests.

Author details

[1]Department of Surgery, Hamad General Hospital (HGH), Doha, Qatar. [2]Clinical Research, Trauma Surgery, Hamad General Hospital, Doha, Qatar. [3]Clinical Medicine, Weill Cornell Medical School, Doha, Qatar. [4]Trauma Surgery Section, Hamad General Hospital, Doha, Qatar. [5]Surgical Intensive Care Unit, HGH, Doha, Qatar.

References

1. Puvanendran R, Huey JC, Pasupathy S. Necrotizing fasciitis. Can Fam Physician. 2009;55:981–7.
2. Yaghoubian A, de Virgilio C, Dauphine C, Lewis RJ, Mathew L. Use of Admission Serum Lactate and Sodium Levels to Predict Mortality in Necrotizing Soft-Tissue Infections. Arch Surg. 2007;142:840–6.
3. Roje Z, Roje Z, Matić D, Librenjak D, Dokuzović S, Varvodić J. Necrotizing fasciitis: literature review of contemporary strategies for diagnosing and management with three case reports: torso, abdominal wall, upper and lower limbs. World J Emerg Surg. 2011;6:46. doi:10.1186/1749-7922-6-46.
4. Magala J, Makobore P, Makumbi T, Kaggwa S, Kalanzi E, Galukande M. The clinical presentation and early outcomes of necrotizing fasciitis in a Ugandan Tertiary Hospital- a prospective study. BMC Research Notes. 2014; 7:476. doi:10.1186/1756-0500-7-476.
5. Kalaivani V, Hiremath BV, Indumathi VA. Necrotising Soft Tissue Infection- Risk Factors for Mortality. J ClinDiagn Res. 2013;7:1662–5.
6. Wall DB, Klein SR, Black S, de Virgilio C. A simple model to help distinguish necrotizing fasciitis from nonnecrotizing soft tissue infection. J Am CollSurg. 2000;191:227–31.
7. Wong CH, Khin LW, Heng KS, Tan KC, Low CO. The LRINEC (laboratory risk indicator for necrotizing fasciitis) score: a tool for distinguishing necrotizing fasciitis from other soft tissue infections. Crit Care Med. 2004;32:1535–41.
8. Huang KF, Hung MH, Lin YS, Lu CL, Liu C, Chen CC, et al. Independent predictors of mortality for necrotizing fasciitis: a retrospective analysis in a single institution. J Trauma. 2011;71:467–73.
9. Hsiao CT, Weng HH, Yuan YD, Chen CT, Chen IC. Predictors of mortality in patients with necrotizing fasciitis. Am J Emerg Med. 2008;26:170–5.
10. Vincent JL, Moreno R, Takala J, Willatts S, De Mendonça A, Bruining H, et al. The SOFA (Sepsis-related Organ Failure Assessment) score to describe organ dysfunction/failure. On behalf of the Working Group on Sepsis-Related Problems of the European Society of Intensive Care Medicine. Intensive Care Med. 1996;22:707–10.
11. Majeski J, Majeski E. Necrotizing fasciitis: improved survival with early recognition by tissue biopsy and aggressive surgical treatment. South Med J. 1997;90:1065–8.
12. Gunter OL, Guillamondegui OD, May AK, Diaz JJ. Outcome of necrotizing skin and soft tissue infections. Surg Infect (Larchmt). 2008;9:443–50.
13. Wang JM, Lim HK. Necrotizing fasciitis: eight-year experience and literature review. Braz J Infect Dis. 2014;18:137–43.
14. Dworkin MS, Westercamp MD, Park L, McIntyre A. The epidemiology of necrotizing fasciitis including factors associated with death and amputation. Epidemiol Infect. 2009;137:1609–14.
15. Elliot DC, Kufera JA, Myers RA. Necrotizing soft tissue infections: risk factors for mortality and strategies for management. Ann Surg. 1996;224:672–83.
16. McHenry CR, Piotrowski JJ, Malangoni MA. Determinants of mortality for necrotizing soft tissue infection. Ann Surg. 1995;221:558–65.
17. Lille ST, Sato TT, Engrav LH, Foy H, Jurkovich GJ. Necrotizing soft tissue infections: obstacles in diagnosis. J Am CollSurg. 1996;182:7–11.
18. Golger A, Ching S, Goldsmith CH, Pennie RA, Bain JR. Mortality in patients with necrotizing fasciitis. PlastReconstr Surg. 2007;119:1803–7.
19. Goh T, Goh LG, Ang CH, Wong CH. Early diagnosis of necrotizing fasciitis. Br JSurg. 2014;101:e119–25. doi:10.1002/bjs.9371.
20. Alva AM, Talwalkar SC, Shah N, Lee N. Necrotising fasciitis: a series of seven cases. Acta Orthop Belg. 2013;79:104–6.
21. Kao LS, Knight MT, Lally KP, Mercer DW. The impact of diabetes in patients withnecrotizing soft tissue infections. Surg Infect (Larchmt). 2005;6:427–38.
22. Cuschieri J. Necrotizing soft tissue infection. Surg Infect (Larchmt). 2008;9: 559–62.
23. Hasham S, Matteucci P, Stanley PR, Hart NB. Necrotising fasciitis. BMJ. 2005; 330:830–3.
24. Shaariyah MM, Marina MB, Razif MYM, Mazita A, Primuharsa Putra SHA. Necrotizing fasciitis of the head and neck: surgical outcomes in three cases. Malays J Med Sci. 2010;17:51–5.

25. Mao JC, Carron MA, Fountain KR, Stachler RJ, Yoo GH, Mathog RH, et al. Craniocervical necrotizing fasciitis with and without thoracic extension: management strategies and outcome. Am J Otolaryngol. 2009;30:17–23.

26. Pessa ME, Howard RJ. Necrotizing fasciitis. SurgGynecol Obstet. 1985;161: 357–61.

27. Urschel JD. Necrotizing soft tissue infections. Postgrad Med J. 1999;75:645–9.

28. Callahan TE, Schecter WP, Horn JK. Necrotizing soft tissue infection masquerading ascutaneous abcess following illicit drug injection. Arch Surg. 1998;133:812–7.

29. Wong CH, Chang HC, Pasupathy S, Khin LW, Tan JL, Low CO. Necrotizing fasciitis: clinical presentation, microbiology, and determinants of mortality. J Bone Joint Surg Am. 2003;85:1454–60.

30. Vosylius S, Sipylaite J, Ivaskevicius J. Sequential organ failure assessment score as the determinant of outcome for patients with severe sepsis. Croat Med J. 2004;45:715–20.

31. Elliott DC, Kufera JA, Myers RA. Necrotizing soft tissue infections. Risk factors for mortality and strategies for management. Ann Surg. 1996;224:672–83.

32. Anaya DA, McMahon K, Nathens AB, Sullivan SR, Foy H, Bulger E. Predictors of mortality and limb loss in necrotizing soft tissue infections. Arch Surg. 2005;140:151–7.

33. Childers BJ, Potyondy LD, Nachreiner R, Rogers FR, Childers ER, Oberg KC, et al. Necrotizing fasciitis: a fourteen-year retrospective study of 163 consecutive patients. Am Surg. 2002;68:109–16.

34. Wong CH, Yam AK, Tan AB, Song C. Approach to debridement in necrotizing fasciitis. Am J Surg. 2008;196:e19–24. doi:10.1016/j.amjsurg.2007. 08.076.

35. Hadeed GJ, Smith J, O'Keeffe T, Kulvatunyou N, Wynne JL, Joseph B, et al. Early Surgical Intervention And Its Impact On Patients Presenting With Necrotizing Soft Tissue Infections: A Single Academic Centre Experience. J Emerg Trauma Shock. 2016;9(1):22–7.

36. Kobayashi L, Konstantinidis A, Shackelford S, Chan LS, Talving P, Inaba K, Demetriades D. Necrotizing soft tissue infections: delayed surgical treatment is associated with increased number of surgical debridements and morbidity. J Trauma. 2011;71(5):1400–5.

37. Yilmazlar T, Ozturk E, Alsoy A, Ozguc H. Necrotizing soft tissue infections: APACHE II score, dissemination, and survival. World J Surg. 2007;31:1858–62.

38. Lee TC, Carrick MM, Scott BG, Hodges JC, Pham HQ. Incidence and clinical characteristics of methicillin-resistant Staphylococcus aureus necrotizing fasciitis in a large urban hospital. Am J Surg. 2007;194:809–12.

39. Yu C-M, Huang W-C, Tung K-Y, Hsiao H-T. Necrotizing Fasciitis Risk Factors in Elderly Taiwan Patients. Int J Gerontology. 2011;5:41–4. doi:10.1016/j.ijge. 2011.01.007.

40. Dahm P, Roland FH, Vaslef SN, Moon RE, Price DT, Georgiade GS, Vieweg J. Outcome analysis in patients with primary necrotizing fasciitis of the male genitalia. Urology. 2000;56(1):31–5. discussion 35–6.

41. Kwan MK, Saw A, Chee EK, Lee CS, Lim CH, Zulkifle NA, Saarey NH, Mohamad Hussien MN. Necrotizing fasciitis of the lower limb: an outcome study of surgical treatment. Med J Malaysia. 2006;61(Suppl A):17–20.

42. Mulla ZD, Gibbs SG, Aronoff DM. Correlates of length of stay, cost of care, and mortality among patients hospitalized for necrotizing fasciitis. Epidemiol Infect. 2007;135(5):868–76. Epub 2006 Nov 3.

43. Bair MJ, Chi H, Wang WS, Hsiao YC, Chiang RA, Chang KY. Necrotizing fasciitis in southeast Taiwan: clinical features, microbiology, and prognosis. Int J Infect Dis. 2009;13(2):255–60. doi:10.1016/j.ijid.2008.04.015. Epub 2008 Oct 15.

44. Kuo Chou TN, Chao WN, Yang C, Wong RH, Ueng KC, Chen SC. Predictors of mortality in skin and soft-tissue infections caused by Vibrio vulnificus. World J Surg. 2010;34(7):1669–75. doi:10.1007/s00268-010-0455-y.

45. Kao LS, Lew DF, Arab SN, Todd SR, Awad SS, Carrick MM, Corneille MG, Lally KP. Local variations in the epidemiology, microbiology, and outcome of necrotizing soft-tissue infections: a multicenter study. Am J Surg. 2011; 202(2):139–45. doi:10.1016/j.amjsurg.2010.07.041. Epub 2011 May 4.

46. Yeung YK, Ho ST, Yen CH, Ho PC, Tse WL, Lau YK, Choi KY, Choi ST, Lam MM, Cheng SH, Wong TC. Factors affecting mortality in Hong Kong patients with upper limb necrotising fasciitis; Hong Kong Society for Surgery of the Hand. Hong Kong Med J. 2011;17(2):96–104.

47. Nisbet M, Ansell G, Lang S, Taylor S, Dzendrowskyj P, Holland D. Necrotizing fasciitis: review of 82 cases in South Auckland. Intern Med J. 2011;41(:543–8. doi:10.1111/j.1445-5994.2009.02137.x. Epub 2009 Dec 4.

48. Krieg A, Dizdar L, Verde PE, Knoefel WT. Langenbecks. Predictors of mortality for necrotizing soft-tissue infections: a retrospective analysis of 64 cases. Arch Surg. 2014;399(3):333–41. doi:10.1007/s00423-014-1162-1. Epub 2014 Jan 11.

49. Lee YC, Hor LI, Chiu HY, Lee JW, Shieh SJ. Prognostic factor of mortality and its clinical implications in patients with necrotizing fasciitis caused by Vibrio vulnificus. Eur J Clin Microbiol Infect Dis. 2014;33(6):1011–8. doi:10.1007/s10096-013-2039-x. Epub 2014 Jan 14.

50. Khamnuan P, Chongruksut W, Jearwattanakanok K, Patumanond J, Yodluangfun S, Tantraworasin A. Necrotizing fasciitis: risk factors of mortality. Risk Manag Healthc Policy. 2015;8:1–7. doi:10.2147/RMHP.S77691. eCollection 2015.

51. Khamnuan P, Chongruksut W, Jearwattanakanok K, Patumanond J, Tantraworasin A. Clinical predictors for severe sepsis in patients with necrotizing fasciitis: an observational cohort study in northern Thailand. Infect Drug Resist. 2015;8:207–16. doi:10.2147/IDR.S85249. eCollection 2015.

52. Arif N, Yousfi S, Vinnard C. Deaths from necrotizing fasciitis in the United States, 2003–2013. Epidemiol Infect. 2016;144(6):1338–44.

18

New Trauma and Injury Severity Score (TRISS) adjustments for survival prediction

Cristiane de Alencar Domingues[1]* ⓘ, Raul Coimbra[2], Renato Sérgio Poggetti[3], Lilia de Souza Nogueira[4] and Regina Marcia Cardoso de Sousa[4]

Abstract

Background: The objective of this study is to propose three new adjustments to the Trauma and Injury Severity Score (TRISS) equation and compare their performances with the original TRISS as well as this index with coefficients adjusted for the study population.

Methods: This multicenter, retrospective study evaluated trauma victims admitted to two hospitals in São Paulo-Brazil and San Diego-EUA between January 1st, 2006, and December 31st, 2010. The proposed models included a New Trauma and Injury Severity Score (NTRISS)-like model that included Best Motor Response (BMR), systolic blood pressure (SBP), New Injury Severity Score (NISS), and age variables; a TRISS peripheral oxygen saturation (SpO_2) model that included Glasgow Coma Scale (GCS), SBP, SpO_2, Injury Severity Score, and age variables; and a NTRISS-like SpO_2 model that included BMR, SBP, SpO_2, NISS, and age variables. All equations were adjusted for blunt and penetrating trauma coefficients. The model coefficients were established by logistic regression analysis. Receiver operating characteristic (ROC) curve analysis was used to evaluate the performance of the models.

Results: The original TRISS (area under the curve (AUC) = 0.90), TRISS with adjusted coefficients (AUC = 0.89), and the new proposals (NTRISS-like, TRISS SpO_2, and NTRISS-like SpO_2) showed no difference in performance (AUC = 0.89, 0.89, and 0.90, respectively).

Conclusions: The new models demonstrated good accuracy and similar performance to the original TRISS and TRISS adjusted for coefficients in the study population; therefore, the new proposals may be useful for the assessments of quality of care in trauma patients using variables that are routinely measured and recorded.

Keywords: Wounds and injuries, Injury Severity Score, Traumatology, Outcome assessment

Background

The quality of trauma care is assessed by the Performance Improvement and Patient Safety (PIPS) Program, based on trauma records and severity indexes [1]. Several severity scoring systems are available; some are universally accepted and reviewed periodically in order to improve their accuracy. These include the Trauma and Injury Severity Score (TRISS), a tool well suited for the evaluation of the quality of care and to propose improvements in trauma care [2]. The predictive value of the TRISS can be maximized by adjusting for coefficients in the population in which it is being applied [3–8].

The TRISS comprises the Revised Trauma Score (RTS) and Injury Severity Score (ISS) indexes as well as the trauma type (blunt or penetrating) and the patient age. Although the TRISS is widely used, it presents limitations which involve, mainly, the RTS and the ISS [9, 10].

Currently, the RTS is difficult to calculate due to increases in the number of rapid-sequence endotracheal intubations performed in prehospital setting, an intervention that makes it impossible to determine the Glasgow Coma Scale (GCS) score and respiratory rate (RR) upon hospital admission, which are necessary for the calculation of the RTS. In addition, the RR is a physiological parameter that requires time to measure during the emergency care of trauma patients. Its normal range is very broad and abnormal values may not be directly related to respiratory function deficits [11].

* Correspondence: crismingues@gmail.com
[1]All Trauma, São Paulo, SP, Brazil
Full list of author information is available at the end of the article

Peripheral oxygen saturation (SpO_2) has gained a place as a respiratory parameter in emergency situations as it allows the evaluation of the tissue perfusion quality in trauma patients and is quick and easy to measure. Regarding the GCS, the literature proposes to replace the total score of the scale with the value of the Best Motor Response (BMR) item [12].

The ISS component has been criticized for not considering more than one lesion in each body region in its calculation, which may underestimate the severity [13–16]. The updated ISS, the New Injury and Severity Score (NISS), considered the three most serious injuries in calculating the severity of the trauma, regardless of the body region affected, thus seeking to increase the sensitivity of the index, as trauma patients can present multiple severe injuries in the same body region [13–16].

As a result of these criticisms, several proposals to modify the TRISS have been published; however, studies that replace the ISS by the NISS or which include the SpO_2 in its components are scarce [12]. The present study presents three new proposals—New Trauma and Injury Severity Score (NTRISS)-like, TRISS SpO_2, and NTRISS-like SpO_2. The first new variation (NTRISS-like) combines the physiological BMR parameters of the GCS, systolic blood pressure (SBP), and the anatomical variable of the NISS. The second and third variations include SpO_2. In the TRISS SpO_2, the RTS is replaced by GCS and SBP values and SpO_2 score; in the NTRISS-like SpO_2, the value assigned to SpO_2 was added to the NTRISS-like index.

Thus, the objective of this study was to compare the accuracy of three proposed variations to the original TRISS index with coefficients adjusted for the study population in predicting survival and to verify the viability of these new proposals as a replacement of the TRISS.

Methods

This multicenter, retrospective cohort study was performed in two reference hospitals for trauma care, one in the city of São Paulo, Brazil (SPBRA), and another in San Diego County, USA (SDEUA).

The study included 10,588 patients, 2416 hospitalized at the SPBRA emergency room and 8172 at the SDEUA trauma center for traumatic and/or penetrating traumatic events, aged 14 years or more between January 1, 2006, and December 31, 2010. The traumatic events were those listed in Chapter XX of the International Statistical Classification of Diseases and Health Related Problems (ICD-10), excluding cases of hanging, suffocation, drowning or near drowning, poisoning, burning, and electrocution. Patients admitted after the first 24 h of the traumatic event or transferred from other hospitals were excluded from the study since the calculation of survival probability by the models requires information from the patient's initial clinical condition.

A total of 300 patients from each of the institutions were randomly selected from the database (10,588 patients), which contained all the information required for the calculation of the indexes of survival probability; this Test Database was used to assess the accuracy of the models. Data from the other patients were grouped in the Derived Database and used to identify the coefficients of the proposed models (NTRISS-like, TRISS SpO_2, and NTRISS-like SpO_2), as well as to adjust the weightings of the TRISS to the study population for both blunt and penetrating trauma.

To ensure that the two hospitals had the same importance in the derivation of the coefficients, a weight of 3.72 was given to each of the SPBRA patients due to the disproportionate distributions of patients from this institution and SDEUA in the Derived Database (2116 versus 7872).

All models of survival probability compared in this study used physiological parameters obtained upon patient hospital admission and were calculated by the equation $Ps = 1/(1 + e^{-b})$, in which:

Ps, probability of survival
e, 2.718282 (base of the Neperian logarithm).
The values of b differed in all three models, as follows:
TRISS

$$b = b_0 + b_1(\text{RTS}) + b_2(\text{ISS}) + b_3(\text{age})$$

RTS, total value of the index (0 to 12)
Age, 0 if age < 55 years and 1 if age ≥ 55 years.
NTRISS-like

$$b = b_0 + b_1(\text{BMR}) + b_2(\text{SBP}) + b_3(\text{NISS}) + b_4 (\text{age})$$

BMR, value attributed to this item in the GCS (1 to 6)
SBP, value assigned to this parameter in the RTS (0 to 4)
Age, 0 if age < 55 years and 1 if age ≥ 55 years.
TRISS SpO_2

$$b = b_0 + b_1(\text{GCS}) + b_2(\text{SBP}) + b_3(SpO_2) + b_4(\text{ISS}) + b_5 (\text{age})$$

GCS and SBP, values assigned to these parameters in the RTS (0 to 4)
SpO_2, according to the following values, 0 or not measurable = 0; 1 to 80 = 1; 81 to 90 = 2; 91 to 95 = 3; 96 to 100 = 4
Age, 0 if age < 55 years and 1 if age ≥ 55 years.
NTRISS-like SpO_2

$$b = b_0 + b_1(\text{BMR}) + b_2(\text{SBP}) + b_3(SpO_2) + b_4(\text{NISS}) + b_5 (\text{age})$$

BMR, used the value attributed to this item on the GCS (1 to 6)
SBP, value assigned to this parameter in the RTS (0 to 4)

SpO$_2$, according to the following values, 0 or not measurable = 0; 1 to 80 = 1; 81 to 90 = 2; 91 to 95 = 3; 96 to 100 = 4.

Age, 0 if age < 55 years and 1 if age ≥ 55 years.

The coefficients of the proposed models and TRISS adjusted to the study population were derived by logistic regression. The diagnostic test receiver operating characteristic (ROC) was used to evaluate the predictive capacity of the new models and the original and adjusted TRISS.

Results

In the sample of 10,588 patients attended between January 1, 2006, and December 31, 2010, was a predominance of males (73.5%). Transportation accidents (44.1%), falls (30.3%), and assaults (18.0%) were the most common external causes. Blunt trauma mechanism was the most common (90.4%). A total of 2736 victims (25.8%) underwent surgical procedures and 4132 patients (39.0%) were admitted to the Intensive Care Unit. The patients remained hospitalized for an average of 5.4 ± 13.3 days and mortality was 5.9% (Table 1).

Considering the physiological variables, 82.8% presented a GCS score between 13 and 15; the mean SBP was 133.7 ± 31.7 mmHg, and the mean RR was 18.1 ± 5.2 breathes per minute. Peripheral oxygen saturation (SpO$_2$) presented an average value of 97.3 ± 8.9%. Only 459 (4.3%) victims did not present GCS or BMR values at hospital admission, and SBP information was missing from 0.9% of the study population. SpO$_2$ and RR data were missing from 29.6 and 8.3% of the victims, respectively. The mean RTS was 7.4 ± 1.4.

The patients presented a mean of 2.1 ± 1.0 injured body regions, the most commonly affected external surfaces being the head (1.6 ± 1.4 injuries) and neck (1.0 ± 1.4 injuries). The mean ISS and NISS values were 9.7 ± 9.6 and 12.8 ± 13.0, respectively. It was not possible to calculate the ISS and NISS in 48 victims (0.5%).

The coefficients for blunt and penetrating trauma of the new models (NTRISS-like, TRISS SpO$_2$, and NTRISS-like SpO$_2$) and adjusted TRISS are shown in Table 2.

Figure 1 shows the ROC curves of the new models. The curves of the three indexes overlap, indicating a similarity between them in the prediction of survival.

The accuracy of all models analyzed in this study was high (area under the curve above 0.89). In addition, the confidence intervals (CIs) of all areas under the ROC curve were similar (95% CI 0.85–0.94) (Table 3).

Discussion

Given the criticism of the component variables of the TRISS, the new proposals included GCS or BMR, SBP, and SpO$_2$ as variables in the models and excluded RTS and RR from the regression equation, as these parameters

Table 1 Descriptive statistics related to trauma and patient gender, age, and clinical variables. São Paulo–San Diego, 2006–2010

Variables	N (%)
Age (years), mean (SD)	41.9 (± 19.9)
Gender	
Male	7798 (73.5)
Female	2790 (26.5)
Mechanism of trauma	
Blunt	9570 (90.4)
Penetrant	1016 (9.6)
No information	2 (0.0)
External causes of morbidity and mortality	
Transportation accidents	4663 (44.1)
Falls	3203 (30.3)
Assault	1908 (18.0)
Intentional self-harm	216 (2.0)
Events with undetermined intent	205 (1.9)
Other	364 (3.4)
No information	29 (0.3)
Surgical procedure	
Yes	2736 (25.8)
No	7852 (74.2)
ICU admission	
Yes	4132 (39.0)
No	6456 (61.0)
Hospital discharge condition	
Survived	9962 (94.1)
Died	626 (5.9)
Hospital length of stay (days), mean (SD)	5.4 (± 13.3)
ISS, mean (SD)	9.7 (± 9.6)
NISS, mean (SD)	12.8 (± 13.0)

ICU Intensive Care Unit, *ISS* Injury Severity Score, *NISS* New Injury Severity Score

exclude the presumably more serious patients from the analysis of survival probability (intubated) [10, 17, 18]. A literature review of comparative studies of the original TRISS with modified models showed an improvement in TRISS performance when the RTS was removed from the model and replaced by the GCS, BMR, SBP, and RR parameters directly in the equation [12].

In view of the indications in the literature that the regression coefficients should be adjusted for the individual site, the results of the present study verified that the adjustment of the weightings to the study population improved the predictive capacity of the TRISS and that this capacity was maintained, as in other studies [6–19].

A literature review of studies that made adjustments to the original TRISS equation and compared the discriminatory capacity of the modified equation with the

Table 2 Coefficients of adjusted TRISS, NTRISS-like, TRISS SpO$_2$, and NTRISS-like SpO$_2$ derived from the Derived Database for blunt and penetrating trauma. São Paulo–San Diego, 2006–2010

Adjusted TRISS
$1/(1 + e^{-b})$, where $b = b_0 + b_1(RTS) + b_2(ISS) + b_3(age)$*

Coefficients	Blunt	Penetrating
b_0	− 1.64790049	− 1.29803310
b_1	0.90535734	0.89538700
b_2	− 0.07845091	− 0.09521947
b_3	− 1.38013670	− 1.27540759

NTRISS-like
$1/(1 + e^{-b})$, where $b = b_0 + b_1(BMR) + b_2(SBP) + b_3(NISS) + b_4 (age)$*

Coefficients	Blunt	Penetrating
b_0	− 1.67602650	− 1.58632944
b_1	0.61944706	0.58883203
b_2	0.89539814	0.96952677
b_3	− 0.07289039	− 0.06659814
b_4	− 1.33088941	− 1.00582810

TRISS SpO$_2$
$1/(1 + e^{-b})$, where $b = b_0 + b_1(GCS) + b_2(SBP) + b_3(SpO_2) + b_4(ISS) + b_5(age)$*

Coefficients	Blunt	Penetrating
b_0	− 2.97523446	− 3.5166820
b_1	0.75773826	0.8515884
b_2	0.58321377	0.3453793
b_3	0.38492625	1.3098071
b_4	− 0.08441861	− 0.1955984
b_5	− 1.59455370	− 4.0353761

NTRISS-like SpO$_2$
$1/(1 + e^{-b})$, where $b = b_0 + b_1(BMR) + b_2(SBP) + b_3(SpO_2) + b_4(NISS) + b_5 (age)$*

Coefficients	Blunt	Penetrating
b_0	− 2.73634921	− 1.5156694
b_1	0.59396868	0.1832071
b_2	0.66226833	1.0209288
b_3	0.56405908	1.1288631
b_4	− 0.06841853	− 0.1138697
b_5	− 1.43274160	− 1.7286860

BMR Best Motor Response, *SBP* systolic blood pressure, *NISS* New Injury Severity Score, *GSC* Glasgow Coma Scale, *ISS* Injury Severity Score, *SpO$_2$* peripheral oxygen saturation
*Age, 0 if < 55 years; 1 if ≥ 55 years

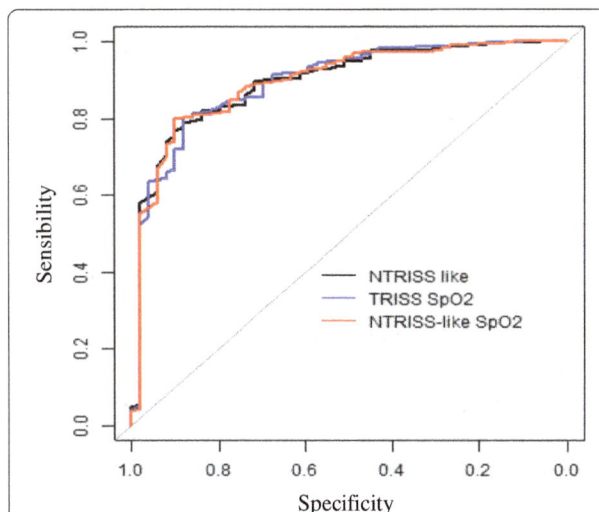

Fig. 1 ROC curves of NTRISS-like, TRISS SpO2, and NTRISS-like SpO2 in predicting survival. São Paulo–San Diego, 2006–2010

original in the prediction of survival showed that adjustments of the coefficients in the index equation were frequent. However, the results showed no trend of improvement in the performance of the models with this type of modification, with a performance improvement reported in only 30% of the analyzed studies [12].

The changes of physiological variables proposed in the new models did not increase the predictive capacity in comparison to the original and adjusted TRISS. The NTRISS-like model, a variation of the TRISS-like model that replaces the ISS was with the NISS, had a similar performance to TRISS. The TRISS-like model was introduced in 1992 [10] and includes only the BMR physiological parameters of the GCS and SBP in order to evaluate potentially more serious patients (intubated) in the calculation of the index; however, this model was criticized in the literature [11, 20] for removing the respiratory parameter from the evaluation of the survival probability. The TRISS-like model also showed a similar performance to the TRISS [10, 17].

The introduction of the SpO$_2$ in the NTRISS-like index (NTRISS-like SpO$_2$) did not improve the performance of the model, indicating that SpO$_2$ as an isolated adjustment did not increase the predictive ability of this model. A study that evaluated the role of the RR and SpO$_2$ in the mortality of trauma patients reported that these two parameters were not good predictors for this outcome when added separately to the TRISS equation (RTS with neutralized RR + ISS + age + RR or RTS with neutralized RR + ISS + age + SpO$_2$) [11].

Table 3 Predictive ability of original TRISS, adjusted TRISS, and new models. São Paulo–San Diego, 2006–2010

	Sens. (%)	Spec. (%)	Cutoff	CI 95%	AUC
TRISS	80.2	83.7	0.97	0.85–0.94	0.90
Adjusted TRISS	82.6	81.6	0.95	0.85–0.94	0.89
NTRISS-like	78.9	87.8	0.96	0.85–0.94	0.89
TRISS SpO$_2$	80.4	87.8	0.96	0.85–0.94	0.89
NTRISS-like SpO$_2$	79.9	89.8	0.97	0.85–0.94	0.90

Sens. sensibility, *Spec.* specificity, *CI* confidence intervals, *AUC* area under the curve

Proposals for replacement of the RTS by physiological parameters such as GCS, BMR, SBP, and RR in the equation resulted, in general, in an equivalent or better performance compared to the original TRISS [12]; in the present study, the substitution of different physiological variables in the models NTRISS-like, TRISS SpO_2, and NTRISS-like SpO_2 also resulted in an equivalent predictive value to that of the original TRISS.

Regarding the anatomical variable, replacement of the ISS by the NISS in the proposed formulas also resulted in a similar performance to that of the original TRISS and the new model that retained the ISS in the equation (TRISS SpO_2). Of four published studies [16, 21–23], which replaced the ISS by the NISS in the TRISS equation, only one [21] showed an improved performance of the index without this adjustment.

The ISS considers the three most serious lesions in different body regions of the victim [24], while the NISS [13] includes the three most serious lesions, regardless of the affected region. Due to the similarity of the performance of the proposed models using the ISS or NISS in the equations and the advantage of the ease of calculation of the NISS, this index is proposed in the survival models.

In this study, the original TRISS with adjusted coefficients and the new proposals had similar performances and accuracies between 89.0 and 90.0%. In the literature, the accuracies of the studies that showed no difference between the predictive power of the TRISS and the new proposals ranged from 85.3 to 96.4% [6, 11, 22, 25]. The studies in which the adjustments of the TRISS resulted in improved predictive ability presented higher accuracies, ranging between 90.1 and 98.1% [4, 6, 16, 25–28].

Although they do not improve the predictive accuracy of the TRISS, the models proposed in this study were equivalent and, given the clinical significance and ease of obtaining information from its components, seem to be good options to estimate the survival probability of trauma victims.

One limitation of this study is that the frequent loss (29.6%) of SpO_2 value may have negatively influenced the predictive capacity of the models that used this parameter (TRISS SpO_2 and NTRISS-like SpO_2). The inclusion of SpO_2 in these models had as a premise the improvement in the performance of the TRISS, considering a probable higher availability of this information compared to the RR and the potential of this parameter to contribute to the estimation of the severity of the physiological conditions of the patient.

Nevertheless, the frequent lack of SpO_2 data may have underestimated its importance in the survival prediction models. While SpO_2 is a procedure performed in emergency services, the results are not always registered; once the inclusion of this variable in the calculation of the indexes is established, the loss of these will likely decrease.

Although they were derived using the variable with the highest degree of data loss, the TRISS SpO_2 and NTRISS-like SpO_2 had equivalent predictive values to that of the other indexes. Thus, the two models that include SpO_2 may also be recommended due to the clinical ease in obtaining SpO_2 and its physiological significance, since they reflect both oxygenation and circulation, while the RR reflects only ventilation [11]. In addition, new analyses of the predictive ability of these adjustments should be made in databases with less loss of SpO_2 data and the new proposals should be validated in trauma systems at different levels of maturity, as well as in patients with penetrating trauma, since in this study this trauma mechanism was infrequent.

Conclusions

This study proposed adjustments to the TRISS, which resulted in three new models of survival probability for trauma victims: NTRISS-like, TRISS SpO_2, and NTRISS-like SpO_2. The new models demonstrated accuracies above 89.0% and similarity of performance among themselves. Moreover, they displayed similar discriminatory capacity compared to that of the original and TRISS adjusted to the study population. These results suggest the potential for professionals to choose a model of survival probability that involves variables that are routinely measured and recorded, as SpO_2. Most importantly, this PIPS tool meets service needs and is easy to use. Since all models have similar accuracy, one could choose the one that contains the variables that make the most sense to the local reality.

Acknowledgements
We thank Dr. Victor Alexandre Percinio Gianvecchio for his valuable contribution in allowing access to necropsy data in the Legal Medical Institute and all the professionals of the Trauma Center at the University of California San Diego, in particular, Dale A. Fortlage, for providing service data.

Funding
Cristiane de Alencar Domingues has received scholarship funds from Coordenação de Aperfeiçoamento de Pessoal de Nível Superior (CAPES).

Authors' contributions
All authors have made substantial contributions to all of the following: (1) the conception and design of the study, or acquisition of data, or analysis and interpretation of data, (2) drafting the article or revising it critically for important intellectual content, (3) final approval of the version to be submitted.

Competing interests

The authors declare that they have no competing interests.

Author details

[1]All Trauma, São Paulo, SP, Brazil. [2]University of California San Diego Medical Center, San Diego, CA, USA. [3]Medical School, University of Sao Paulo, São Paulo, SP, Brazil. [4]School of Nursing, University of Sao Paulo, São Paulo, SP, Brazil.

References

1. American College of Surgeons Committee on Trauma. Resource for the optimal care of the injured patient. Illinois: American College of Surgeons Committee on Trauma; 2014.
2. Champion HR, Copes WS, Sacco WJ, Lawnick MM, Keast SL, Bain LW Jr, Flanagan ME, Frey CF. The major trauma outcome study: establishing national norms for trauma care. J Trauma. 1990;30:1356–65.2.
3. Cinelli SM, Brady P, Rennie CP, Tuluca C, Hall TS. Comparative results of trauma scoring systems in fatal outcomes. Conn Med. 2009;73:261–5.
4. Bouamra O, Wrotchford A, Hollis S, Vail A, Woodford M, Lecky F. Outcome prediction in trauma. Injury. 2006;37:1092–7.
5. Kilgo PD, Meredith JW, Osler TM. Incorporating recent advances to make the TRISS approach universally available. J Trauma. 2006;60:1002–8.
6. Bergeron E, Rossignol M, Osler T, Clas D, Lavoie A. Improving the TRISS methodology by restructuring age categories and adding comorbidities. J Trauma. 2004;56:760–7.
7. Lane PL, Doig G, Mikrogianakis A, Charyk ST, Stefanits T. An evaluation of Ontario trauma outcomes and the development of regional norms for Trauma and Injury Severity Score (TRISS) analysis. J Trauma. 1996;41:731–4.
8. Millham FH, LaMorte WW. Factors associated with mortality in trauma: re-evaluation of the TRISS method using the National Trauma Data Bank. J Trauma. 2004;56:1090–6.
9. Moore L, Lavoie A, Turgeon AF, Abdous B, Le Sage N, Emond M, et al. Improving trauma mortality prediction modeling for blunt trauma. J Trauma. 2010;68:698–705.
10. Offner PJ, Jurkovich GJ, Gurney J, Rivara FP. Revision of TRISS for intubated patients. J Trauma. 1992;32:32–5.
11. Raux M, Thicoïpé M, Wiel E, Rancurel E, Savary D, David JS, et al. Comparison of respiratory rate and peripheral oxygen saturation to assess severity in trauma patients. Intensive Care Med. 2006;32:405–12.
12. Domingues CA, Nogueira LS, Sttervall CHC, Sousa RMC. Performance of Trauma and Injury Severity Score (TRISS) adjustments: an integrative review. Rev Esc Enferm USP. 2015;49:138–46.
13. Osler T, Baker SP, Long W. A modification of the injury severity score that both improves accuracy and simplifies scoring. J Trauma. 1997;43:922–5.
14. Brenneman FD, Boulanger BR, McLellan BA, Redelmeier DA. Measuring injury severity: time for a change? J Trauma. 1998;44:580–2.
15. Sutherland AG, Johnston AT, Hutchison JD. The new injury severity score: better prediction of functional recovery after muscoloskeletal injury. Value Health. 2006;9:24–7.
16. Domingues CA, Sousa RMC, Nogueira LS, Poggetti RS, Fontes B, Muñoz D. The role of the New Trauma and Injury Severity Score (NTRISS) for survival prediction. Rev Esc Enferm USP. 2011;45:1353–8.
17. Garber BG, Hebert PC, Wells G, Yelle JD. Differential performance of TRISS-like in early and late blunt trauma deaths. J Trauma. 1997;43:1–5.
18. Lane PL, Doig G, Stewart TC, Mikrogianakis A, Stefanits T. Trauma outcome analysis and the development of regional norms. Accid Anal Prev. 1997;29:53–6.
19. Voskresensky IV, Rivera-Tyler T, Dossett LA, Riordan WP Jr, Cotton BA. Use of scene vital signs improves TRISS predicted survival in intubated trauma patients. J Surg Res. 2009;154:105–11.
20. Champion HR, Sacco WJ, Hannan DS, Lepper RL, Atzinger ES, Copes WS, et al. Assessment of injury severity: the triage index. Crit Care Med. 1980;8:201–8.
21. Moini M, Rezaishiraz H, Zafarghandi MR. Characteristics and outcome of injured patients treated in urban trauma centers in Iran. J Trauma. 2000;48:503–7.
22. Aydin SA, Bulut M, Ozgüç H, Ercan I, Türkmen N, Eren B, et al. Should the New Injury Severity Score replace the Injury Severity Score in the Trauma and Injury Severity Score? Ulus Travma Acil Cerrahi Derg. 2008;14:308–12.
23. Fraga GP, Mantovani M, Magna LA. Índices de trauma em doentes submetidos à laparotomia. Rev Col Bras Cir. 2004;31:299–306.
24. Baker SP, O'Neill B, Haddon W Jr, Long WB. The injury severity score: a method for describing patients with multiple injuries and evaluating emergency care. J Trauma. 1974;14:187–96.
25. Kimura A, Nakahara S, Chadbunchachai W. The development of simple survival prediction models for blunt trauma victims treated at Asian emergency centers. Scand J Trauma Resusc Emerg Med. 2012;20:9.
26. Kimura A, Chadbunchachai W, Nakahara S. Modification of the Trauma and Injury Severity Score (TRISS) method provides better survival prediction in Asian blunt trauma victims. World J Surg. 2012;36:813–8.
27. Schluter PJ. Trauma and Injury Severity Score (TRISS): is it time for variable re-categorisations and re-characterisations? Injury. 2011;42:83–9.
28. Schluter PJ. The Trauma and Injury Severity Score (TRISS) revised. Injury. 2011;42:90–6.

19

Preventive transarterial embolization in upper nonvariceal gastrointestinal bleeding

Aleksejs Kaminskis[1*], Aina Kratovska[2], Sanita Ponomarjova[2], Anna Tolstova[1], Maksims Mukans[1], Solvita Stabiņa[1], Raivis Gailums[1], Andrejs Bernšteins[2], Patricija Ivanova[2], Viesturs Boka[3] and Guntars Pupelis[4]

Abstract

Background: Transarterial embolization (TAE) is a therapeutic option for patients with a high risk of recurrent bleeding after endoscopic haemostasis. The aim of our prospective study was a preliminary assessment of the safety, efficacy, and clinical outcomes following preventive TAE in patients with non-variceal acute upper gastrointestinal bleeding (NVUGIB) with a high risk of recurrent bleeding after endoscopic haemostasis.

Methods: Preventive visceral angiography and TAE were performed after endoscopic haemostasis on patients with NVUGIB who were at a high risk of recurrent bleeding (PE+ group). The comparison group consisted of similar patients who only underwent endoscopic haemostasis, without preventive TAE (PE– group). The technical success of preventive TAE, the completeness of haemostasis, the incidence of rebleeding and the need for surgical intervention and the main outcomes were compared between the groups.

Results: The PE+ group consisted of 25 patients, and the PE– group of 50 patients, similar in age (median age 66 vs. 63 years), gender and comorbid conditions. The ulcer size at endoscopy was not significantly different (median of 152 mm vs. 127 mm). The most frequent were Forest II type ulcers, 44% in both groups. The distribution of the Forest grade was even. The median haemoglobin on admission was 8, 2 g/dl vs. 8,7 g/dl, $p = 0,482$, erythrocyte count was $2,7 \times 10^{12}$/L vs. $2,9 \times 10^{12}$/L, $p = 0,727$. The shock index and Rockall scores were similar, as well as and transfusion – on average, four units of packed red blood cells for the majority of patients in both groups, however, significantly more fresh frozen plasma was transfused in the PE– group, $p = 0,013$. The rebleeding rate was similar, while surgical treatment was needed notably more often in the PE- group, 8% vs. 35% accordingly, $p = 0,012$. The median ICU stay was 3 days, hospital stay – 6 days vs. 9 days, $p = 0.079$. The overall mortality reached 20%; in the PE+ group it was 4%, not reaching a statistically significant difference.

Conclusion: Preventive TAE is a feasible, safe and effective minimally invasive type of haemostasis decreasing the risk of repeated bleeding and preparing the patient for the definitive surgical intervention when indicated.

Keywords: Nonvariceal upper gastrointestinal bleeding, Transarterial, Preventive embolization

Background

Rebleeding is one of the most serious complications of endoscopic haemostasis in patients with NVUGIB. The prevention of rebleeding is, therefore, crucial in the treatment of NVUGIB due to a considerable increase in mortality in case of failure.

Over the past two decades, TAE has become the first-line therapy for the management of upper gastrointestinal bleeding that is refractory to endoscopic haemostasis [1]. Despite conservative medical treatment or endoscopic intervention severe rebleeding occurs in 5–10% of patients, requiring surgery or TAE [2], and TAE has been increasingly used as an alternative to surgery in the upper NVUGIB refractory to endoscopic therapy. The method has been associated with a lower mortality and complication rate compared to surgery [3, 4]. Although early aggressive endoscopic haemostasis is generally the first choice of treatment in the cohort of patients who are at a high risk of rebleeding, additional methods of haemostasis may be needed to achieve a favourable outcome. Due to

* Correspondence: Aleksejs.kaminskis@aslimnica.lv
[1]Department of General and Emergency Surgery, Riga East University Hospital, 2 Hipokrata Str. Riga, Riga LV 1038, Latvia
Full list of author information is available at the end of the article

former evidence that in the situation of acute bleeding, it is not always possible to perform TAE successfully as an additional method of haemostasis, the preventive mode of TAE was proposed as one of the possible ways to achieve complete haemostasis, decrease the rebleeding rate, the need for surgical intervention, complications and mortality. A possible benefit of using TAE as a preventive measure in patients who are considered to have a high risk of rebleeding after endoscopic haemostasis has never been properly examined. One of the main arguments in favour of preventive TAE is speculation that rebleeding after a temporarily successful endoscopic therapy might be caused by an inadequate endoscopic treatment resulting in a residual arterial flow beneath the ulcer. In this subgroup of patients, preventive TAE performed shortly after endoscopic haemostasis is achieved, could result in a decreased rate of rebleeding and reduced mortality thereby [5]. The aim of our prospective study was a preliminary assessment of the safety, efficacy, and clinical outcomes following preventive TAE in NVUGIB patients with a high risk of recurrent bleeding after endoscopic haemostasis.

Methods

The preparation of the study included an analysis of the medical charts of 379 patients who were emergently admitted to the Riga East University Hospital with NVUGIB in the period from 2010 to 2013, (Fig. 1). The results suggested that the patients with NVUGIB who were at a high risk of rebleeding after emergent endoscopic haemostasis had Forrest I-IIb type of ulcer and the Rockall score ≥ 5. These two criteria were important for further grouping and inclusion of patients in the prospective study. Informed consent was obtained from the patients who underwent endovascular treatment. Preventive visceral angiography and TAE were performed on patients with acute NVUGIB who were considered to be at a high risk of recurrent bleeding after endoscopic haemostasis according to the evidence of Forest I-IIb ulcer and Rockall score ≥ 5 (PE+ group). The comparison group consisted of similar patients who underwent only endoscopic haemostasis, patients who did not agree to undergo preventive TAE with a similar prognosis of high rebleeding risk after endoscopic hemostasis and similar comorbid conditions (PE– group). The exclusion criterion was terminal end stage renal

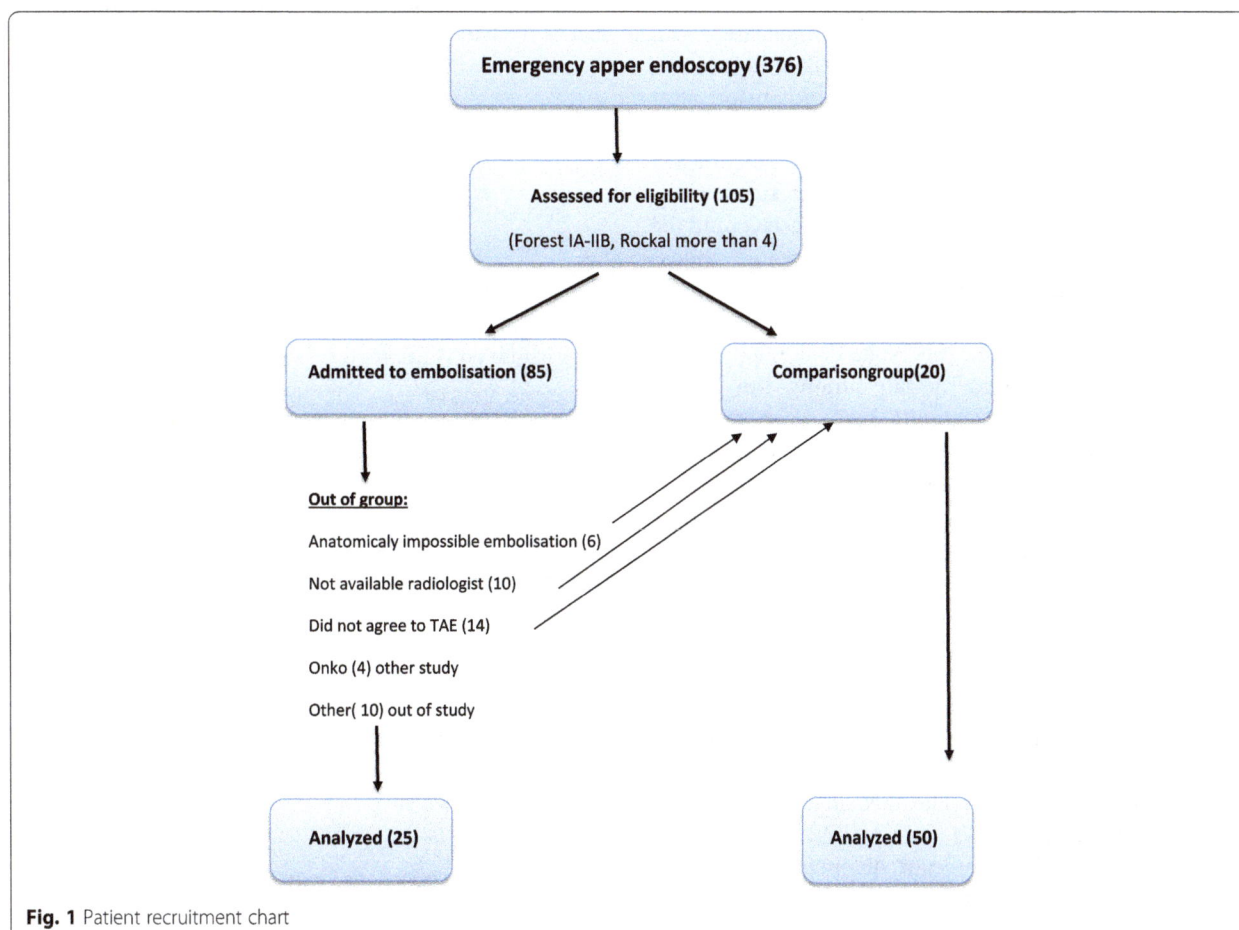

Fig. 1 Patient recruitment chart

disease. The participants were enrolled and assigned to their treatment by the consensus among the consultant surgeon, consultant radiologist and duty endoscopy specialist. Endoscopic combination therapy (injection of diluted adrenaline 1:10,000, treatment with a heater probe, and/or hemoclip) followed by a 72-h infusion of esomeprazole (80 mg bolus followed by 8 mg/h) was applied to all patients. Blood transfusion was given if haemoglobin was lower than 9.7 g/dl. Patients were closely monitored at ICU.

Technical approach

The technical goal was preventive embolization of the left gastric artery or the gastroduodenal artery (depending on the ulcer localization) within 24 h of endoscopic haemostasis, achieving a decrease of the arterial flow in the tissue beneath the ulcer. Usually, proximal embolization of the left gastric artery with coil and/or sandwich type TAE embolization of the gastroduodenal artery was used. In cases with the ulcer localized in the smaller or greater curvature or the gastric fundus – the left gastric artery was obliterated; in gastric antral, pyloric or duodenal ulcers – the gastroduodenal artery was embolized. Rebleeding was defined as a presence of hematemesis, blood from the nasogastric tube, or melena associated with a fall in haemoglobin of more than 0.8 g/dl (not explained by hemodilution) or arterial hypotension after primary endoscopy. If the therapeutic endoscopy were insufficient to comparison haemorrhage (technically difficult primary therapeutic endoscopy or signs of exsanguination), TAE or surgical haemostasis could be performed without being preceded by repeated endoscopy. The complication rate, recurrence of bleeding, and the need for repeat endoscopic therapy or surgery were the variables for the statistical analysis in groups. In-hospital mortality rate among the groups was analysed, and the patients who were excluded from the study. The study was approved by the local research ethics committee and followed the declaration of Helsinki [Helsinki declaration]. All authors had access to the study data and have reviewed and approved the final manuscript.

Results

During the 32-month period of inclusion 75 patients received endoscopic haemostasis for acute high-risk NVU-GIB and were evaluated according to the inclusion criteria. The PE+ group consisted of 25 patients, and the PE– group of 50 patients. The median age of patients was 66 years (IQR 74–57) vs. 63 (IQR 75–52) years without a statistically significant difference. There was no difference in gender and comorbid conditions, including the presence of cancer, liver and pulmonary

diseases, which were rare in both groups, Table 1. Endoscopic findings were not different, with the median ulcer size of 152 mm (IQR 400–79) vs. 127 mm (IQR 225–79). The bleeding site was similar in both groups. Gastric ulcer was the cause of bleeding in 52% of patients from the PE + group, and 54% of patients from the PE– group, $p = 0,870$. Duodenal ulcer was the cause of bleeding in 48 and 46% of patients respectively. The most commonly found ulcers were Forest II type in 44% of cases in both groups. The distribution of the Forest grade was even, Table 1. The median haemoglobin level on admission was 8,2 g/dl (IQR 11–7) vs. 8,7 g/dl (IQR 10–5,8), $p = 0,482$ and the erythrocyte count was $2,7 \times 1012/L$ (IQR 3,5–2,1) vs. $2,9 \times 1012/L$ (IQR 3,7–2,1), $p = 0,727$ including similar shock index and Rockall scores for both groups. The Rockall score values and shock index values were evenly distributed in the groups, Table 2. The use of anticlotting drugs in the groups was also similar, Table 3. Transfusion support was needed for the majority of patients, using, on average, four units of packed red blood cells (PRBC) in both groups and significantly more fresh frozen plasma (FFP) in the PE– group, $p = 0,013$. The rebleeding rate was similar, however, surgical treatment in patients who did not undergo embolization was needed significantly more often, 8% vs. 35,4%, $p = 0,012$. The median ICU stay was 3 days, and

Table 1 Patient characteristics

Variables	PE+ n = 25	PE– n = 50	p
Age, years, median (IQR)	66 (74-57)	63 (75-52)	0,393
Gender/Male, no. of patients	16 (64%)	34 (68%)	0,797
Comorbidities, no. of patients	18 (72%)	35 (70%)	0,858
Heart disease, no. of patients	13 (52%)	30 (60%)	0,509
Kidney disease, no. of patients	3 (12%)	6 (12%)	1,000
Liver disease, no. of patients	2 (8%)	4 (8%)	1,000
Cancer, no. of patients	1 (4%)	1 (2%)	1,000
Metabolic disease, no. of patients	4 (16%)	10 (20%)	0,763
Respiratory disease, no. of patients	2 (8%)	4 (8%)	1,000
Cerebral disease, no. of patients	6 (24%)	11 (22%)	0,881
Ulcer size, mm, median (IQR)	152 (400-79)	127 (225-79)	0,737
Forrest IA, no. of patients	5 (20%)	11 (22%)	0,937
Forrest IB, no. of patients	4 (16%)	7 (14%)	0,937
Forrest IIA, no. of patients	11 (44%)	22 (44%)	0,937
Forrest IIB, no. of patients	5 (20%)	10 (20%)	0,937
HGB, g/dl, median (IQR)	8,2 (11-7)	8,7 (10-5,8)	0,482
ERY, ×10¹²/L, median (IQR)	2,7 (3,5-2,1)	2,9 (3,7-2,1)	0,727
INR, ratio, median (IQR)	1,07 (1,25-1)	1,16 (1,34-1)	0,318
Shock index, median (IQR)	0,93 (1,2-0,67)	0,86	0,567
Rockall score, points, median (IQR)	6 (5-7)	6	0,608

Table 2 Median Rockall score and shock index

Scores	PE+ n = 25	PE– n = 50	p
Rockall score 3	3/12%	7/14%	1.000
Rockall score 4–5	4/16%	11/22%	0.761
Rockall score 6–7	13/52%	21/42%	0.412
Rockall score 8–9	4/16%	10/20%	0.763
Rockall score 10–11	1/4%	1/2%	1.000
Shock index 0,1 >	0/0	3/6%	0.546
Shock index 0,5 >	6/24%	12/24%	1.000
Shock index 0,7 >	9/36%	15/30%	0.600
Shock index 1 >	10/40%	20/40%	1.000

the hospital stay did not differ either, 6 (IQR 10–6) vs. 9 (IQR 11–6), $p = 0,079$. Mortality for all patients reached 20%, however, in the PE+ group it was 4%, though not reaching a statistically significant difference. The main outcomes are displayed in Table 4.

Discussion

Management of the upper gastrointestinal bleeding is still a challenge despite the recognized leading role of endoscopic hemostasis [6]. All improvements in the medical and endoscopic treatment are not sufficiently effective in treating the aging population with comorbid conditions that often has concomitant treatment with nonsteroidal anti-inflammatory or anti-clotting drugs [1]. The risk of rebleeding increases when Forest I-II ulcers diagnosed during endoscopic hemostasis is associated with different comorbid conditions and medication that interferes with the clotting system [7–9]. When rebleeding happens, several options are recommended – emergent repeated endoscopy, emergent TAE or surgical intervention [7, 10]. Preventive TAE is an additional option to decrease the rebleeding rate after an endoscopic hemostasis attempt. Nevertheless, the exact criteria for the selection of indications and strong evidence supporting the rational to use this method of hemostasis are insufficient [11]. Advances in catheter-based techniques and newer embolic agents, as well as the recognition of the efficiency of minimally invasive treatment options have expanded the role of interventional radiology in the management of hemorrhage for a variety of indications, such as peptic ulcer bleeding, malignant diseases,

hemorrhagic Dieulafoy lesions and iatrogenic or trauma bleeding [1, 6]. The technical aspects of TAE in the current study were performed following the recommendations described in the publication of Scandinavian authors, providing diagnostic angiography within 24 h of endoscopic hemostasis. The branches of the celiac trunk and the superior mesenteric artery, and the artery related to the peptic ulcer were identified according to the hemoclip placed during the endoscopic procedure. Microcatheter technique and coils were used routinely, and the blind technique in exclusive cases only [12].

Risk assessment

The assessment of the medical charts of the patients with acute NVUGI bleeding who were admitted to our institution revealed a group of patients who experienced rebleeding episodes after emergent endoscopic haemostasis. The most frequent endoscopic finding in this cohort was Forrest I-IIb type ulcers and the Rockall score ≥ 5. A further prospective study confirmed this observation complying with the reports from literature including the observation that the patient's age of over 60 years may be a risk factor. The other criteria, except for blood pressure and heart rate, like haemoglobin levels are reported as insufficiently sensitive in determining the severity of the upper gastrointestinal bleeding [13, 14]; however, patients from both groups who experienced rebleeding in our study had a median haemoglobin level of 8.2–8.7 g/dl before repeated haemostasis. The majority of reports emphasize that patients undergoing a transarterial procedure for the evaluation and management of haemorrhage are often poor surgical candidates due to the hemodynamic instability, comorbid conditions and coagulopathy [1, 7, 8]. In the current study, the patient condition in both groups was quite similar before repeated haemostasis, including the incidence of comorbid conditions, level of blood loss, shock index and coagulation status complying with the recommendations [1, 7, 8]. The total need for transfusion was not different among the

Table 3 Anticlotting agents

Drugs	PE+ n = 25	PE– n = 50	p
Anticoagulants	2/8%	5/10%	1.000
Antiaggregants	6/24%	13/26.5%	0.814
NSAID (excluding Aspirine)	3/12%	12/24%	0.359

Table 4 Main outcomes

Outcomes	PE+	PE–	p
ICU needed	25 (100%)	40 (82%)	0,024
ICU stay, days, median (IQR)	3 (3-2)	3 (5-2)	0,352
Transfusion needed, no of patients	22 (88%)	40 (80%)	0,524
PRBC, units	4 (5-3)	4 (5-2)	0,399
FFP, units, (IQR)	2 (2-2)	3 (4-2)	0,013
Surgery, no of patients	2 (8%)	17 (35%)	0,012
Re-bleeding, no of patients	3 (12%)	11 22,4%	0,358
Hospital stay, days (IQR)	6 (10-6)	9 (11-6)	0,079
Mortality, no of patients	1 (4%)	8 16,3%	0,258

groups, including the transfused amount of PRBC units, while significantly more FFP units were needed for patients who did not undergo preventive TAE. The strategy was preventive and the decision to perform prophylactic preventive TAE was the decision of the duty personnel in consensus with the consultant surgeon, consultant radiologist and duty endoscopy specialist. This strategy allowed to perform preventive TAE shortly after the inclusion criteria were established and indirectly supported the evidence that early TAE is associated with lower morbidity and mortality [2, 15, 16]. It is difficult to pinpoint the author of the idea of preventive embolization, however, a large part of clinical data and tactical recommendations are published by Scandinavian authors [1, 2, 15, 16]. The current study supports the reported positive experience with preventive TAE. Both patient groups were at a high risk of rebleeding after endoscopic hemostasis, and even if the ICU and hospital stay was not different, the need for surgical intervention was significantly higher in patients who did not undergo preventive TAE. Even more, mortality was also higher, albeit not significantly, probably due to a small sample size. The weak points of our study were the relatively small sample size and unpowered statistics. All the same, as in other reports, the uncertain selection of criteria for inclusion and the need for a larger cohort of patients were the weaknesses of the study. The advantages included the availability of the duty stuff for the definition of the inclusion criteria and the rather short time span for performing preventive TAE.

Conclusion

Preventive TAE is a feasible, safe and effective minimally invasive type of haemostasis, decreasing the risk of repeated bleeding and preparing the patient for the definitive surgical intervention when indicated. The availability of the duty stuff and the performance of TAE soon after the indications are defined increase the efficiency of the procedure.

Abbreviations
ICU: Intensive care unit; IQR: Inter quartile range; NVUGIB: Nonvariceal upper gastrointestinal bleeding; PE: Preventive embolization; TAE: Transcatheter arterial embolization

Acknowledgements
Not applicable.

Funding
No funding to declare.

Authors' contributions
AK, GP conducted the research/study, analyzed the data, and wrote the manuscript. AKr, SP, PI, AB performed the radiologic assessment and TAE. AT, MM, RG, SS conducted the research/study and analyzed the data. AK designed the study and interpreted the results. All authors have read and approved the final manuscript.

Competing interests
The authors declare that they have no competing interests.

Author details
[1]Department of General and Emergency Surgery, Riga East University Hospital, 2 Hipokrata Str. Riga, Riga LV 1038, Latvia. [2]Department of Interventional Radiology, Riga East University Hospital, Riga, Latvia. [3]Riga East University Hospital, Riga, Latvia. [4]Surgical Department, Riga East University Hospital, Riga, Latvia.

References
1. Loffroy RF, Abualsaud BA, Lin MD, Rao PP. Recent advances in endovascular techniques for management of acute nonvariceal upper gastrointestinal bleeding. World J Gastrointest Surg. 2011;3:89–100.
2. Loffroy R, Rao P, Ota S, De Lin M, Kwak BK, Geschwind JF. Embolization of acute nonvariceal upper gastrointestinal hemorrhage resistant to endoscopic treatment: results and predictors of recurrent bleeding. Cardiovasc Intervent Radiol. 2010;33:1088–100.
3. Eriksson LG, Ljungdahl M, Sundbom M, Nyman R. Transcatheter arterial embolization versus surgery in the treatment of upper gastrointestinal bleeding after therapeutic endoscopy failure. J Vasc Interv Radiol. 2008;19: 1413–8.
4. Wong TC, Wong KT, Chiu PW, Teoh AY, Yu SC, Au KW, et al. A comparison of angiographic embolization with surgery after failed endoscopic hemostasis to bleeding peptic ulcers. Gastrointest Endosc. 2011;73:900–8.
5. Laursen SB, Hansen JM, Andersen PE, Schaffalitzky de muckadell OB. Supplementary arteriel embolization an option in high-risk ulcer bleeding–a randomized study. Scand J Gastroenterol. 2014;49:75–83.
6. Andersen PE, Duvnjak S. Endovascular treatment of nonvariceal acute arterial upper gastrointestinal bleeding. World J Radiol. 2010;2:257–61.
7. Gralnek IM, Dumonceau JM, Kuipers EJ, Lanas A, Sanders DS, Kurien M, et al. Diagnosis and management of nonvariceal upper gastrointestinal hemorrhage: European Society of Gastrointestinal Endoscopy (ESGE) Guideline. Endoscopy. 2015;47:a1–a46.
8. Hearnshaw SA, Logan RF, Lowe D, Travis SP, Murphy MF, Palmer KR. Acute upper gastrointestinal bleeding in the UK: patient characteristics, diagnoses and outcomes in the 2007 UK audit. Gut. 2011;60:1327–35.
9. Biecker E. Diagnosis and therapy of non-variceal upper gastrointestinal bleeding. World J Gastrointest Pharmacol Ther. 2015;6:172–82.
10. National Clinical Guideline Centre (UK). Acute Upper Gastrointestinal Bleeding: Management. In: National Institute for Health and Clinical Excellence: Guidance. London: Royal College of Physicians (UK); 2012.
11. Beggs AD, Dilworth MP, Powell SL, Atherton H, Griffiths EA. A systematic review of transarterial embolization versus emergency surgery in treatment of major nonvariceal upper gastrointestinal bleeding. Clin Exp Gastroenterol. 2014;7:93–104.
12. Craenen EM, Hofker HS, Peters FT, Kater GM, Glatman KR, Zijlstra JG. An upper gastrointestinal ulcer still bleeding after endoscopy: what comes next? Neth J Med. 2013;71(7):355–8.
13. Barkun AN, Bardou M, Kuipers EJ, Sung J, Hunt RH, Martel M, et al. International Consensus Upper Gastrointestinal Bleeding Conference Group International consensus recommendations on the management of patients with nonvariceal upper gastrointestinal bleeding. Ann Intern Med. 2010;152:101–13.
14. Laine L. Upper Gastrointestinal Bleeding Due to a Peptic Ulcer. N Engl J Med. 2016;374:2367–76.
15. Loffroy R, Guiu B, D'Athis P, Mezzetta L, Gagnaire A, Jouve JL, et al. Arterial embolotherapy for endoscopically unmanageable acute gastroduodenal hemorrhage: predictors of early rebleeding. Clin Gastroenterol Hepatol. 2009;7:515–23.
16. Hoon Shin J. Refractory Gastrointestinal Bleeding: Role of Angiographic Intervention. Clin Endosc. 2013;46:486–91.

20

Proceedings of resources for optimal care of acute care and emergency surgery consensus summit Donegal

M. Sugrue[1*] [iD], R. Maier[2,3], E. E. Moore[4], M. Boermeester[5], F. Catena[6], F. Coccolini[7], A. Leppaniemi[8], A. Peitzman[9], G. Velmahos[10], L. Ansaloni[11], F. Abu-Zidan[12], P. Balfe[13], C. Bendinelli[14], W. Biffl[15], M. Bowyer[16], M. DeMoya[17], J. De Waele[18], S. Di Saverio[19], A. Drake[20], G. P. Fraga[21], A. Hallal[22], C. Henry[23], T. Hodgetts[24], L. Hsee[25], S. Huddart[26], A. W. Kirkpatrick[27], Y. Kluger[28], L. Lawler[29], M. A. Malangoni[30], M. Malbrain[31], P. MacMahon[32], K. Mealy[33], M. O'Kane[34], P. Loughlin[35], M. Paduraru[36], L. Pearce[37], B. M. Pereira[38], A. Priyantha[39], M. Sartelli[40], K. Soreide[41,46], C. Steele[42], S. Thomas[43], J. L. Vincent[44] and L. Woods[45]

Abstract

Background: Opportunities to improve emergency surgery outcomes exist through guided better practice and reduced variability. Few attempts have been made to define optimal care in emergency surgery, and few clinically derived key performance indicators (KPIs) have been published. A summit was therefore convened to look at resources for optimal care of emergency surgery. The aim of the Donegal Summit was to set a platform in place to develop guidelines and KPIs in emergency surgery.

Methods: The project had multidisciplinary global involvement in producing consensus statements regarding emergency surgery care in key areas, and to assess feasibility of producing KPIs that could be used to monitor process and outcome of care in the future.

Results: Forty-four key opinion leaders in emergency surgery, across 7 disciplines from 17 countries, composed evidence-based position papers on 14 key areas of emergency surgery and 112 KPIs in 20 acute conditions or emergency systems.

Conclusions: The summit was successful in achieving position papers and KPIs in emergency surgery. While position papers were limited by non-graded evidence and non-validated KPIs, the process set a foundation for the future advancement of emergency surgery.

Keywords: Emergency surgery, Optimal care, Performance indicators, Surgical outcomes

Background

Optimal consistent emergency surgery care presents a major health challenge worldwide [1–3]. Patients requiring urgent surgical care are often critically ill with significant pre-existing comorbidities [4]. While there is a wide spectrum of potential presenting surgical conditions, there is a predictable pattern because the top seven emergency surgery conditions account for nearly 80% of presentations [5]. Modern surgical care requires a multi-disciplinary approach and streamlined acute pathways are critical to ensure optimal outcomes [6].

Historically, it is not uncommon to manage emergency surgical patients interspersed with daily elective activities within a given hospital system [7]. The lack of timely appropriate access to emergency surgical care is often multi-factorial and may include shortage of emergency surgeons, inadequate access to the operating room, lack of a dedicated team, and a paucity of clinical pathways [8].

Over the past decade, the importance of a comprehensive system in managing emergency surgical care has become evident, resulting in training bodies and health

* Correspondence: michaelesugrue@gmail.com
[1]Department of Surgery, Letterkenny University Hospital and Donegal Clinical Research Academy, Donegal, Ireland
Full list of author information is available at the end of the article

ministries publishing multiple consensus papers and statements on this topic [6, 9–13].

Monitoring emergency surgery performance and outcomes is essential and clinicians themselves need to be involved in determining key performance indicators (KPIs). KPIs in emergency surgery have not been widely developed. For this reason, under the leadership of the World Society of Emergency Surgery, with support from the Abdominal Compartment Society and Donegal Clinical Research Academy key opinion leaders in the field of emergency surgery care across many disciplines were invited to contribute to a Performance Summit in Donegal in 2016.

The Emergency Surgery Performance Summit aimed to develop key performance indicators in clinical and systems delivery that would lay the foundation for future optimal surgery development.

Methods

Common aspects of emergency surgery were identified into 14 categories (Table 1), 44 key opinion leaders were invited to participate and co-author individual chapters. There were 14 position papers and 20 topics for KPI development (Table 2). A review of published articles and consensus statements relating to the establishment and design of emergency, acute care surgery, and emergency general services was performed. Emergency surgery position statements from the surgical colleges, surgical institutions and key government organisations were assessed. The key performance indicators were proposed according to a standardised pro forma (Table 3). Each KPI had to be easily measured and reproducible. Due to the extent and complexity of topics and number of authors, the original intent to grade level was not uniform and thus reporting was confined to consensus opinion.

Table 1 Key position topics for summit

Resources and designation of emergency surgery
Acute care unit structure
Reception and triage
Data systems, registry and evaluation
Rural emergency care and transfer
Paediatric emergency care
Geriatric emergency care
Interaction and laboratory, radiology, ICU gastroenterology
Quality assurance and performance improvement
Sepsis control in emergency room
Research in acute care surgery
Education in emergency surgery
Accreditation review and consultative program
Patient related outcomes measures

Table 2 Key performance indicators topics

Appendicitis
Cholecystitis
Pancreatitis
Perforated ulcer
Gastrointestinal bleeding
Bowel obstruction
Diverticulitis
Mesenteric ischaemia
Abdominal vascular emergencies
Coagulation
Complex pneumothorax and empyema
Septic shock in emergency; ICU
Fluid resuscitation in septic shock
Abdominal compartment syndrome
Geriatric care
Triage; ICU admission
Laboratory
Wound care
Emergency theatre
Health care systems

Results

The summit was held in Lough Eske Castle Donegal Ireland on 25 July 2016, attended by 80 people of which 44 contributed to writing the Proceeding's chapters, and associated KPIs. The key opinion leaders were from seven disciplines, predominantly surgery, but also including critical care, internal medicine, emergency medicine, radiology and nursing. There were 119 KPIs

Table 3 Example of KPI of 1 of the 112 KPI generated

Title	Negative appendectomy rate
Description	Percentage of negative appendectomies performed
Rationale	It is an indicator of diagnostic efficiency. In order to avoid unnecessary surgery and decrease costs and complications.
Target	< 10% appendixes removed are normal
KPI collection frequency	Annually
KPI reporting frequency	Annually
KPI calculation	Numerator divided by denominator expressed as a percentage Numerator: number of patients underwent appendectomy with negative appendectomy Denominator: number of all patients underwent appendectomy
Reporting aggregation	Hospital, hospital group
Data source(s)	OR registry, medical records, patients chart, hospital discharge data, emergency surgery database

described for the 20 conditions, a sample is shown in Table 3. The entire proceedings for the summit are available on line [14]. The summit provided a platform for discussion and agreed consensus on the key position topics. Future resources for advancing systems, clinical care, research and reporting were debated and supported. Consensus was reached that the KPIs for use in emergency surgery care needed to be simple, with a small number for each major condition.

Discussion

Globally, there is increasing interest in improving emergency surgery outcomes by health providers, learned societies, colleges and health departments [15–17]. Over a decade ago, it was estimated that more than 230 million surgical procedures were performed and within that workload, emergency general surgery accounts for a significant part [18]. In addition, emergency surgery has one of the greatest overall associated mortalities of any medical discipline [19]. It is estimated that 890,000 patients die during their emergency surgical care annually [20]. Patients undergoing laparotomy have variable mortality depending on their diagnosis, treatment and location of service provision [1, 2, 4, 21]. The American College of Surgeons National Surgical Quality Improvement Program database identified that emergency surgery patients have significantly more postoperative complications (23 vs 14%; $P < .0001$) as well as greater mortality rates (6 vs 1%; $P < .0001$) compared with non-emergency general surgery patients [22]. Ingraham recently reported that an expert panel ranked quality indicators in certain emergency surgery conditions [23]. They reviewed historic compliance with select quality indicators for four procedures (cholecystectomy, appendectomy, colectomy, small bowel resection) at four academic centres and concluded that potential adherence to quality indicators may improve the quality of emergency general surgery care provided for which current outcomes are potentially modifiable [23]. The summit reported KPIs in a much larger group, incorporating 20 conditions and sectors of health care provision.

To improve outcomes, we must not just develop quality benchmarks and standards but also understand prevalence and significance of complications [24, 25]. While there are limitations to many new systems being developed [26, 27]. It is only through engagement with all the disciplines involved in emergency surgery that care will evolve and improve. The Donegal Summit on resources for optimal care included not just surgeons, but also emergency physicians, anaesthetists, critical care, internal medicine, gastroenterology, radiology and nursing. While the summit developed and reported potential key performance indicators and outlines of basic resources required for functioning part of emergency

surgery systems, it had limitations. There was inadequate patient forum representation. The process was consensus-based and did not use a formal statistical or Delphi approach for the development of KPIs. The KPIs would in time need to be validated.

The summit and this proceedings paper have however set a process in place to facilitate concepts and benchmarks in resourcing emergency surgery. It has mirrored that international desire to improve outcomes [24].

Over the last decade there has been increasing development of Acute Care Surgical Units. Some of these have developed and reported limited KPIs [7]. Trauma care has been to the forefront of KPI development in acute care. In other areas of surgery, KPIs are widely reported. This summit was unique in having many key opinion leaders in attendance and discussing the process.

Conclusion

In conclusion, the Summit on Resources for Optimal Care of Acute Care and Emergency Surgery Consensus Summit successfully identified key aspects of emergency surgery that need to be tackled to outline optimal strategy of care and definitive KPIs. Future work needs to expand on the work achieved here and in other forums, to define optimum care and robust, meaningful measurement tools of process and outcome. The WSES will lead the process in standardised KPI development. The summit acknowledged superb efforts to enhance emergency surgery care by others but felt an international collaboration and commitment was needed to implement and monitor these systems as soon as possible.

Acknowledgements
World Society of Emergency Surgery. World Society of Abdominal Compartment. Donegal Clinical Research Academy. A project supported by the EU's INERREGVA Programme managed by the Special EU Programmes Body (SEUPB).

Funding
Donegal Clinical Research Academy. It donated 10,000 euros to help run the meeting and had no influence on outcomes.

Authors' contributions
Each author contributed to writing a chapter on either position statement or key performance indicators. All authors read and approved the final manuscript.

Competing interests
Michael Sugrue Consultant Smith and Nephew. Jan J. De Waele—consultancy for Cubist, AtoxBio, Pfizer, Smith & Nephew, KCI, Bayer Healthcare and MSD.

Author details

[1]Department of Surgery, Letterkenny University Hospital and Donegal Clinical Research Academy, Donegal, Ireland. [2]Department of Surgery, University of Washington, Seattle, USA. [3]Harborview Medical Center, Seattle, USA. [4]University of Colorado, Denver, USA. [5]Department of Surgery, Academic Medical Center, Amsterdam, Netherlands. [6]Department of Emergency Surgery, Maggiore Hospital, Parma, Italy. [7]Department of Emergency, General and Transplant Surgery, Papa Giovanni XXIII Hospital, Bergamo, Italy. [8]Abdominal Center, University Hospital Meilahti, Helsinki, Finland. [9]Department of Surgery, University of Pittsburgh School of Medicine, Pittsburgh, PA, USA. [10]Department of Trauma, Emergency Surgery and Surgical Critical Care, Massachusetts General Hospital, Boston, MA, USA. [11]General Surgery Department, Papa Giovanni XXIII Hospital, Bergamo, Italy. [12]Department of Surgery, College of Medicine and Health Sciences, UAE University, Al-Ain, United Arab Emirates. [13]Department of Surgery, St. Luke's Hospital, Kilkenny, Ireland. [14]Department of Surgery, John Hunter Hospital, Newcastle, NSW, Australia. [15]Acute Care Surgery, The Queens Medical Center, Honolulu, HI, USA. [16]Department of Surgery, Uniformed Services University and Walter Reed National Military Medical Center, Bethesda, MD, USA. [17]Department of Trauma/Critical Care, Massachusetts General Hospital, Boston, MA, USA. [18]Department of Critical Care Medicine, Ghent University Hospital, Ghent, Belgium. [19]Maggiore Hospital of Bologna, AUSL, Bologna, Italy. [20]Letterkenny University Hospital and Donegal Clinical Research Academy, Donegal, Ireland. [21]Division of Trauma Surgery, Department of Surgery, School of Medical Sciences, University of Campinas, Campinas, Brazil. [22]Department of Surgery, American University of Beirut Medical Center, Beirut, Lebanon. [23]National Clinical Advisor for the Acute Hospitals Division, Health Service Executive, Dublin, Ireland. [24]Trauma Governance, UK Defence Medical Services, Lichfield, UK. [25]Department of Trauma and Acute Care Surgery, Auckland City Hospital, Auckland, New Zealand. [26]Department of Anaesthesiology, Royal Surrey County Hospital, Guildford, UK. [27]Department of Surgery, Critical Care Medicine and Regional Trauma Service, Foothills Medical Centre, Calgary, AB, Canada. [28]Department of General Surgery, Division of Surgery, Rambam Health Care Campus, Haifa, Israel. [29]Department of Radiology, Mater Misericordiae University Hospital, Dublin, Ireland. [30]American Board of Surgery, Philadelphia, PA, USA. [31]Intensive Care Unit and High Burn Unit, ZNA "Ziekenhuis Netwerk Antwerpen" Stuivenberg and ZNA St-Erasmus hospitals, Antwerp, Belgium. [32]Department of Radiology, Mater Misericordiae University Hospital, Dublin, Ireland. [33]Department of Surgery, Wexford University Hospital, Wexford, Ireland. [34]Department of Pathology, Altnagelvin Hospital, Londonderry, UK. [35]Department of Surgery, Altnagelvin Hospital, Londonderry, UK. [36]Milton Keynes University Hospital NHS Foundation Trust, Milton Keynes, UK. [37]Northwest Research Collaborative, Manchester, UK. [38]Division of Trauma Surgery, Department of Surgery, School of Medical Sciences, University of Campinas, Campinas, Brazil. [39]Department of Gastroenterology, Teaching Hospital, South, Colombo, Sri Lanka. [40]Department of Surgery, Macerata Hospital, Macerata, Italy. [41]Department of Clinical Medicine, University of Bergen, Bergen, Norway. [42]Department of Gastroenterology, Letterkenny University Hospital and Donegal Clinical Research Academy, Donegal, Ireland. [43]Department of Trauma Services, Memorial Hospital of South Bend, Indiana, USA. [44]Department of Intensive Care, Erasme Hospital, Université libre de bruxelles, Brussels, Belgium. [45]Department of Acute Hospitals, Health Services Executive, Dublin, Ireland. [46]Department of Gastrointestinal Surgery, Stavanger University Hospital, Stavanger, Norway.

References

1. Tan BH, Mytton J, Al-Khyatt W, Aquina CT, Evison F, Fleming FJ, Griffiths E, Vohra RS. A comparison of mortality following emergency laparotomy between populations from New York state and England. Annals Surgery. 2017;266(2):280–6.

2. The Second Patient Report of the National Emergency Laparotomy Audit (NELA) December 2014 to November 2015 July 2016 http://www.nela.org.uk/reports accessed 23 Feb 2017.

3. Santry HP, Madore JC, Collins CE, Ayturk MD, Velmahos GC, Britt LD, et al. Variations in implementation of acute care surgery: results from a national survey of university-affiliated hospitals. J Trauma Acute Care Surg. 2015; 78(1):60–7.

4. Tolstrup MB, Watt SK, Gögenur I. Morbidity and mortality rates after emergency abdominal surgery: an analysis of 4346 patients scheduled for emergency laparotomy or laparoscopy. Langenbeck's Arch Surgery. 2016;9:1–9.

5. Scott JW, Olufajo OA, Brat GA, Rose JA, Zogg CK, Haider AH, SalimA HJM. Use of national burden to defineoperative emergency general surgery. JAMA Surg. 2016;151(6):e160480.

6. Royal College of Surgeons in Ireland. Model of care for acute surgery: National Clinical Programme in Surgery [Internet]. RCSI; 2013. Available at http://www.rcsi.ie/files/surgery/20131216021838_Model%20of%20Care%20for%20Acute%20Surger.pdf. Accessed 12 Apr 2017.

7. Hsee L, Devaud M, Middleberg L, Jones W, Civil I. Acute surgical unit at Auckland City Hospital: a descriptive analysis. ANZ J Surg. 2012;82(9): 588–91.

8. Association of Surgeons of Great Britain and Ireland. Emergency general surgery: the future a consensus statement [Internet]. ASGBI. Available at http://www.asgbi.org.uk/consensus-statements/ accessed 12 Apr 2017.

9. Sorelli PG, El-Masry NS, Dawson PM, Theodorou NA. The dedicated emergency surgeon: towards consultant-based acute surgical admissions. Ann R Coll Surg Engl. 2008;90:104–8.

10. Hameed SM, Brenneman FD, Ball CG, Pagliarello J, Razek T, Parry N, et al. General surgery 2.0: the emergence of acute care surgery in Canada. Can J Surg. 2010;53(2):79–83.

11. Royal Australasian College of Surgeons. The case for the separation of elective and emergency surgery [Internet]. RACS; 2011. Available at http://www.surgeons.org/media/college-advocacy/submission-to-the-council-of-australian-government's-expert-panel-on-the-case-for-the-separation-of-elective-and-emergency-surgery/ accessed 12 Apr 2017.

12. The Royal College of Surgeons of England. Separating emergency and elective surgical care: recommendations for practice [Internet]. RCSENG Professional Standards and Regulation; 2007. Available https://www.rcseng.ac.uk/library-and-publications/college-publications/year/ accessed 12 Apr 2017.

13. Professional Standards and Regulation Directorate: Royal College of Surgeons of England. Standards for Unscheduled Surgical Care: Guidance for providers, commissioners and service planners [Internet]. Publications Department, The Royal College of Surgeons of England; 2011. Available at: https://www.rcseng.ac.uk/library-and-publications/college-publications/year/ accessed 12 Apr 2017.

14. Resources for optimal care of emergency surgery Letterkenny 2016 978-0-09926109-9-9 Available http://dcra.ie/images/Resources_2016_Emergency_Surgery.pdf accessed 12 Apr 2017.

15. Royal Australasian College of Surgeon (2015) Position paper of emergency surgery. Available at: https://www.surgeons.org/media/311630/2015-05-20_pos_fes-pst-050_emergency_surgery.pdf accessed 5 Oct 2017.

16. General Surgeon Association of Australia (2010) 12-Point plan on emergency surgery. Available at: https://www.generalsurgeons.com.au/media/files/Publications/PLN%202010-09-19%20GSA%2012%20Point%20Plan.pdf. Accessed 5 Oct 2017.

17. Ministry of Health New Zealand (2011) Targeting emergencies: shorter stays in emergency departments. Available at: https://www.health.govt.nz/search/results/Targeting%20emergencies%3A%20shorter%20stays%20in%20emergency%20department. Accessed 5 Oct 2017.

18. Stewart B, Khanduri P, McCord C, Ohene-Yeboah M, Uranues S, Vega Rivera F, Mock C. Global disease burden of conditions requiring emergency surgery. BJS. 2014;101:e9–e22.

19. Tolstrup MB, Watt SK, Gögenur I. Morbidity and mortality rates after emergency abdominal surgery: an analysis of 4346 patients scheduled for emergency laparotomy or laparoscopy. Langenbeck's Arch Surg. 2017;402(4):615–23.

20. Scott JW, Olufajo OA, Brat GA, Rose JA, Zogg CK, Haider AH, Salim A, Havens JM. Use of national burden to define operative emergency general surgery. JAMA surgery. 2016;151(6):e160480.

21. Ogola GO, Haider A, Shafi S. Hospitals with higher volumes of emergency general surgery patients achieve lower mortality rates: a case for establishing designated centers for emergency general surgery. J Trauma Acute Care Surg. 2017;82(3):497–504.

22. Becher RD, Hoth JJ, Miller PR, Mowery NT, Chang MC, Meredith JW. A critical assessment of outcomes in emergency versus nonemergency general surgery using the American College of Surgeons National Surgical Quality Improvement Program database. Am Surg. 2011;77:951–9.

23. Ingraham A, Nathens A, Peitzman A, Bode A, Dorlac G, Dorlac W, Miller P, Sadeghi M, Wasserman DD, Bilimoria K. Assessment of emergency general surgery care based on formally developed quality indicators. Surgery. 2017;162:397–407.

24. Clavien PA, Puhan MA. Measuring and achieving the best possible outcomes in surgery. Br J Surg. 2017;104:1121–2.

25. Scarborough JE, Schumacher J, Pappas TN, McCoy CC, Englum BR, Agarwal SK, Greenberg CC. Which complications matter most? Prioritizing quality improvement in emergency general surgery. J Am Coll Surg. 2016;222(4):515–24.

26. Nathan H, Dimick JB. Quality accounting: understanding the impact of multiple surgical complications. Ann Surgery. 2017;265(6):1051–2.

27. Quiney N, Aggarwal G, Scott M, Dickinson M. Survival after emergency general surgery: what can we learn from enhanced recovery programmes? World J Surg. 2016;40(6):1283–7.

21

Circulation first – the time has come to question the sequencing of care in the ABCs of trauma; an American Association for the Surgery of Trauma multicenter trial

Paula Ferrada[1][*][†], Rachael A. Callcut[2][†], David J. Skarupa[3], Therese M. Duane[4], Alberto Garcia[5], Kenji Inaba[6], Desmond Khor[6], Vincent Anto[7], Jason Sperry[7], David Turay[8], Rachel M. Nygaard[9], Martin A. Schreiber[10], Toby Enniss[11], Michelle McNutt[12], Herb Phelan[13], Kira Smith[13], Forrest O. Moore[14], Irene Tabas[15], Joseph Dubose[16] and AAST Multi-Institutional Trials Committee

Abstract

Background: The traditional sequence of trauma care: Airway, Breathing, Circulation (ABC) has been practiced for many years. It became the standard of care despite the lack of scientific evidence. We hypothesized that patients in hypovolemic shock would have comparable outcomes with initiation of bleeding treatment (transfusion) prior to intubation (CAB), compared to those patients treated with the traditional ABC sequence.

Methods: This study was sponsored by the American Association for the Surgery of Trauma multicenter trials committee. We performed a retrospective analysis of all patients that presented to trauma centers with presumptive hypovolemic shock indicated by pre-hospital or emergency department hypotension and need for intubation from January 1, 2014 to July 1, 2016. Data collected included demographics, timing of intubation, vital signs before and after intubation, timing of the blood transfusion initiation related to intubation, and outcomes.

Results: From 440 patients that met inclusion criteria, 245 (55.7%) received intravenous blood product resuscitation first (CAB), and 195 (44.3%) were intubated before any resuscitation was started (ABC). There was no difference in ISS, mechanism, or comorbidities. Those intubated prior to receiving transfusion had a lower GCS than those with transfusion initiation prior to intubation (ABC: 4, CAB:9, $p = 0.005$). Although mortality was high in both groups, there was no statistically significant difference (CAB 47% and ABC 50%). In multivariate analysis, initial SBP and initial GCS were the only independent predictors of death.

Conclusion: The current study highlights that many trauma centers are already initiating circulation first prior to intubation when treating hypovolemic shock (CAB), even in patients with a low GCS. This practice was not associated with an increased mortality. Further prospective investigation is warranted.

Trial registration: IRB approval number: HM20006627. Retrospective trial not registered.

Keywords: Trauma resuscitation, Circulation first, Effects of intubation, Resuscitation in trauma, Trauma, Resuscitation, Circulation, Hypovolemia and hypotension, Hypotension in trauma, Hypotension and resuscitation

* Correspondence: pferrada@mcvh-vcu.edu
[†]Equal contributors
[1]Trauma, Emergency surgery and Critical Care, Virginia Commonwealth University, 417 N 11th St, Richmond, VA 23298, Richmond, VA 23298-0454, USA
Full list of author information is available at the end of the article

Background

The evidence supporting the systematic Airway, Breathing, and Circulation (ABC) approach to injured patients is based on expert consensus with little literature to support the clinical application of the order in which this sequence should be applied [1]. Early intubation can result in deleterious effects in adult and pediatric patients with traumatic brain injury [2–6]. There are many physiological explanations why intubation in hypovolemic shock might result in worse perfusion [2–6]. After rapid sequence intubation (RSI), there is a vasodilatory response placing the hypovolemic patient at very high risk for more pronounced hypotension and decreased perfusion [7–11]. Shafi et al. previously published an analysis of the national trauma data bank showing how pre-hospital intubations resulted in further hypotension in hypovolemic patients [12]. In addition to the vasodilation following RSI, positive pressure ventilation decreases venous return and therefore cardiac output resulting in further decreased perfusion [13]. This event is critical in hypovolemic patients that are dependent on venous return and adrenergic response to maintain perfusion [14–17].

In the medical literature, while treating patients with cardiorespiratory arrest, the focus of the protocols have moved from acquiring an airway first, to prioritizing perfusion by initiating chest compressions expeditiously [14, 15, 18, 19]. This has resulted in better outcomes [14, 15, 18, 19]. This practice has not been previously investigated in the trauma population.

The objective of this study is to investigate if there are differences in outcome when following the traditional sequence of ABC versus starting transfusion and resuscitation first (CAB). We hypothesized that patients in hypovolemic shock would have at least comparable outcomes with initiation of bleeding treatment (transfusion) prior to intubation, compared to those patients treated with the traditional ABC sequence.

Methods

The present study was sponsored by the American Association for the Surgery of Trauma (AAST) multicenter trials committee, and 12 level one trauma centers contributed patients to the study. The study was approved by the Institutional Review Board of each participating site. We performed a retrospective analysis of all patients that presented to trauma centers with presumptive hypovolemic shock (report of pre-hospital hypotension or confirmed hypotension on arrival to the emergency department) and required intubation in the trauma bay from January 1, 2014 to July 1, 2016.

Data collected included demographics, comorbidities (hypertension, chronic obstructive pulmonary disease, history of stroke, congestive heart failure, diabetes, chronic renal failure, others), pre-hospital intravenous fluids, timing of intubation, vital signs before and after intubation, and the order of initiation of blood products to intubation. Patients were classified in the ABC group if they were intubated before packed red blood cell transfusion was started. Patients were considered in the CBA group if transfusion was begun before intubation medications were given. Massive transfusion was defined as receiving 10 units of packed red blood cells in the first 24 h. Univariate and multivariate predictors of mortality were determined using mixed effects logistic regression controlling for center effect. Univariate predictors at the $p < 0.05$ level of significance and clinically significant variables were considered in the multivariate models. Subset analysis was performed of all patients with a confirmed systolic blood pressure of 90 mmHg or less in the emergency department prior to intubation, penetrating mechanism, initial GCS < =8, and need for massive transfusion. Continuous variables are reported as medians (interquartile range). All analyses were conducted with STATA v14.2 (College Station, TX).

Results

Twelve centers were included in the study, including an international trauma program. During the study period, 440 patients met inclusion criteria of either a reported hypotensive episode in the field or confirmed hypotension in the emergency department and need for intubation. The cohort median age was 39 (26–54) with 33.6% suffering from penetrating mechanisms. The group was severely injured with a median initial emergency department SBP (systolic blood pressure) of 80 mmHg (59–98 mmHg), initial GCS 6 [3–14], and a median injury severity score (ISS) of 25 (16–38). Comorbidities were common with 42.1% of the cohort having one or more known comorbidities. Median hospital length of stay was 6 days [1–20]. Overall mortality was 49.1%.

The CAB group consisted of 245 (55.7%) who received intravenous blood product resuscitation first, and the ABC group, 195 (44.3%), representing those intubated before any resuscitation was started. There was no difference in age, ISS, mechanism, or comorbidities between the groups (Table 1). Patients in the CAB group had an average GCS of 9 compared with 4 in the ABC group, $p = 0.0005$ (Table 1).

The percentage of patients receiving pre-hospital IVFs (intravenous fluids) and the amount received were similar (CAB 500 mL vs. ABC 800 mL, $p = 0.13$; Table 2). The only difference in hemodynamic parameters prior to intubation was a lower initial emergency department diastolic blood pressure in the CAB group (48 vs 51 mmHg, $p = 0.03$). Pre-intubation SBP (systolic blood pressure) and DBP (diastolic blood pressure) were the same (Table 2). Although only half of the cohort had a

Table 1 Demographics of the CAB vs. ABC group

	n	CAB	ABC	p value
Median age (years, IQR)	440	41 (28–56)	37 (25–53)	0.26
Median ISS (IQR)	440	25 (16–38)	25 (17–38)	0.99
Penetrating mechanism	440	30.8%	35.5%	0.3
Hypertension	440	11.8%	10.6%	0.7
COPD	440	1.5%	2.0%	0.7
CAD	440	1.0%	3.3%	0.1
CVA	440	0.0%	2.0%	0.05
CHF	440	0.5%	1.2%	0.44
DM	440	5.6%	3.7%	0.33
CRF	440	0.0%	1.2%	0.12
Other comorbidity	440	33.3%	33.5%	0.98
No comorbidities	440	56.9%	58.0%	0.83
Initial GCS	434	9 (3–15)	4 (3–13)	0.0005

Abbreviations: *CAB* Transfusion prior to intubation, *ABC* Intubation prior to transfusion, *ISS* injury severity score, *IQR* Interquartile range, *COPD* Chronic obstructive pulmonary disease, *CAD* Coronary artery disease, *CVA* Stroke, *CHF* Congestive heart failure, *DM* Diabetes mellitus, *CRF* Chronic renal failure, *GCS* Glasgow coma score

Table 3 Outcomes of the CAB and ABC groups

	n	CAB	ABC	p value
Transfusion in first 24 h	440	62.1%	69.4%	0.11
Massive transfusion	440	34.4%	29.4%	0.27
ICU admission	440	72.8%	67.8%	0.25
LOS*	440	8 (0–22)	4 (1–20)	0.24
Mortality	440	47.7%	50.0%	0.63

*Median (interquartile range)
ICU Intensive care unit, *LOS* Length of stay

In mixed effects logistic regression controlling for center effect ($n = 416$ patients), initial GCS (OR 0.76, 0.72–0.80, $p < 0.0001$) and emergency department SBP were the only independent predictors of death (0.97, 0.96–0.98, $p < 0.0001$). Intubation before initiation of transfusion ($p = 0.13$) and emergency department DBP ($p = 0.17$) were not independent predictors of mortality. In the subset analyses of patients with confirmed initial hypotension (SBP ≤ 90 mmHg) in the emergency department, penetrating mechanism, initial GCS ≤ 8, or requiring massive transfusion, intubation before transfusion (ABC) was not an independent predictor of mortality (Table 4).

pre-intubation lactate obtained, there was no difference between the groups (Table 2). Following intubation, there was no difference in blood pressure or lactate between the two groups (Table 2).

Both groups had a similar percentage of patients that received blood transfusion overall (CAB 62.1% vs. ABC 69.4% $p = 0.11$) and there was no difference in those receiving massive transfusion (Table 3). There was no statistical difference regarding those surviving to ICU admission with 72.8 and 67.8% admitted initially to the ICU in each group (Table 3). The median LOS in the CAB was slightly longer at 8 days compared with 4 days, but the difference did not reach statistical significance ($p = 0.24$). There was also no statistically significant difference in mortality between groups (CAB 47% and ABC 50%, $p = 0.63$).

Discussion

For patients in extremis including those suffering cardiac arrest, airway, then breathing, followed by circulation have been the priorities established in resuscitative algorithms including the Advanced Trauma Life Support ATLS course. However, more recent data in non-trauma patients have found that prioritizing perfusion over airway has been associated with better outcomes in patients with a primary cardiac event [15, 18–20]. There are a number of potential explanations including the phenomenon of agonal breaths or gasping that happens

Table 2 Pre-hospital and emergency department fluids, vital signs, and labs

	n	CAB	ABC	p value
IVF pre-hospital	440	53.9%	55.1%	0.79
IVF volume pre-hospital (mL)	151	500 (250–1010)	800 (300–1800)	0.13
SBP initial	440	80 (50–95)	82 (62–99)	0.1
DBP initial	422	48 (0–64)	51 (25–68)	0.03
SBP pre-intubation	440	84 (54–101)	85 (62–99)	0.3
DBP pre-intubation	430	50 (0–66)	53 (0–76)	0.07
SBP post-intubation	439	92 (42–114)	90 (62.5–113.5)	0.53
DBP post-intubation	434	52.5 (20–73)	58 (32–79)	0.11
Lactate pre-intubation	222	0 (0–3)	0 (0–2)	0.5
Lactate post-intubation	325	3 (0–6)	2 (0–5)	0.12

All values represent medians (interquartile range)
Abbreviations: *IVF* Intravenous fluids, *mL* Milliliter, *SBP* Systolic blood pressure, *DBP* Diastolic blood pressure

Table 4 Independent predictors of mortality in subset analysis

	Subset of interest							
	Initial SBP ≤ 90		Penetrating		Initial GCS ≤ 8		Massive transfusion	
	(n = 302)		(n = 140)		(n = 246)		(n = 126)	
Variable	OR (95% CI)	p value	OR (95% CI)	p value	OR (95% CI)	p value	OR (95% CI)	p value
Initial SBP	0.97 (0.96–0.99)	< 0.001	0.99 (0.96–1.01)	0.456	0.98 (0.97–0.99)	0.008	0.97 (0.95–0.99)	0.008
Initial DBP	1.00 (0.99–1.02)	0.644	0.98 (0.95–1.02)	0.377	1.00 (0.99–1.02)	0.603	1.02 (1.00–1.04)	0.061
Initial GCS	0.77 (0.72–0.82)	< 0.001	0.65 (0.56–0.75)	< 0.001	0.57 (0.46–0.70)	< 0.001	0.79 (0.72–0.87)	< 0.001
ABC	0.57 (0.29–1.13)	0.108	0.79 (0.22–2.9)	0.721	0.57 (0.28–1.16)	0.120	0.52 (0.20–1.36)	0.183

in patients in extremis which has been shown to increase cardiac output and perfusion [21–23].

The idea of prioritizing circulation over airway in the trauma cohort has not been previously investigated. In part, this is difficult to study in a prospective fashion as it is well established that even brief periods of hypoxemia portend a poor prognosis in brain-injured patients or those with a secondary brain injury from cardiac arrest or profound hypotension [4, 20]. Most importantly, it is difficult in the first moments of emergency department evaluation to determine if a patient in extremis, especially a bluntly injured patient, has both significant bleeding and traumatic brain injury. However, the risk of intubation in hypovolemic patients is worsening hypotension which also has deleterious effects especially in the brain-injured patient.

During intubation, administration of sedative and neuromuscular relaxants result in vasodilation counteracting the very much needed adrenergic response keeping the patient in profound hypovolemic shock alive [7–11]. Even if a patient does not experience a hemodynamic collapse after this vasodilation, then the positive pressure ventilation can further decrease the venous return and cardiac output resulting in cardiac arrest [13, 17]. It is plausible that there may be a benefit to redefining the classic ABC sequence taught in ATLS for the patient felt to be presenting in shock as intubation and positive pressure ventilation can result in further physiological insult [24]. Prioritizing resuscitation, or at least not causing further physiological challenges, can be desirable to ensure perfusion [12, 24].

In this retrospective study, it was surprising with the emphasis on ABC in ATLS to find that the use of transfusion prior to intubation occurred in the majority of patients (55.7%). In a retrospective study, it is impossible to understand clinician decision making regarding why these patients were resuscitated with a CAB sequence rather than ABC. However, it is likely this is a reflection of the evolution of massive transfusion protocols and practices that have become wide spread in the last 5–10 years. It is now well established that time to initiation of massive transfusion protocols in those patients

suffering from hemorrhagic shock is a major determinant of outcome. As a result, it is now common place in level one trauma centers to have rapid and immediate access to blood products including some centers storing these products directly in the trauma bay or emergency department. This allows for extremely early initiation of transfusion without delaying intubation.

Our results have demonstrated that initiation of transfusion prior to intubation is associated with equivalent mortality outcome compared with the concept of airway first (ABC). It is plausible that those patients in the CAB group had more obvious signs of hypovolemic shock that were not possible to ascertain using retrospective data. Thus, transfusion was begun in rapid fashion which preceded intubation. In an effort to further elucidate if particular types of patients were more or less likely to benefit from CAB, multiple subset analyses were undertaken. There was no difference in outcome demonstrated for those with hypotension on arrival to the emergency department, those suffering an initial decreased GCS, penetrating trauma, or those receiving massive transfusion. The concept of simultaneous ABCs might not be possible in places where one provider is responsible for the entire care of a bleeding trauma patient [25, 26]. It also might not be clear for clinicians working in areas in which trauma is not a prevalent disease. Especially, since the international guidelines for trauma care traditionally teach that the sequence of ABC is life saving and should be followed systematically on the strict order airway, breathing, circulation [27].

Limitations

The present series has several limitations including the use of retrospective data; this fact can offer obvious bias. Extraction of data from medical records review did not allow identification of reasoning for transfusion before intubation. We aimed to include patients with hypotension due to hypovolemia, not patients with hypotension for other reasons such as pneumothorax, blunt cardiac injury, or pericardial tamponade.

Furthermore, pre-hospital vital sign records were not universally available, and therefore, patients were included in the study if they were called hypotensive in the field or had hypotension in the emergency department. Given that a number of patients were not hypotensive on arrival to the emergency department, a subset analysis of those with an initial SBP ≤ 90 mmHg was performed. These results remained unchanged compared with the entire cohort results. It was also not possible to determine the neurologic outcome of patients surviving to discharge, and therefore, we cannot determine if CAB had a negative impact on functional outcome.

The mortality rate of 47.7 and 50% for an ISS of 25 (median) is high for both groups due to the degree of injury and the rate of penetrating trauma (> 30% in both groups). Given the lack of inferiority of CAB compared with the ABC group for mortality outcome, early initiation of transfusion while not delaying intubation may have promise for improving trauma outcomes further. However, to ideally understand the true impact of intubation on hypovolemic patients a prospective observational trial needs to be developed to fully elucidate if CAB offers an advantage similar to that seen in medical patients experiencing cardiac arrest.

Conclusions

In this retrospective review, national and international centers are already addressing circulation first before airway in bleeding trauma patients. A prospective, multicenter trial should be the next step to understand the physiological challenges of intubation in hypovolemic patients.

Acknowledgements
We thank Jinfeng Han our research assistant and Luke Wolfe for performing a secondary review of the data. We want to acknowledge Carlos Brown for his participation in the study as a local investigator at the Dell Medical School, University of Texas at Austin

Funding
This project was not funded.

Authors' contributions
PF conceived the study. PF and RC wrote the manuscript. RC performed all the statistical analysis. All authors contributed with the patients as well as participated in the critical review of the manuscript. All authors read and approved the final manuscript.

Competing interests
The authors' declare no competing interests with the current work.

Author details
¹Trauma, Emergency surgery and Critical Care, Virginia Commonwealth University, 417 N 11th St, Richmond, VA 23298, Richmond, VA 23298-0454, USA. ²University of California San Francisco, San Francisco, USA. ³University of Florida College of Medicine, Gainesville, USA. ⁴John Peter Smith Hospital Network, Fort Worth, USA. ⁵Centro de Investigaciones Clínicas, Fundación Valle del Lili Hospital, Cali, Colombia. ⁶University of Southern California, California, USA. ⁷University of Pittsburg, Pittsburg, USA. ⁸Loma Linda University, Loma Linda, USA. ⁹Hennepin County Medical Center, Minneapolis, USA. ¹⁰Oregon Health & Science University, Portland, USA. ¹¹University of Utah School Medicine, Salt Lake City, USA. ¹²McGovern Medical School at the University of Texas Health Science Center at Houston, Houston, USA. ¹³University of Texas-Southwestern Medical Center, Dallas, USA. ¹⁴Chandler Regional Medical Center, Chandler, USA. ¹⁵Dell Medical School, University of Texas at Austin, Austin, USA. ¹⁶Shock Trauma Centre, University of Maryland, Baltimore, USA.

References
1. Thim T, Krarup NH, Grove EL, Rohde CV, Lofgren B. Initial assessment and treatment with the airway, breathing, circulation, disability, exposure (ABCDE) approach. Int J Gen Med. 2012;5:117–21.
2. Bochicchio GV, Ilahi O, Joshi M, Bochicchio K, Scalea TM. Endotracheal intubation in the field does not improve outcome in trauma patients who present without an acutely lethal traumatic brain injury. J Trauma. 2003;54(2):307–11.
3. Davis DP, Hoyt DB, Ochs M, Fortlage D, Holbrook T, Marshall LK, et al. The effect of paramedic rapid sequence intubation on outcome in patients with severe traumatic brain injury. J Trauma. 2003;54(3):444–53.
4. Karch SB, Lewis T, Young S, Hales D, Ho CH. Field intubation of trauma patients: complications, indications, and outcomes. Am J Emerg Med. 1996; 14(7):617–9.
5. Murray JA, Demetriades D, Berne TV, Stratton SJ, Cryer HG, Bongard F, et al. Prehospital intubation in patients with severe head injury. J Trauma. 2000; 49(6):1065–70.
6. Sokol KK, Black GE, Azarow KS, Long W, Martin MJ, Eckert MJ. Prehospital interventions in severely injured pediatric patients: rethinking the ABCs. J Trauma Acute Care Surg. 2015;79(6):983–9. discussion 9-90
7. Capuzzo M, Verri M, Alvisi R. Hemodynamic responses to laryngoscopy and intubation: etiological or symptomatic prevention? Minerva Anestesiol. 2010; 76(3):173–4.
8. Kovac AL. Controlling the hemodynamic response to laryngoscopy and endotracheal intubation. J Clin Anesth. 1996;8(1):63–79.
9. Min JH, Chai HS, Kim YH, Chae YK, Choi SS, Lee A, et al. Attenuation of hemodynamic responses to laryngoscopy and tracheal intubation during rapid sequence induction: remifentanil vs. lidocaine with esmolol. Minerva Anestesiol. 2010;76(3):188–92.
10. Pepe PE, Raedler C, Lurie KG, Wigginton JG. Emergency ventilatory management in hemorrhagic states: elemental or detrimental? J Trauma. 2003;54(6):1048–55. discussion 55-7
11. Rackelboom T, Marcellin L, Benchetrit D, Mignon A. Anesthesiologists at the initial stage of postpartum hemorrhage. J Gynecol Obstet Biol Reprod. 2014; 43(10):1009–18.
12. Shafi S, Gentilello L. Pre-hospital endotracheal intubation and positive pressure ventilation is associated with hypotension and decreased survival in hypovolemic trauma patients: an analysis of the National Trauma Data Bank. J Trauma. 2005;59(5):1140–5. discussion 5-7
13. Cournand A, Motley HL, Werko L. Mechanism underlying cardiac output change during intermittent positive pressure breathing (IPP). Fed Proc. 1947;6(1 Pt 2):92.
14. Olasveengen TM, Wik L, Steen PA. Standard basic life support vs. continuous chest compressions only in out-of-hospital cardiac arrest. Acta Anaesthesiol Scand. 2008;52(7):914–9.
15. Ong ME, Ng FS, Anushia P, Tham LP, Leong BS, Ong VY, et al. Comparison of chest compression only and standard cardiopulmonary resuscitation for out-of-hospital cardiac arrest in Singapore. Resuscitation. 2008;78(2):119–26.
16. Woda RP, Dzwonczyk R, Bernacki BL, Cannon M, Lynn L. The ventilatory effects of auto-positive end-expiratory pressure development during cardiopulmonary resuscitation. Crit Care Med. 1999;27(10):2212–7.

17. Downs JB, Douglas ME, Sanfelippo PM, Stanford W, Hodges MR. Ventilatory pattern, intrapleural pressure, and cardiac output. Anesth Analg. 1977;56(1): 88–96.

18. Iwami T, Kawamura T, Hiraide A, Berg RA, Hayashi Y, Nishiuchi T, et al. Effectiveness of bystander-initiated cardiac-only resuscitation for patients with out-of-hospital cardiac arrest. Circulation. 2007;116(25):2900–7.

19. Iwami T, Kitamura T, Kawamura T, Mitamura H, Nagao K, Takayama M, et al. Chest compression-only cardiopulmonary resuscitation for out-of-hospital cardiac arrest with public-access defibrillation: a nationwide cohort study. Circulation. 2012;126(24):2844–51.

20. Ewy GA, Zuercher M, Hilwig RW, Sanders AB, Berg RA, Otto CW, et al. Improved neurological outcome with continuous chest compressions compared with 30:2 compressions-to-ventilations cardiopulmonary resuscitation in a realistic swine model of out-of-hospital cardiac arrest. Circulation. 2007;116(22):2525–30.

21. Noc M, Weil MH, Sun S, Tang W, Bisera J. Spontaneous gasping during cardiopulmonary resuscitation without mechanical ventilation. Am J Respir Crit Care Med. 1994;150(3):861–4.

22. Xie J, Weil MH, Sun S, Yu T, Tang W. Spontaneous gasping generates cardiac output during cardiac arrest. Crit Care Med. 2004;32(1):238–40.

23. Yang L, Weil MH, Noc M, Tang W, Turner T, Gazmuri RJ. Spontaneous gasping increases the ability to resuscitate during experimental cardiopulmonary resuscitation. Crit Care Med. 1994;22(5):879–83.

24. Ruchholtz S, Waydhas C, Ose C, Lewan U, Nast-Kolb D. Working group on multiple trauma of the German trauma S. prehospital intubation in severe thoracic trauma without respiratory insufficiency: a matched-pair analysis based on the trauma registry of the German Trauma Society. J Trauma. 2002;52(5):879–86.

25. Mock C, Nguyen S, Quansah R, Arreola-Risa C, Viradia R, Joshipura M. Evaluation of trauma care capabilities in four countries using the WHO-IATSIC guidelines for essential trauma care. World J Surg. 2006;30(6):946–56.

26. Tabiri S, Nicks BA, Dykstra R, Hiestand B, Hildreth A. Assessing trauma care capabilities of the health centers in northern Ghana. World J Surg. 2015; 39(10):2422–7.

27. Mayglothling J, Duane TM, Gibbs M, McCunn M, Legome E, Eastman AL, et al. Emergency tracheal intubation immediately following traumatic injury: an Eastern Association for the Surgery of Trauma practice management guideline. J Trauma Acute Care Surg. 2012;73(5 Suppl 4):S333–40.

22

Triple diagnostics for early detection of ambivalent necrotizing fasciitis

Falco Hietbrink[1*] ⓘ, Lonneke G. Bode[2], Louis Riddez[3], Luke P. H. Leenen[1] and Marijke R. van Dijk[4]

Abstract

Background: Necrotizing fasciitis is an uncommon, rapidly progressive and potential lethal condition. Over the last decade time to surgery decreased and outcome improved, most likely due to increased awareness and more timely referral. Early recognition is key to improve mortality and morbidity. However, early referral frequently makes it a challenge to recognize this heterogeneous disease in its initial stages. Signs and symptoms might be misleading or absent, while the most prominent skin marks might be in discrepancy with the position of the fascial necrosis. Gram staining and especially fresh frozen section histology might be a useful adjunct.

Methods: Retrospective analysis of 3 year period. Non-transferred patients who presented with suspected necrotizing fasciitis are included. ASA classification was determined. Mortality was documented.

Results: In total, 21 patients are included. Most patients suffered from severe comorbidities. In 11 patients, diagnoses was confirmed based on intra-operative macroscopic findings. Histology and/or microbiotic findings resulted in 6/10 remaining patients in a change in treatment strategy. In total, 17 patients proved to suffer necrotizing fasciitis. In the cohort series 2 patients died due to necrotizing fasciitis

Conclusion: In the early phases of necrotizing fasciitis, clinical presentation can be ambivalent. In the present cohort, triple diagnostics consisting of an incisional biopsy with macroscopic, histologic and microbiotic findings was helpful in timely identification of necrotizing fasciitis.

Keywords: Necrotizing fasciitis, Early recognition, Triple diagnostics, Histology, Fresh frozen section

Background

Necrotizing fasciitis is a relatively rare disease, which describes a group of infections that comprises skin, soft tissue and muscle and swiftly can spread through fascial planes [1–3]. The disease can be rapidly progressive and can have devastating outcome with many patients not surviving the infection (up to 70 % mortality rate reported in past series) [2]. Early diagnosis followed by immediate and thorough surgical debridement of affected tissue is necessary to prevent mortality and curb the systemic effects from resultant sepsis. However, diagnosis in the early stages can be challenging [4, 5]. Patients with necrotizing fasciitis might be brought to the ICU because of their sepsis without known cause and later prove unresponsive to resuscitation therapy [6, 7]. In a systematic review, a close correlation between the percentage of

initially missed cases and the mortality rate in the presented cohort series has been described [8]. A 75 % mortality reduction has been reported if operated within 12 h after onset [9–13]. Moreover, a mismatch between external signs and affected fascia has been mentioned. Thus, early recognition, timely surgery and thorough initial debridement are mandatory for survival [6, 8].

Over the last decade, mortality rate has decreased to 20-40 % in reported series [14–17]. Some have attributed this to the improved awareness for necrotizing fasciitis at general practitioners and ED-physicians, probably due to the attention that has been given to this disease in medical journals and general media [18]. Due to this improved awareness, patients are presented to the different surgical specialties in more early stages of their disease. This is a challenge for the treating surgeon, as local signs can be minimal and only become more prominent as the disease progresses [19]. In these early stages of necrotizing fasciitis, triple diagnostics is suggested to be a

* Correspondence: F.Hietbrink@umcutrecht.nl
[1]Department of surgery, University Medical Center Utrecht, Utrecht, The Netherlands
Full list of author information is available at the end of the article

useful adjunct in obtaining a diagnosis [20]. We provide an algorithm that contributes in the early phases of these patients in which a fresh frozen section and Gram staining can be of paramount importance to the treating surgeon. Implementation of this algorithm was analysed.

Methods

Patients

A retrospective analysis was performed of all non-transferred patients, presented to the emergency department of the University Medical Centre Utrecht with suspected necrotizing fasciitis. Inclusion criteria were age >18 and incisional biopsy or operation performed under the suspicion of necrotizing fasciitis. No exclusion criteria were formulated. A waiver was granted by the Ethical Committee for retrospective data collection.

Comorbidity severity was scored according to the ASA (American Society for Anesthesiologists) classification. Patients are scored grade 1–4 in our hospital describing the pre-hospital situation, with the addendum that grade 5 and 6 (created for emergency surgery settings) are not used in our hospital as all critical ill patients will be in those categories upon presentation. Mortality was recorded.

Deep tissue pain, hypoesthesia, purple skin changes, ecchymotic changes of intact skin indicate neural and vascular involvement and signify the need for immediate operative intervention without biopsy [19]. All other patients undergo incisional biopsy. Macroscopic findings that are suggestive for necrotizing fasciitis are summarized in Table 1. Findings that are suggestive for necrotizing fasciitis in fresh frozen sections or Gram stain are listed (Table 1). Only few studies describe their results on triple diagnostics, which makes a meta-analysis of this procedure not possible [20, 21]. To endorse the usefulness of triple diagnostics in necrotizing fasciitis, we questioned in what frequency its use had led to an altered treatment strategy in our hands.

Triple diagnostics: macroscopic findings

When necrotizing fasciitis is suspected, an incisional biopsy over the most suspected area is obtained via an longitudinal or incision in the Langer lines [6, 22, 23]. Classical signs indicative for necrotizing fasciitis are swollen tissue, dull grey necrotic tissue, grey fascia, lack of bleeding, small vessel thrombosis, "dishwater"

pus, non-contracting muscle fibres and a positive "finger test" [24–26]. These macroscopic findings are pathognomonic and should prompt aggressive surgical debridement (Table 1). However, especially in the early phases of necrotizing fasciitis or immunocompromised patients, classical signs may not be present during biopsy at all or are present on a distant site from the external signs [27]. Merely oedema is no reason for thorough debridement. In these cases, triple diagnostics by biopsy might be an adjunct for both diagnosis and treatment. This was first coined in the early eighties for ambivalent cases of necrotizing fasciitis [19, 20]. Since then, it has been mentioned occasionally, but has not been given the place in diagnostics it deserves and even neglected in recent guidelines due to lack of large scale studies [26]. In ambivalent cases microbiological findings by urgent Gram staining and histopathological analysis by fresh frozen section of soft tissue should be obtained [6, 20, 22]. The sample should contain infected subcutaneous tissue, fascia and muscle of the affected area.

Triple diagnostics: Gram staining

Fascia biopsy material is transported to the lab in a sterile container. For Gram staining, the tissue is fixed to a glass slide by alcohol or heating. For microscopy, x1,000 magnification (using an oil immersion objective lens (100×)) is used to assess the presence, Gram staining, characteristic arrangements and morphology of microorganisms.

Group A Streptococci (GAS, also called Streptococcus pyogenes) are Gram positive spherical cocci. In clinical specimens such as fascia biopsy material, they may appear as pairs or short chains. However, when they are grown in liquid media, they form the typical long chains. Polymicrobial infections are usually mixtures of aerobic and anaerobic bacteria, and therefore, many morphologically different microorganisms can be seen. Gram staining may even show more different microorganisms than are cultured eventually, as culturing anaerobic bacteria can be difficult due to specific growth requirements. Antibiotic therapy can be modulated according to the results of the Gram stain.

Gram staining and microscopy can be performed rapidly after arrival of the tissue in the lab, with a turn-around-time of approximately 30 min depending on the techniques used in the lab and the skills of the microscopist. Negative

Table 1 Characteristic findings suggestive for necrotizing fasciitis. Typical findings that can indicate necrotizing fasciitis during incision biopsy for macroscopic findings and findings on the fresh frozen section and Gram staining

Macroscopy	Fresh frozen section	Gram stain
• Dishwater pus	• Necrosis of superficial fascia	• Microbes
• Lack of bleeding	• Polymorphonuclear infiltration of the deep dermis and fascia	• With or without leukocytes
• Lack of tissue resistance	• Fibrinous trombi of arteries and veins passing through the fascia	• Group A Streptococci
• Grey necrotic tissue	• Angiitis with fibrinoid necrosis of vessel walls	• Clostridium perfringens
• Non-contracting muscles	• Microorganisms within the destroyed fascia and dermis	• Vibrio species
• Fascial oedema		
• Purple blisters on skin		

microscopy does not rule out the presence of microorganisms in tissue however; tissue should therefore be cultured as well. This also facilitates antimicrobial susceptibility testing on the causative microorganisms. Special care should be given to anaerobic microbes.

Triple diagnostics: fresh frozen section

Especially in cases with only peri-fascial oedema and absence of macroscopic necrosis, a fresh frozen section is of the upmost importance. Fresh, non-fixed tissue from a true cut section including fascia is embedded in gel and frozen rapidly to about –20° C. With a cryostat sections of 6 to 9 micrometer are produced and stained with hematoxylin and eosin (H&E). This procedure takes 10 to 15 min. The most specific predictive finding is necrosis of the superficial fascia with fibrinous trombi of arteries and veins located in the fascia. The vessels walls can show signs of angiitis with fibrinoid necrosis of the walls. Both the fascia and the deep dermis often show infiltration of polymorphonuclear cells. If bacteria are present in large numbers, they can often be seen in the H&E staining [20, 28]. In macroscopically obvious cases of necrotic fascia, histology will only demonstrate non-specific necrosis and is not indicated. No data is available about under and over diagnosis using this method and microbiology and pathology findings should not replace clinical parameters. Nevertheless, the combination

of the 3 modalities might provide the surgeon sufficient data to identify the correct patients as early as possible or to extent the exploration of the suspected area.

Suggested approach

A treatment algorithm that might help in the management of these patients with ambivalent cases is postulated (Fig. 1). When there is a suspicion of necrotizing fasciitis, skin lesions are marked, blood cultures are drawn and laboratory tests are performed. Thereafter, broad spectrum antibiotics are initiated and should cover *Streptococcus* (Penicillin or 2nd/3rd generation Cephalosporin), Clindamycin (as toxin scavenger) and Gentamicin. The surgeon is consulted. Sepsis is treated immediately according to the Surviving Sepsis Campaign guidelines [29]. If clinical signs and symptoms in combination with laboratory tests are not suspicious, the patient is re-examined on set time points. However, if necrotizing fasciitis is suspected or cannot be ruled out, the patients consent is obtained for all possible scenario's (debridement, amputation, intensive care and ventilator support and dialysis) and the patient is brought to the operation room for biopsy as soon as possible [30].

An incision is made over the most prominent skin marks or spot that is most painful. If during this procedure the diagnosis can be confirmed macroscopically, this prompts aggressive debridement. An incision biopsy for Gram stain

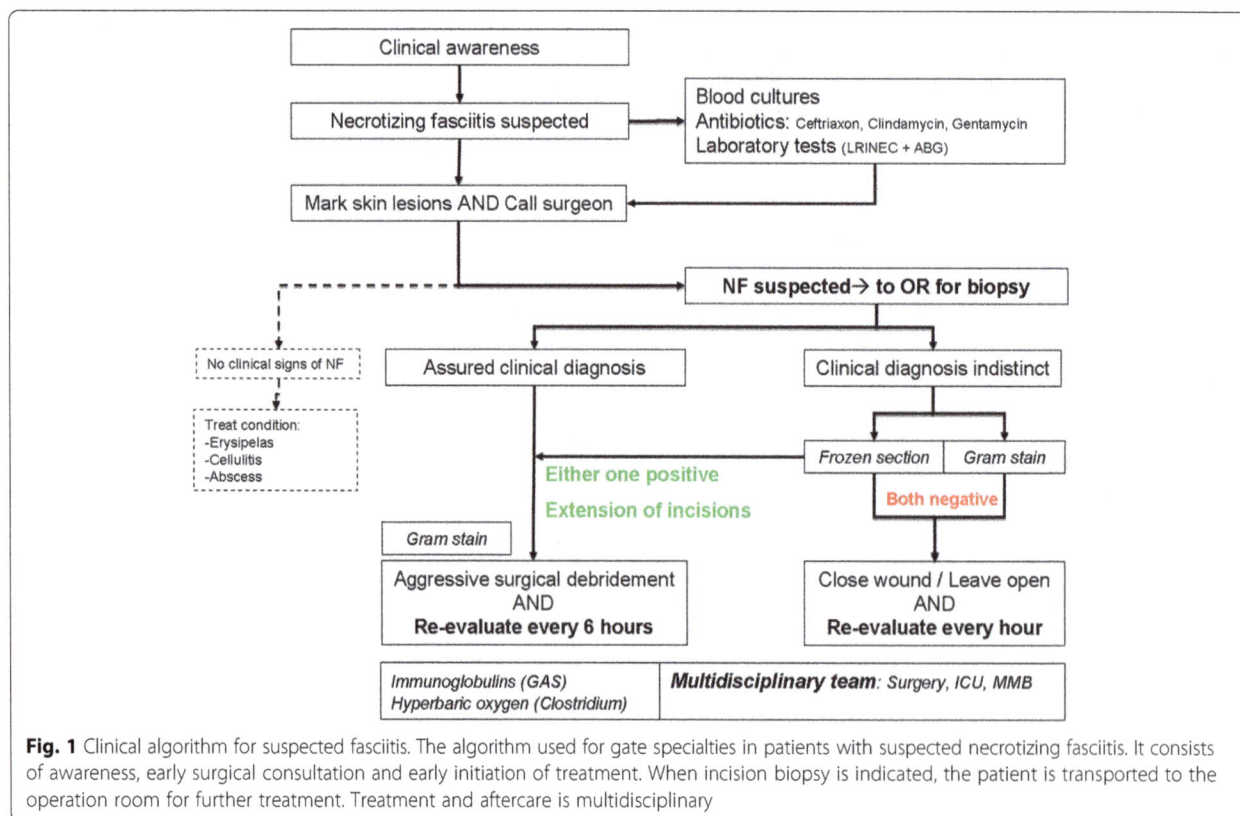

Fig. 1 Clinical algorithm for suspected fasciitis. The algorithm used for gate specialties in patients with suspected necrotizing fasciitis. It consists of awareness, early surgical consultation and early initiation of treatment. When incision biopsy is indicated, the patient is transported to the operation room for further treatment. Treatment and aftercare is multidisciplinary

is obtained, but should not delay further surgical control of the tissue when there are macroscopic findings of necrosis. Macroscopic necrosis frequently hampers the interpretation of histology and fresh frozen section is considered less useful in these cases.

However, if the diagnosis is indistinct by macroscopic findings (i.e. merely oedema), the biopsy is used for a Gram stain and fresh frozen section. If either one of them is suggestive for necrotizing fasciitis this prompts longitudinal extension of the incision. Skin marks can be misleading and necrotic lesions of the fascia can be found at distance after extension of the incision(s). When indicated by findings on histology of microbiology, aggressive debridement should follow of the entire affected area. Because either a positive or ambivalent macroscopic finding prompts further surgery, we prefer to perform the incision biopsy in the operation room.

After debridement, the wounds are left open, the patient is transported to the ICU for resuscitation and re-evaluated at set time points. When there are no indications for necrotizing fasciitis by macroscopy, Gram stain and fresh frozen section, the wound is either closed or left open when there is reasonable doubt. Re-evaluation takes place at set time points. Supportive therapeutic measures are initiated when indicated and based on mainly the Gram stain, such as immunoglobulins for GAS and hyperbaric oxygen in clostridium. Thereafter the patient is further treated by a multidisciplinary team, consisting of a surgeon, intensivist, microbiologist, physiotherapist, social worker, dietician and additional specialties depending on the location of the disease (i.e. plastic surgery,

ophthalmologist, ENT-physician) [31]. When progression of necrosis is controlled, wounds are usually covered by vacuum devices until closure can be achieved.

Results

In a three year period, 21 non-transferred cases were presented to the emergency department who underwent incision biopsy or operative debridement. Their average age was 53 (range 34–75) and most patients suffered from severe comorbidities (6 ASA I, 4 ASA II, 2 ASA III and 9 (47 %) ASA IV patients). In 11 patients, diagnoses was confirmed based on intra-operative macroscopic findings of fascial necrosis. There were 10 ambivalent cases with only macroscopic peri-fascial oedema or necrosis of the subcutaneous fatty tissue, in which fresh frozen section and Gram staining resulted in a change in treatment strategy in six patients. Based on macroscopic findings the surgeon would have ended the surgical procedure, but instead extended the incisional area and focal necrosis was found at a distant side in all 6 patients. Follow-up proved that 4/21 patients did not have necrotizing fasciitis (Fig. 2). Group A Streptococcus were found in 8 of the 17 patients with confirmed necrotizing fasciitis. Mortality due to necrotizing fasciitis was the outcome in two patients (12.5 %) and 2 additional patients died within the first 30 days after admission due to other pre-existing conditions (25 % total 30 day mortality).

Discussion

In this cohort series we present the results of an algorithm which uses triple diagnostics for ambivalent cases of

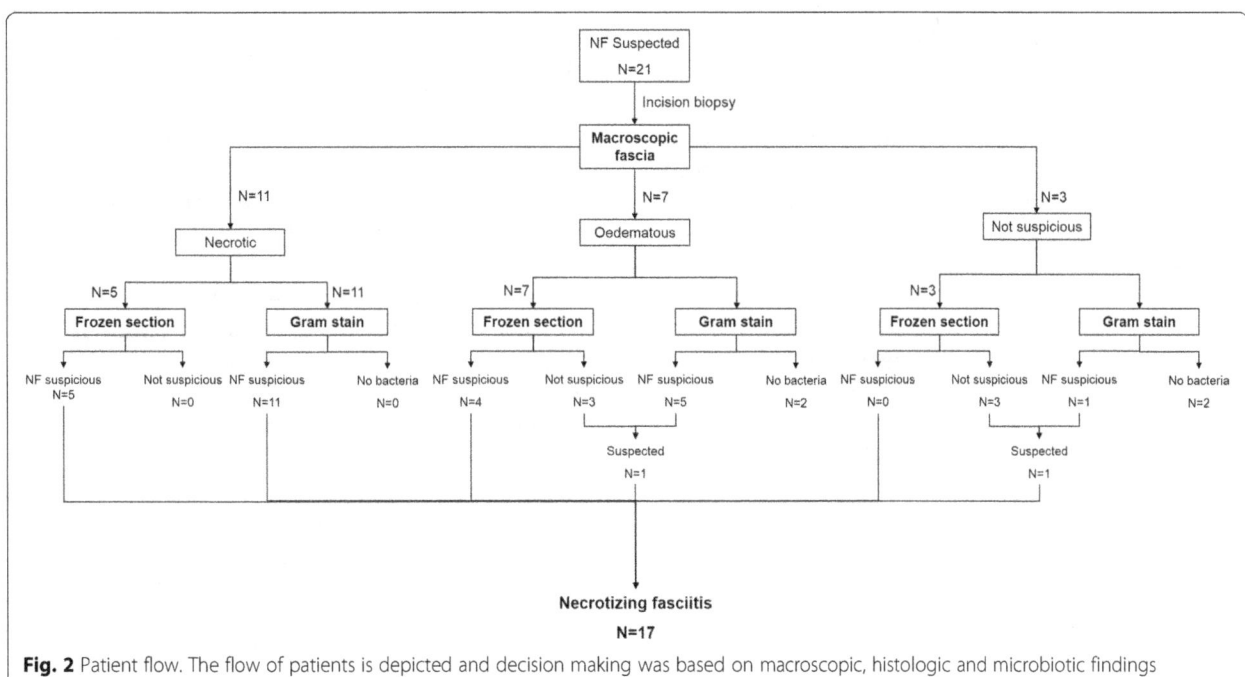

Fig. 2 Patient flow. The flow of patients is depicted and decision making was based on macroscopic, histologic and microbiotic findings

necrotizing fasciitis in the very early stages of the disease. In patients with an ambivalent presentation and no clear macroscopic necrosis of the fascia during incisional biopsy, the combination of a fresh frozen section and Gram staining altered treatment in 60 % of the cases. All of which later proved to be necrotizing fasciitis based on clinical follow-up. Mortality due to necrotizing fasciitis in this series was 12.5 % and overall mortality was 25 %, which is a fair result considering the large number of ASA IV classified patients.

The mortality rate in the present series is identical to the first report (12.5 %) on the use of histology in necrotizing fasciitis [20]. It was discussed if the relative low mortality was the result of the early operative debridement or could be attributed to the histology [19]. We feel that the use of histology and Gram staining results in more timely decision making and therefore early debridement and source control.

Necrotizing fasciitis is rare and heterogeneous in its presentation for body region as it can occur in every fascia and mimic many other infectious and non-infectious diseases. As a result, numbers per treating physician and expertise gained with this disease are often limited. In addition, physicians frequently find it a "scary" disease, because of its rapid progression and the necessary thorough debridement that might result in bad function and appearance [24].

Awareness is advocated in patients with sudden onset and rapid progression of a suspected infectious disease. Disproportional pain is often referred to as the common denominator in this disease and should trigger further investigation. More classical symptoms for necrotizing fasciitis, such as erythema, oedema, blisters, crepitus, and skin necrosis have been described in only 10–40 % of the cases and are seldom seen within the first 24 h [22, 32, 33]. The difficulty in recognition is further stretched by underlying conditions, for instance trauma, vascular disease, diabetic wounds or drug abuse [24]. Co-morbidities are found in nearly 50 % of patients with necrotizing fasciitis and frequently some form of trauma (blunt or penetrating) preceded symptoms. In the present series 55 % suffered severe co-morbidities such as congestive heart failure, renal insufficiency or acute leukemia. Although heterogeneous in its presentation, the philosophy of early identification and aggressive holistic treatment is uniform. This is often referred to as the "search and destroy" strategy [7, 21, 31, 34, 35]. In the presented cohort, a total of 4 patients were brought to the operation room based on clinical suspicion, who did not prove to have necrotizing fasciitis, This demonstrates the low threshold for incisional biopsy when necrotizing fasciitis is suspected, leading to a relative over treatment of patients with a less severe condition (i.e. erysipelas).

Proposed classifications are universal and either based on location or microbiology [36, 37]. Locations which are often affected are the trunk, extremities and the maxillofacial region. Frequently encountered specific locations include Fournier (perineum), Ludwig's angina (submandibular) and Meleney's synergistic gangrene (abdominal wall and/or post-operative) [24, 25, 38].

Classification by microbiology covers all locations, although some locations are more associated with a specific type than others. Type 1 accounts for 55–90 % of all cases and consists of a polymicrobial flora [24, 26, 38, 39]. Fournier is often associated with type 1 necrotizing fasciitis. Type 2 consists of a mono-microbial flora, of which necrotizing fasciitis with Group A Haemolytic Streptococcus (GAS, also called *Streptococcus pyogenes*) is the most important one. Other suggested classification groups are type 3 for virulent Gram negative bacilli (i.e. *Vibrio species*) and type 4 for fungi and yeasts (i.e. *Cryptococcus* or *Candida species*) [40]. Microbiological findings, and thus classification types, are highly geographically dependant. For instance, *Vibrio species* is mostly situated in Asia, while methicillin-resistant *Staphylococcus aureus* (MRSA) is seldom seen in the northern region of Europe [41, 42]. In order to combine multiple aetiologies, it has been proposed to integrate all types of necrotizing fasciitis like entities in the diagnose of severe necrotizing soft tissue disease as therapy is similar [43]. In addition, the potential whole body presentation causes many different medical specialties to be confronted with necrotizing fasciitis, resulting in more scattered experience. This stretches the need for a universal treatment algorithm [34, 44, 45].

To aid in the identification of patients with necrotizing fasciitis, several adjuncts have been described. A large base deficit or high Laboratory Risk Indicator for Necrotizing Fasciitis (LRINEC) score have been suggested to increase the possibility of a patient having necrotizing fasciitis, however, they are not tools to provide a definitive diagnosis [16, 32, 33, 46, 47]. Their values may provide insight in the severity of disease, however, sensitivity remains low [7, 48, 49].

Imaging studies might provide additional information. Although air in the fascial planes is seldom present in the early stages and fascial fluid collections are not always seen. Moreover, CT-scanning might provide information about underlying conditions in cases for necrotizing fasciitis in the maxillo-facial area or trunk (Fournier), such as diverticulitis or abscesses. Some clinics have incorporated CT-scanning in their standard work-up for hemodynamic stable patients with fasciitis to screen for underlying pathology. In certain cases CT helps to evaluate the extent of tissue infection showing swelling, inflammation and gas formation.

MRI scanning proves to have the highest sensitivity and specificity [50]. However, MRI scanning may not be desirable in all patients or available in all hospitals. Furthermore, the exact contribution of imaging modalities in the early stages of necrotizing fasciitis is still under debate and should always be correlated with the clinical presentation [48, 51, 52]. In more advanced cases treatment should not be delayed for imaging. Taken together, clinical suspicion should outweigh both laboratory and imaging adjuncts for the diagnosis of necrotizing fasciitis, especially in the early stages of the disease, where the therapeutic yield of debridement is the greatest [9]. Clinical suspicion can be supported by fresh frozen section and Gram staining during incisional biopsy and might result in more timely identification of this life threatening condition.

Conclusion

With improved awareness, a challenge arises with the early and correct identification of necrotizing fasciitis. Signs and symptoms might be absent or misleading, as prominent skin marks might not be the place of fascial necrosis. This emphasizes the importance of adequate algorithms and treatment protocols for *all* medical specialties that might encounter necrotizing fasciitis. Identification and debridement as soon as possible and aggressive enough are the major contributors for survival. Therefore, triple diagnostics which include a fresh frozen section and Gram staining might be an important adjunct in early ambivalent stages of suspected necrotizing fasciitis.

Acknowledgements
Not applicable

Funding
No funding was obtained for this manuscript.

Authors' contributions
FH, MvD and LB prepared the first draft. FH analysed database. FH, MvD, LB, LL, LR critically reviewed and drafted the manuscript until its final version. All authors read and approved the final manuscript.

Competing interests
All authors declare to have no financial or non-financial conflict of interest.

Author details
[1]Department of surgery, University Medical Center Utrecht, Utrecht, The Netherlands. [2]Department of Medical Microbiology, University Medical Center Utrecht, Utrecht, The Netherlands. [3]Department of Surgery, Karolinska Institutet, Solna, Sweden. [4]Department of Pathology, University Medical Center Utrecht, Utrecht, The Netherlands.

References
1. Low DE, McGeer A. Skin and soft tissue infection: necrotizing fasciitis. Curr Opin Infect Dis. 1998;11:119–23.
2. Lancerotto L, Tocco I, Salmaso R, Vindigni V, Bassetto F. Necrotizing fasciitis: classification, diagnosis, and management. J Trauma Acute Care Surg. 2012;72:560–6.
3. Dixon B. Fasciitis continues to surprise. Lancet Infect Dis. 2008;8:279–3099.
4. Anaya DA, McMahon K, Nathens AB, Sullivan SR, Foy H, Bulger E. Predictors of mortality and limb loss in necrotizing soft tissue infections. Arch Surg. 2005;140:151–7.
5. Anaya DA, Dellinger EP. Necrotizing soft-tissue infection: diagnosis and management. Clin Infect Dis. 2007;44:705–10.
6. Tsitsilonis S, Druschel C, Wichlas F, Haas NP, Schwabe P, Bail HJ, et al. Necrotizing fasciitis: is the bacterial spectrum changing? Langenbecks ArchSurg. 2013;398:153–9.
7. Hakkarainen TW, Kopari NM, Pham TN, Evans HL. Necrotizing soft tissue infections: review and current concepts in treatment, systems of care, and outcomes. Curr Probl Surg. 2014;51:344–62.
8. Goh T, Goh LG, Ang CH, Wong CH. Early diagnosis of necrotizing fasciitis. Br J Surg. 2014;101:e119–25.
9. Lille ST, Sato TT, Engrav LH, Foy H, Jurkovich GJ. Necrotizing soft tissue infections: obstacles in diagnosis. J Am Coll Surg. 1996;182:7–11.
10. Mok MY, Wong SY, Chan TM, Tang WM, Wong WS, Lau CS. Necrotizing fasciitis in rheumatic diseases. Lupus. 2006;15:380–3.
11. Ustin JS, Malangoni MA. Necrotizing soft-tissue infections. Crit Care Med. 2011;39:2156–62.
12. McHenry CR, Piotrowski JJ, Petrinic D, Malangoni MA. Determinants of mortality for necrotizing soft-tissue infections. Ann Surg. 1995;221:558–63.
13. Hussein QA, Anaya DA. Necrotizing soft tissue infections. Crit Care Clin. 2013;29:795–806.
14. Hodgins N, Damkat-Thomas L, Shamsian N, Yew P, Lewis H, Khan K. Analysis of the increasing prevalence of necrotising fasciitis referrals to a regional plastic surgery unit: a retrospective case series. J Plast Reconstr Aesthet Surg. 2015;68:304–11.
15. Nordqvist G, Wallden A, Brorson H, Tham J. Ten years of treating necrotizing fasciitis. Infect Dis (Lond). 2015;47:319–25.
16. Swain RA, Hatcher JC, Azadian BS, Soni N, De SB. A five-year review of necrotising fasciitis in a tertiary referral unit. AnnRCollSurgEngl. 2013;95:57–60.
17. van Stigt SF, de VJ, Bijker JB, Mollen RM, Hekma EJ, Lemson SM e.a. Review of 58 patients with necrotizing fasciitis in the Netherlands. World J.Emerg. Surg. 2016; 11:21. doi: 10.1186/s13017-016-0080-7. eCollection@2016.: 21–0080.
18. Garssen FP, Goslings JC, Bouman CS, Beenen LF, Visser CE, de Jong VM. [Necrotising soft-tissue infections: diagnostics and treatment]. NedTijdschrGeneeskd. 2013;157:A6031.
19. Pruitt Jr BA. Biopsy diagnosis of surgical infections. N Engl J Med. 1984;310:1737–8.
20. Stamenkovic I, Lew PD. Early recognition of potentially fatal necrotizing fasciitis. The use of frozen-section biopsy. N Engl J Med. 1984;310:1689–93.
21. Majeski J, Majeski E. Necrotizing fasciitis: improved survival with early recognition by tissue biopsy and aggressive surgical treatment. South Med J. 1997;90:1065–8.
22. Misiakos EP, Bagias G, Patapis P, Sotiropoulos D, Kanavidis P, Machairas A. Current concepts in the management of necrotizing fasciitis. Front Surg. 2014;1:36. doi:10.3389/fsurg.2014.00036. eCollection@2014.: 36.
23. Gibson T. Karl Langer (1819–1887) and his lines. Br J Plast Surg. 1978;31:1–2.
24. Sartelli M, Malangoni MA, May AK, Viale P, Kao LS, Catena F, et al. World Society of Emergency Surgery (WSES) guidelines for management of skin and soft tissue infections. World J Emerg Surg. 2014;9:57–9.
25. Mallikarjuna MN, Vijayakumar A, Patil VS, Shivswamy BS. Fournier's gangrene: current practices. ISRN Surg. 2012;2012:942437. doi:10.5402/2012/942437. Epub@2012 Dec 3.: 942437.
26. Stevens DL, Bisno AL, Chambers HF, Dellinger EP, Goldstein EJ, Gorbach SL, et al. Practice guidelines for the diagnosis and management of skin and soft tissue infections: 2014 update by the infectious diseases society of America. Clin Infect Dis. 2014;59:147–59.
27. Keung EZ, Liu X, Nuzhad A, Adams C, Ashley SW, Askari R. Immunocompromised status in patients with necrotizing soft-tissue infection. JAMA Surg. 2013;148:419–26.
28. Tocco I, Lancerotto L, Pontini A, Voltan A, Azzena B. "Synchronous" multifocal necrotizing fasciitis. J Emerg Med. 2013;45:e187–91.

29. Dellinger RP, Levy MM, Rhodes A, Annane D, Gerlach H, Opal SM, et al. Surviving sepsis campaign: international guidelines for management of severe sepsis and septic shock: 2012. Crit Care Med. 2013;41:580–637.

30. Kluger Y, Ben-Ishay O, Sartelli M, Ansaloni L, Abbas AE, Agresta F, et al. World society of emergency surgery study group initiative on Timing of Acute Care Surgery classification (TACS). World J Emerg Surg. 2013;8:17–8.

31. Majeski JA, Alexander JW. Early diagnosis, nutritional support, and immediate extensive debridement improve survival in necrotizing fasciitis. Am J Surg. 1983;145:784–7.

32. Wong CH, Khin LW. Clinical relevance of the LRINEC (Laboratory Risk Indicator for Necrotizing Fasciitis) score for assessment of early necrotizing fasciitis. Crit Care Med. 2005;33:1677.

33. Wong CH, Khin LW, Heng KS, Tan KC, Low CO. The LRINEC (Laboratory Risk Indicator for Necrotizing Fasciitis) score: a tool for distinguishing necrotizing fasciitis from other soft tissue infections. Crit Care Med. 2004;32:1535–41.

34. Tu GW, Hwabejire JO, Ju MJ, Yang YF, Zhang GJ, Xu JW, et al. Multidisciplinary intensive care in extensive necrotizing fasciitis. Infection. 2013;41:583–7.

35. Bilton BD, Zibari GB, McMillan RW, Aultman DF, Dunn G, McDonald JC. Aggressive surgical management of necrotizing fasciitis serves to decrease mortality: a retrospective study. Am Surg. 1998;64:397–400.

36. Anaya DA, Bulger EM, Kwon YS, Kao LS, Evans H, Nathens AB. Predicting death in necrotizing soft tissue infections: a clinical score. Surg Infect (Larchmt). 2009;10:517–22.

37. Lee CY, Kuo LT, Peng KT, Hsu WH, Huang TW, Chou YC. Prognostic factors and monomicrobial necrotizing fasciitis: gram-positive versus gram-negative pathogens. BMC Infect Dis. 2011;11:5. doi:10.1186/1471-2334-11-5. 5–11.

38. Lamb LE, Sriskandan S, Tan LK. Bromine, bear-claw scratch fasciotomies, and the Eagle effect: management of group A streptococcal necrotising fasciitis and its association with trauma. Lancet Infect Dis. 2015;15:109–21.

39. Bucca K, Spencer R, Orford N, Cattigan C, Athan E, McDonald A. Early diagnosis and treatment of necrotizing fasciitis can improve survival: an observational intensive care unit cohort study. ANZ J Surg. 2013;83:365–70.

40. Ho SW, Ang CL, Ding CS, Barkham T, Teoh LC. Necrotizing Fasciitis Caused by Cryptococcus gattii. Am J Orthop (BelleMead NJ). 2015;44:E517–22.

41. Bode LG, Wertheim HF, Kluytmans JA, Bogaers-Hofman D, Vandenbroucke-Grauls CM, Roosendaal R, et al. Sustained low prevalence of meticillin-resistant Staphylococcus aureus upon admission to hospital in The Netherlands. J Hosp Infect. 2011;79:198–201.

42. Kuo YL, Shieh SJ, Chiu HY, Lee JW. Necrotizing fasciitis caused by Vibrio vulnificus: epidemiology, clinical findings, treatment and prevention. Eur J Clin Microbiol Infect Dis. 2007;26:785–92.

43. Dellinger EP. Severe necrotizing soft-tissue infections. Multiple disease entities requiring a common approach. JAMA. 1981;246:1717–21.

44. Muhammad JK, Almadani H, Al Hashemi BA, Liaqat M. The value of early intervention and a multidisciplinary approach in the management of necrotizing fasciitis of the neck and anterior mediastinum of odontogenic origin. J Oral Maxillofac Surg. 2015;73:918–27.

45. Tambe K, Tripathi A, Burns J, Sampath R. Multidisciplinary management of periocular necrotising fasciitis: a series of 11 patients. Eye (Lond). 2012;26:463–7.

46. Wong CH, Wang YS. The diagnosis of necrotizing fasciitis. Curr Opin Infect Dis. 2005;18:101–6.

47. Chao WN, Tsai SJ, Tsai CF, Su CH, Chan KS, Lee YT, et al. The laboratory risk indicator for necrotizing fasciitis score for discernment of necrotizing fasciitis originated from vibrio vulnificus infections. J Trauma Acute Care Surg. 2012;73:1576–82.

48. Kim KT, Kim YJ, Won LJ, Kim YJ, Park SW, Lim MK, et al. Can necrotizing infectious fasciitis be differentiated from nonnecrotizing infectious fasciitis with MR imaging? Radiology. 2011;259:816–24.

49. Hakkarainen TW, Burkette IN, Bulger E, Evans HL. Moving beyond survival as a measure of success: understanding the patient experience of necrotizing soft-tissue infections. J Surg Res. 2014;192:143–9.

50. Malghem J, Lecouvet FE, Omoumi P, Maldague BE, Vande Berg BC. Necrotizing fasciitis: contribution and limitations of diagnostic imaging. Joint Bone Spine. 2013;80:146–54.

51. Ali SZ, Srinivasan S, Peh WC. MRI in necrotizing fasciitis of the extremities. Br J Radiol. 2014;87:20130560.

52. Chaudhry AA, Baker KS, Gould ES, Gupta R. Necrotizing fasciitis and its mimics: what radiologists need to know. AJR Am J Roentgenol. 2015;204:128–39.

23

Treating patients in a trauma room equipped with computed tomography and patients' mortality: a non-controlled comparison study

Shintaro Furugori[1][*] , Makoto Kato[2], Takeru Abe[1], Masayuki Iwashita[1] and Naoto Morimura[3]

Abstract

Background: To improve acute trauma care workflow, the number of trauma centers equipped with a computed tomography (CT) machine in the trauma resuscitation room has increased. The effect of the presence of a CT machine in the trauma room on a patient's outcome is still unclear. This study evaluated the association between a CT machine in the trauma room and a patient's outcome.

Methods: Our study included all trauma patients admitted to a trauma center in Yokohama, Japan, between April 2014 and March 2016. We compared 140 patients treated using a conventional resuscitation room with 106 patients treated in new trauma rooms equipped with a CT machine.

Results: For the group treated in a trauma room with a CT machine, the Injury Severity Score (13.0 vs. 9.0; $p = 0.002$), CT scans of the head (78.3 vs. 66.4%; $p = 0.046$), CT scans of the body trunk (75.5 vs. 58.6%; $p = 0.007$), intubation in the emergency department (48.1 vs. 30.7%; $p = 0.008$), and multiple trauma patients (47.2 vs. 30.0%; $p = 0.008$) were significantly higher and Trauma and Injury Severity Score probability of survival (96.75 vs. 97.80; $p = 0.009$) was significantly lower than the group treated in a conventional resuscitation room. In multivariate analysis and propensity score matched analysis, being treated in a trauma room with a CT machine was an independent predictor for fewer hospital deaths (odds ratio 0.002; 95% CI 0.00–0.75; $p = 0.04$, and 0.07; 0.00–0.98, respectively).

Conclusions: Equipping a trauma room with a CT machine reduced the time in decision-making for treating a trauma patient and subsequently lowered the mortality of trauma patients.

Keywords: Acute care, Trauma resuscitation room, CT

Background

Trauma is the leading cause of death among young people around the world [1] and in those aged < 45 years in Japan [2]. In addition, approximately 23,000 trauma deaths occur each year in Japan [2]. Trauma has a negative impact on the lives of people and is a risk for social welfare [1]. Improving therapeutic procedures and diagnostic evaluations for trauma patients is necessary to increase their survival and improve public health.

In recent years, computed tomography (CT) has provided faster operations and more detailed images and can be made easily available in acute trauma care. CT scanning in the early diagnostic phase of trauma care is critical and has become an essential part of a trauma diagnostic work-up. In previous studies, CT scanning contributed to a change of treatment without obvious external signs of injuries [3–5], gained time benefits compared with a conventional resuscitation [6–9], and had potential survival benefits for trauma patients, especially when total-body CT scanning (TBCT) was performed [10–15]. To improve acute trauma care workflow, the number of trauma centers equipped with a CT machine in the trauma resuscitation room has

* Correspondence: shintarou0420@yahoo.co.jp
[1]Department of Emergency Medicine, Yokohama City University, 4-57 Urafunecho, Minamiku, Yokohama City, Kanagawa Prefecture 232-0024, Japan
Full list of author information is available at the end of the article

increased [6, 7, 16–20]. Equipping a CT machine in a trauma room is expensive, and the effect of a CT machine in the trauma room compared with a conventional resuscitation room on a patient's outcome is still unclear because of the inconsistency in previous findings [6, 18–22]. Thus, we conducted a before and after comparison study to evaluate the association between the presence of a CT machine in the trauma resuscitation room and a patient's outcome.

Methods

The Yokohama City University Medical Center (YCUMC), Yokohama, Japan, has recently equipped a trauma room with a CT machine and has been functioning as a designated, regional trauma center since April 2015. Yokohama City has approximately 3.7 million inhabitants. In April 2015, a prehospital-to-hospital care protocol was introduced. In the protocol, emergency medical services were used to transport severe trauma patients, such as those suffering from shock from a blunt trauma, penetrating injuries to the neck, or two or more proximal long-bone fractures, to a designated trauma center. Regarding pre-hospital care system in Japan, a regional medical control council (MC council) determines treatment and delivery protocols, depending on a patient's conditions. In this system, a local ambulance transfers severe trauma patients to a tertiary medical facility, and an emergency and critical care center admits the patient. Yokohama City designated two hospitals as regional severe-trauma centers, based on a criteria indicated by the Japanese Association for The Surgery of Trauma, and YCUMC is one of them. Such designations in Yokohama City are the first attempt by a local administration in the country. At the same time, YCUMC placed a CT machine in a new trauma resuscitation room in the emergency department (ED) (Fig. 1). A trauma team was established, consisting of well-trained staffs to provide

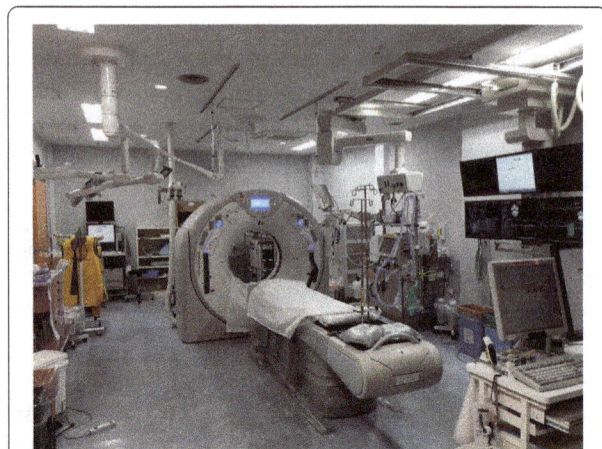

Fig. 1 The new trauma resuscitation room at the Yokohama City University Medical Center

patients with a trauma survey and treatment. The trauma team has a leader, who is a trauma surgeon or an emergency physician. After the establishment of the new trauma resuscitation room, a patient is directly transferred to the trauma resuscitation room and onto a CT carbon table. Any life-saving procedures, including airway management, chest tube replacement, or emergency laparotomy, can be performed on the CT table. After the life-saving procedures, each leader decides whether or not to perform a CT scan immediately during the primary survey for patients whose vital signs are within an acceptable range, such as percutaneous oxygen saturation (SaO_2), 90%; heart rate (HR), 130 bpm; and systolic blood pressure (SBP), 70 mmHg. The patient undergoes a CT scan without transfer because the CT table can slide. The CT machine is an 80-slice multidetector device, PRIME Aquilion®, manufactured by Toshiba. The team leader can call a general surgeon, an anesthesiologist, a radiologist, an orthopedic surgeon, a plastic surgeon, or a neurosurgeon within 30 min any time during the day, if necessary. The leader decides whether to perform TBCT or selective CT on the trauma patient, not dependent on previous protocols presented [23–25]. This reduces the number of unnecessary scans for the patient receiving a head CT scan, preventing a disturbance of consciousness or head trauma.

Before the protocol was introduced, a patient received a conventional resuscitation room and trauma care based on the guidelines of the Japan Advanced Trauma Evaluation and Care program by the Advanced Trauma Life Support [2, 26]. Briefly, in the primary survey, the trauma care team begins with priority-oriented resuscitation. The team performs a focused assessment with sonography for trauma (FAST) with chest and pelvic X-ray examinations for diagnosis during the primary survey. In addition, if available in the facility, a selective CT scan is performed before emergency bleeding control is initiated. Each team leader decides whether or not to perform the CT scan if life-threatening problems are clearly detected in the FAST and X-ray images or if patient transfer is difficult because of hemodynamic instability. The CT machine is located on the same floor as the resuscitation room, approximately 50 m away. The time required to perform the CT scan, including patient transfer time, is approximately 20 min.

This observational study utilized data from all trauma patients admitted to YCUMC. Our study included all trauma patients admitted to YCUMC between April 2014 and March 2016. Inclusion criteria consisted of all adult trauma patients (aged ≥ 18 years). Exclusion criteria included the following: patients with traumatic cardiopulmonary arrest on arrival, burn patients, patients who were < 18 years, and those who were transferred from other hospitals. We categorized the patients into two groups: patients treated using the conventional resuscitation room and patients treated in the CT-equipped trauma room.

The following data were retrospectively obtained from the patients' medical records: sex; age; Abbreviated Injury Score (AIS); Injury Severity Score (ISS); Revised Trauma Score (RTS); probability of survival (Ps); initial vital signs upon arrival to the hospital, including HR, SBP, the Glasgow Coma Scale (GCS), respiratory rates, and body temperature; CT scans of the head and body trunk; initial laboratory data, including lactate, base excess, hemoglobin, fibrinogen, activated partial thromboplastin time, international normalized ratio of prothrombin time (PT-INR), fibrin degradation products, and D-dimer levels; injury mechanisms; intubation in ED; chest tube placement in ED; use of the resuscitative endovascular balloon for occlusion of the aorta in ED; transcatheter arterial embolization (TAE); need for large transfusions defined as transfused red blood cells of 10 units or more within 24 h after arrival to ED; ED stay, which was the time from arrival to transfer to the operation room, the angiography room, or the intensive care units (ICUs); time to CT scan, which was the time from arrival to the start of the CT scan; time to emergency operations to control bleeding, which was the time from arrival to the initiation of the operation; time to TAE, which was the time from arrival to the start of TAE; length of hospital stay (LOS; in days); and the length of ICU stay (in days). The types of trauma were categorized as blunt or penetrating. RTS was calculated using a formula described by Champion et al. [26, 27]. Ps was calculated using the Trauma and Injury Severity Score (TRISS) methods [28]. Hypotension was defined as SBP below 90 mmHg at arrival. Isolated traumatic brain injury was defined as having a GCS score of below 9 and an AIS head score of 3 or above without non-head region AIS score of greater than 1. Patients with multiple traumas were defined as those with an ISS of 16 or above.

The primary outcome measure was hospital mortality. Secondary outcome measures included LOS, length of ICU stay, need for large transfusions, time from the CT scan to the initiation of surgeries for controlling bleeding, time from the CT scan to the start of TAE, and the length of ED stay.

Data were analyzed for all eligible patients. Data were presented as median and interquartile ranges for not normally distributed values or number with percentages as appropriate. Continuous variables were compared between the two patient groups using the Mann–Whitney U test. Categorical variables were analyzed using Fisher's exact test. Predictive survival rates (TRISS Ps), actual survival rates, and their ratios were calculated for the two groups: a patient group treated in the trauma room with CT and treated in the conventional resuscitation room. In order to compare predicted survival rate and actual survival rate by each group, Z statistic was calculated. M statistic was calculated to compare the difference from the standard severity distribution by Major Trauma Outcome

Study (MTOS) [28]. As subgroup analysis, we calculated predictive survival rate, actual survival rate, Z statistic, and M statistic for multiple trauma patients, defined as ISS ≥ 16. In addition, we compared the two groups in terms of clinical and basic characteristics, such as mortality, age, and sex, to acknowledge the difference between the included and excluded samples.

Multivariate logistic regression analysis was used to control for potentially confounding variables, identified as prior to locating the CT in the trauma resuscitation room. Based on clinical reasoning and avoiding multicollinearity within variables, the following variables were entered in the model: CT machine in the trauma room, age, gender, ISS, RTS, lactate, PT-INR, and time to CT scan.

Furthermore, to minimize the effect of confounding variables due to a non-randomized study in evaluating the effect of locating a CT machine in the trauma resuscitation room on mortality, propensity scores were calculated with locating the CT machine or not as a dependent variable and ISS, RTS, sex, PT-INR, fibrinogen, and performing CT as independent variables. We used optimal methods to create 1:1-matched study groups with a 0.05 caliper width. After adjusting for these confounding variables, we performed both univariate and multivariate logistic regression analyses with a forward selection, in which $p < 0.10$ was set as a criterion to include in the model for evaluating the effect of locating the CT machine in the trauma resuscitation room on mortality.

A p value of < 0.05 was considered to indicate statistical significance. All statistical analyses were performed using EZR, which is a graphical user interface for R (version 3.1.2, The R Foundation for Statistical Computing, Vienna, Austria) [29] and IBM SPSS Statistics, Version 22.0 (IBM Corp, Armonk, NY, USA).

Results

During the study period, 381 trauma patients were admitted to YCUMC. We found a total of 246 trauma patients who were meeting the inclusion criteria (Fig. 2). We compared the included patient group with the excluded group. Compared to the included samples, the excluded samples had significantly higher mortality (34.8 vs. 5.7%; $p < 0.001$) and younger age [51 (36–69) years (median, IQR) vs. 45 (17–61); $p < 0.001$)]. We found no significant difference in sex ($p = 0.482$) between the groups.

Baseline characteristics of the included patients are summarized in Table 1. TRISS was applied to all 246 patients. In a total of 246 patients, the median age was 51 (36–69) years and the ISS was 10 (4–18). In total, 206 patients (83.7%) underwent CT and 15 died (6.1%). In the standard work-up group, one patient could not undergo a CT scan because of hemodynamic instability. The group with patients treated using the standard work-up included 140 patients, and the group with those treated in the trauma

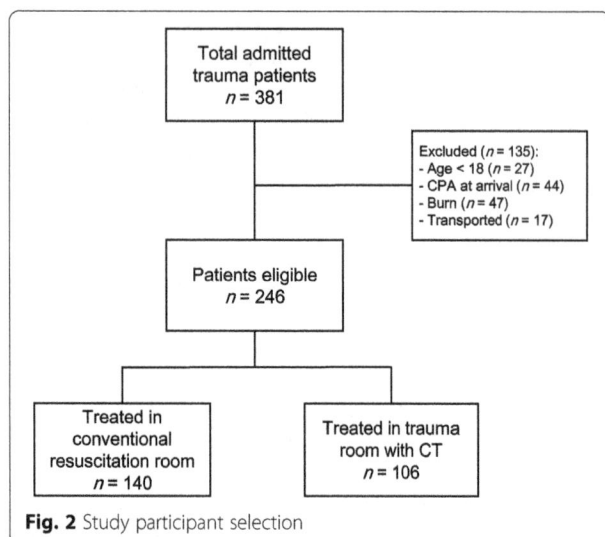

Fig. 2 Study participant selection

rooms equipped with a CT machine included 106 patients. There were no statistically significant differences in age, arrival status without GCS, type of trauma, isolated TBI using REBA, and urgent operations to control bleeding between the two groups. ISS (13.0 vs. 9.0; $p = 0.002$), CT scan of the head (78.3 vs. 66.4%; $p = 0.046$), CT scan of the body trunk (75.5 vs. 58.6%; $p = 0.007$), intubation in ED (48.1 vs. 30.7%; $p = 0.08$), and multiple trauma patients (47.2 vs. 30.0%; $p = 0.08$) were significantly higher in the group treated in the CT-equipped trauma room compared with the group treated using the standard work-up, respectively. There were no statistically significant differences in the hospital mortality. The median time to CT scan was significantly shorter after installation of the CT machine (23 vs. 37 min, $p < 0.001$). The median time in ED was significantly shorter in the group treated in the trauma room with a CT machine (72 vs. 91 min, $p = 0.044$). The median time to urgent operations to control bleeding and the time to TAE were not statistically different between the groups. LOS and the need for large transfusions were not significantly different between the two groups. TRISS Ps (96.75 vs. 97.80; $p = 0.009$) was significantly lower in the group treated in the CT-equipped trauma room (Table 1). The survival ratio in the main analysis was significantly higher in the CT trauma room group. The severity distribution was found far from the standard distribution of MTOS both in all patients and multiple trauma patients in the CT in the trauma room group (M statistic 0.78 and 0.39 respectively).

Multivariate logistic regression analysis was applied to control for potentially confounding variables. Being treated in the CT-equipped trauma room was an independent predictor for fewer hospital deaths ($p = 0.04$). Age, ISS, RTS, lactate, and time to CT scan were also independent predictors for hospital deaths (Table 2). Being treated in the trauma room with the CT machine was not a predictor for ICU stay (over 3 days), hospital stay

(over 16 days), or the need for large transfusions. ISS was an independent predictor for ICU stay, hospital stay, and the need for large transfusions. RTS was an independent predictor for hospital stay and massive transfusions. Lactate was an independent predictor for massive transfusions. Details on the logistic regression results for ICU stay, hospital stay, and the need for large transfusions are provided (Fig. 3).

After propensity score matching of patients treated using CT or not in the trauma room, we obtained 88 patients for each group with a total of 176 trauma patients. We found no significant differences in baseline characteristics, except for the time to perform CT and ED stay between the two matched study groups (Table 3). There were no statistically significant differences in hospital mortality on univariate analysis with the propensity score-matched samples. Furthermore, multivariate logistic regression analysis of the matched samples demonstrated that being treated in a CT-equipped trauma room was a significant factor and resulted in fewer hospital deaths [odds ratio (OR) 0.07, 95% confidence interval 0.00–0.98, $p = 0.0478$]. Age, ISS, and RTS were also significant independent predictors for hospital death ($p < 0.001$, $p = 0.024$, and $p < 0.001$, respectively; Table 4). Details of the results of logistic regression analysis after propensity score matching of ICU stay, hospital stay, and the need for large transfusions are shown in Fig. 3.

Discussion

Our study showed for the first time that a CT machine in the trauma room had a significantly positive effect on mortality. Patient mortality in the room with a CT machine was higher than that treated with the standard work-up; however, there were no statistically significant differences in hospital mortality after univariate analysis. This was after YCUMC was designated as a trauma center with more severe patients, higher ISS, and lower Ps. However, multivariate logistic regression analysis of the entire sample and the samples after propensity score matching showed positive effect on mortality. This significant association might attribute to a reduced time in decision-making. Equipping a trauma room with a CT machine allows clinicians quicker access to the machine to provide clinical decisions to treat faster with greater accuracy than a standard work-up. This speed with accuracy in the decision-making likely contributes to a lower mortality.

In addition, we had prepared and conducted series of simulation training in advance using the new trauma room with staffs involved in acute trauma care such as doctors, nurses, and laboratory technicians. Improvement of workflow through these simulation trainings might contribute to lower mortality for the trauma room with the CT group.

We did not find other significant associations in the secondary outcomes, such as the length of ICU stay and

Table 1 Characteristics and outcome differences between patients treated in a trauma room with CT and a conventional resuscitation room (n = 246)

		Total (n = 246) n (%)/median (IQR)	Conventional resuscitation room (n = 140) n (%)/median (IQR)	Trauma room with CT (n = 106) n (%)/median (IQR)	p value
Gender	Male	181 (73.6)	93 (66.4)	88 (83.0)	0.004
	Female	65 (26.4)	47 (33.6)	18 (17.0)	
Age		51 (36, 69)	50 (35, 70)	54 (38, 69)	0.769
Initial vital signs	GCS	14 (13, 15)	15 (14, 15)	14 (10, 15)	0.017
	Heart rate	88 (72, 103)	87 (72, 99)	89 (73, 105)	0.249
	Systolic pressure	141 (118, 162)	143 (121, 164)	139 (113, 159)	0.541
	Respiratory rate	20 (17, 24)	20 (17, 24)	20 (18, 24)	0.243
	Temperature	36.4 (36.1, 36.9)	36.4 (36.0, 36.9)	36.4 (36.1, 36.9)	0.618
CT performed		206 (83.7)	113 (80.7)	93 (87.7)	0.164
	For head	176 (71.5)	93 (66.4)	83 (78.3)	0.046
	For body trunk	162 (65.9)	82 (58.6)	80 (75.5)	0.007
Intubation in ER		94 (38.2)	43 (30.7)	51 (48.1)	0.008
Use REBOA		7 (2.8)	1 (0.7)	6 (5.7)	0.045
Arterial embolization		25 (10.2)	10 (7.1)	15 (14.2)	0.089
Place chest tube in ER		18 (7.5)	6 (4.5)	12 (11.3)	0.052
Type of Trauma	Blunt	209 (85.0)	118 (84.2)	91 (85.8)	0.857
	Penetrate	37 (15.0)	22 (15.7)	15 (14.1)	
Isolated TBI		21 (8.5)	12 (8.6)	9 (8.5)	1.000
Polytrauma		92 (37.4)	42 (30.0)	50 (47.2)	0.008
Hypotension		29 (11.8)	14 (10.0)	15 (14.2)	0.324
TAC INR > 1.3		16 (3.9)	5 (3.6)	11 (10.4)	0.038
ISS category	1–8	89 (36.2)	58 (41.4)	31 (29.2)	0.011
	9–15	65 (26.4)	40 (28.6)	25 (23.6)	
	16–24	54 (22.0)	29 (20.7)	25 (23.6)	
	≥ 25	38 (15.4)	13 (9.3)	25 (23.6)	
ISS		10 (4, 18)	9 (4, 16)	13 (5, 22)	0.002
RTS		7.84 (6.90, 7.84)	7.84 (7.48, 7.84)	7.84 (6.38, 7.84)	0.015
Ps		97.6 (92.2, 99.3)	97.8 (94.2, 99.4)	96.8 (81.3, 99.2)	0.009
Lactate		2.0 (1.3, 2.9)	2.0 (1.3, 2.9)	1.9 (1.3, 3.0)	0.876
BE		−0.20 (−2.62, 1.33)	−0.30 (−2.6, 1.2)	−0.10 (−2.8, 1.5)	0.807
Hg		13.2 (11.4, 14.4)	13.2 (11.6, 14.5)	13.2 (11.2, 14.0)	0.439

Table 1 Characteristics and outcome differences between patients treated in a trauma room with CT and a conventional resuscitation room (*n* = 246) (*Continued*)

		Total (*n* = 246)	Conventional resuscitation room (*n* = 140)	Trauma room with CT (*n* = 106)	*p* value
		n (%)/median (IQR)	*n* (%)/median (IQR)	*n* (%)/median (IQR)	
Fbg		286 (230, 336)	298 (257, 353)	260 (208, 314)	< 0.001
APTT		26.4 (24.1, 28.8)	26.4 (24.1, 28.5)	26.9 (24.3, 29.4)	0.283
PT-INR		1.04 (0.97, 1.12)	1.02 (0.95, 1.10)	1.06 (0.99, 1.15)	0.001
FDP		13.7 (3.6, 53.2)	10.8 (3.2, 30.9)	18.4 (4.7, 87.0)	0.025
D-dimer		7.6 (1.4, 29.4)	6.6 (1.2, 21.4)	9.7 (1.7, 46.1)	0.043
Transfusion	RBC	0 (0, 6)	0 (0, 4)	0 (0, 8)	0.009
	FFP	0 (0, 4)	0 (0, 0)	0 (0, 10)	0.002
Mortality	In-hospital	15 (6.1)	6 (4.3)	9 (8.5)	0.189
	24 h	6 (2.4)	2 (1.4)	4 (3.8)	0.407
RBC ≥ 10 U/24 h		39 (15.9)	17 (12.1)	22 (20.8)	0.079
Time to CT (min)		30 (23, 42)	37 (30, 48)	23 (18, 28)	< 0.001
Time to TAE (min)		81 (67, 93)	81 (56, 97)	80 (73, 87)	0.856
Time to operation (min)		94 (61, 122)	97 (7, 123)	83 (68, 121)	0.687
ED staying (min)		81 (58, 117)	91 (61, 122)	72 (53, 113)	0.044
ICU stay (day)		3 (2, 7)	3 (2, 7)	3 (2, 6)	0.811
Hospital stay (day)		16 (5, 35)	15 (5, 34)	17 (5, 37)	0.975

TAC traumatic acute coagulopathy, *ISS* Injury Severity Score, *RTS* Revised Trauma Score, *Ps* probability of survival

Table 2 Multivariate logistic regression analysis on mortality with associated factors (n = 246)

Factors		Odds ratio	(95% CI)	p value
Age		1.16	(1.02–1.33)	0.028
Gender	(reference: female)	1.65	(0.10–26.60)	0.720
ISS		1.20	(1.02–1.42)	0.029
RTS		0.11	(0.03–0.42)	0.002
Lactate		1.80	(1.04–3.11)	0.034
PT-INR		463	(0.51–42 × 10⁴)	0.077
Time to CT		0.84	(0.71–0.99)	0.037
Treated in trauma room with CT	(reference: treated in conventional resuscitation room)	0.002	(0.00–0.75)	0.040

hospital stay. Our results suggest that the quality of care for patients will improve in a trauma room with a CT machine, independent of the severity of the trauma.

Previous studies with a pre–post study design showed inconsistent findings on the association between a CT machine in the trauma resuscitation room and an improvement in clinical outcomes [6, 17–19]. A randomized

control trial, the RACT1 trial, compared a CT machine in the trauma room to the conventional resuscitation room in two Dutch trauma centers (n = 1124) and found no significant effects of the CT machine in the trauma room on patient mortality [21]. Recently, a multicenter randomized control trial to examine the effect of immediate TBCT scanning, the REACT 2 trial, conducted in several trauma centers found no significance in the reduction of mortality [30]; however, not all the trauma centers conducting the immediate TBCT had a CT machine in the trauma room. Stefan Huber-Wagner et al. compared the distance of the CT machine from the trauma resuscitation room with survival from several trauma centers [14]. Our study was the first to identify the significant and positive effect of a trauma room equipped with a CT machine on patient mortality.

Our study also showed that a CT machine in the trauma room reduced the time to the start of CT scan by 20 min (from 37 to 23 min) and the length of the ED stay by 19 min (from 91 to 72 min). In selected samples after propensity score matching, time to start CT scan was reduced by 18 min (from 40 to 22 min) and the length of the ED stay reduced by 25.5 min (from 94.5 to 69 min). This

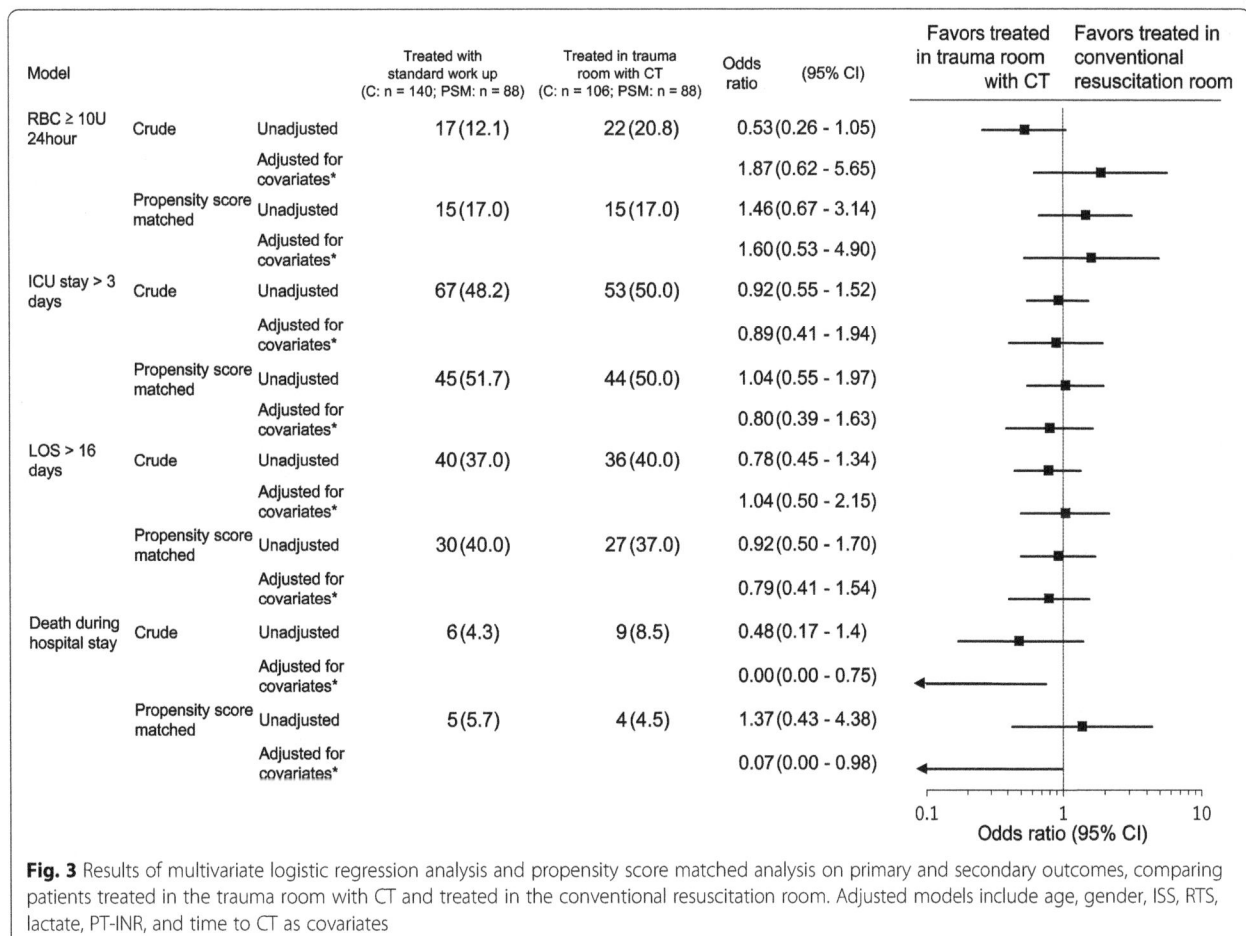

Fig. 3 Results of multivariate logistic regression analysis and propensity score matched analysis on primary and secondary outcomes, comparing patients treated in the trauma room with CT and treated in the conventional resuscitation room. Adjusted models include age, gender, ISS, RTS, lactate, PT-INR, and time to CT as covariates

Table 3 Characteristics and outcome differences between patients treated in trauma room with CT and conventional resuscitation room after propensity score matching (n = 176)

		Total (n = 176)	Conventional resuscitation room (n = 88)	Trauma room with CT (n = 88)	p value
		n (%)/median (IQR)	n (%)/median (IQR)	n (%)/median (IQR)	
Gender	Male	145 (82.4)	72 (81.8)	73 (83.0)	1.000
	Female	31 (17.6)	16 (18.2)	15 (17.0)	
Age		50 (35.8,67.2)	49 (33, 68.3)	52.5 (36, 67)	0.726
Initial vital signs	GCS	14 (13, 15)	14 (13, 15)	14 (13.8, 15)	0.931
	Heart rate	88 (72, 103)	88 (72, 102.3)	89 (72.5, 103.1)	0.877
	Systolic pressure	142 (120, 162)	143 (117.8, 164.8)	140 (120, 159)	0.747
	Respiratory rate	20 (17, 24)	20 (17, 24)	20 (17, 24)	0.366
	Temperature	36.4 (36, 36.9)	36.4 (35.9, 36.8)	36.4 (36.1, 36.9)	0.537
CT performed		152 (86.4)	77 (87.5)	93 (85.2)	0.826
	For head	127 (72.2)	61 (69.3)	83 (75.0)	0.501
	For body trunk	122 (69.3)	58 (65.9)	80 (72.7)	0.414
Intubation in ER		72 (40.9)	34 (38.6)	38 (43.2)	0.646
Use REBOA		5 (2.8)	1 (1.1)	4 (4.5)	0.364
Arterial embolization		20 (11.4)	9 (10.2)	11 (12.5)	0.812
Place chest tube in ER		15 (8.5)	6 (6.8)	9 (10.2)	0.589
Type of trauma	Blunt	147 (83.5)	73 (83.0)	74 (84.1)	1.000
	Penetrate	29 (16.5)	15 (17.0)	14 (15.9)	
Isolated TBI		12 (6.8)	8 (9.1)	4 (4.5)	0.370
Polytrauma		69 (39.2)	35 (39.8)	34 (38.6)	1.000
Hypotension		20 (11.4)	10 (11.4)	10 (11.4)	1.000
TAC INR > 1.3		9 (5.1)	5 (5.7)	4 (4.5)	1.000
ISS category	1–8	62 (35.2)	32 (36.4)	30 (34.1)	0.696
	9–15	45 (25.6)	21 (23.9)	24 (27.3)	
	16–24	45 (22.2)	22 (25.0)	17 (19.3)	
	≥ 25	30 (17.0)	13 (14.8)	17 (19.3)	
ISS		10 (4.8, 20)	10 (4.8, 17.3)	10 (4.8, 20)	0.709
RTS		7.84 (6.90, 7.84)	7.84 (6.90, 7.84)	7.84 (7.06, 7.84)	0.873
Ps		97.7 (92.1, 99.3)	97.7 (92.1, 99.2)	97.6 (91.5, 99.3)	0.781
Lactate		2 (1.3, 2.9)	2 (1.4, 3.2)	1.9 (1.3, 2.7)	0.245
BE		−0.3 (−2.6, 1.5)	−0.5 (−2.9, 1.1)	0.15 (−2, 1.9)	0.082
Hg		13.3 (11.4, 14.6)	13.3 (11.2, 14.7)	13.3 (11.4, 14.3)	0.537
Fbg		280 (229, 327)	289 (246, 332)	268 (222, 317)	0.278
APTT		26.4 (24.1, 28.7)	26.2 (24.1, 28.6)	26.7 (24.1, 28.9)	0.771
PT-INR		1.04 (0.97, 1.12)	1.02 (0.95, 1.12)	1.06 (0.98, 1.12)	0.096
FDP		14 (3.9, 47.3)	15.3 (4.3, 37.8)	12.7 (3.9, 67.9)	0.858
D-dimer		7.6 (1.5, 25.8)	8.5 (1.5, 23.3)	7.1 (1.6, 35.6)	0.955
Transfusion	RBC	0 (0, 6)	0 (0, 6)	0 (0, 6)	0.909
	FFP	0 (0, 6)	0 (0, 4)	0 (0, 6)	0.727
Mortality	In-hospital	9 (5.1)	5 (5.7)	4 (4.5)	1.000
	24 h	3 (1.7)	2 (2.3)	1 (1.1)	1.000
RBC ≥ 10 U/24 h		30 (17.0)	15 (17.0)	15 (17.0)	1.000
Time to CT (min)		30 (22, 43)	40 (30, 52)	22 (17, 28)	< 0.001

Table 3 Characteristics and outcome differences between patients treated in trauma room with CT and conventional resuscitation room after propensity score matching (n = 176) (Continued)

	Total (n = 176)	Conventional resuscitation room (n = 88)	Trauma room with CT (n = 88)	p value
	n (%)/median (IQR)	n (%)/median (IQR)	n (%)/median (IQR)	
Time to TAE (min)	81 (81, 100)	77 (56, 98)	81 (78, 91)	0.438
Time to operation (min)	75 (60, 122)	99 (60, 127)	83 (70, 118)	0.842
ED staying (min)	74 (56, 103)	91 (65, 115)	68 (52, 83)	< 0.001
ICU stay (day)	3 (2, 7)	3 (2, 9)	3 (2, 6)	0.401
Hospital stay (day)	17 (5, 39)	17 (5.5, 40)	17 (5, 37)	0.534

TAC traumatic acute coagulopathy, ISS Injury Severity Score, RTS Revised Trauma Score, Ps probability of survival

reduction was comparable or larger than that described in previous studies [7, 18, 20–22, 30]. This time saved could improve the workflow in a trauma care center and has a beneficial effect for the department staff. Previous studies have shown that the diagnostic work-up time was significantly longer in patients undergoing a conventional resuscitation [7, 18, 20–22, 30]. A rapid overview of all threatened body regions can be obtained, which increased decision-making and treatment times, leading to a lower mortality.

The presence of a CT machine in a trauma resuscitation room also has the following potential benefits. Installing a CT machine in a trauma room reduces the number of transfers to a CT room. Patient transfers can be time-consuming and laborious as the patient has to be moved to a transport stretcher and then back to a CT table. In a previous study, it was dangerous to transfer patients with hemodynamic instability to a CT room, which was called the tunnel of death [31]. These hemodynamically unstable patients could undergo a CT scan using the CT machine located in the trauma room. In our study, there were no patients who were unable to receive a CT scan because of hemodynamic instability in the group of patients treated in the trauma room with a CT machine. Installing a CT machine in a trauma room may resolve decision-making dilemmas in acute trauma care in patients without an obvious primary source or potentially multiple sources of hemorrhage. Such patients would benefit the most from CT scan information, as well as the reduced time to treatment.

We acknowledge several limitations of our study. First, this was a retrospective study; therefore, it was impossible to perform a sample size calculation. The current sample size would justify the utilization of a regression model with given proportions of outcomes [32]. Second, significant differences in baseline, including ISS and RTS, were observed between the two groups, which suggest heterogeneity in patients and raise concerns regarding the inability to control the effects of confounding factors. Thus, we employed a valid multivariate model to control these differences in our analysis. In addition, to overcome the bias, we further performed propensity score matching analysis because randomly allocating a patient into use or non-use of a trauma room with a CT machine could be difficult in certain clinical situations. Third, we also conducted a single-center study. There could be selection bias and a limitation in generalizability. Patients admitted to our hospital might be treated with a shorter time to transfer compared to those admitted in hospitals in a rural region. To evaluate the effects of a CT machine in the trauma room, our study design would be still appropriate. Fourth, we excluded pediatric patients and patients with CPA. This exclusion might affect the generalization of our study findings. Lastly, there was selection bias due to potential differences in decisions on performing the CT scan made by each trauma leader. The leaders were trained in YCUMC, and daily conferences by the trauma team could guarantee equality in decision-making.

Table 4 Multivariate logistic regression analysis after propensity score matching on mortality with associated factors (n = 176)

Factors		Odds ratio	(95% CI)	p value
Age		1.14	(1.04–1.25)	< 0.001
ISS		1.16	(1.02–1.31)	0.024
RTS		0.09	(0.02–0.37)	< 0.001
Lactate		1.28	(0.979–1.67)	0.07
Treated in trauma room with CT	(reference: treated in conventional resuscitation room)	0.065	(0.00–0.985)	0.0487

Conclusions

In conclusion, our study showed the effects on mortality using a CT-equipped trauma room. Our study also showed the time benefits of placing a CT machine in the trauma room. This time benefit could be critical in severe trauma patients, allowing life-threatening problems to be detected and allowing earlier critical decision-making. Installing a CT machine in the trauma room could reduce time for decision-making in treating a trauma patient and subsequently lower the mortality of trauma patients.

Abbreviations

AIS: Abbreviated Injury Score; APTT: Activated partial thromboplastin time; CT: Computed tomography; ED: Emergency department; FAST: Focused assessment with sonography for trauma; Fbg: Fibrinogen; FDP: Fibrin degradation products; GCS: Glasgow Coma Scale; HR: Heart rate; ICUs: Intensive care units; ISS: Injury Severity Score; LOS: Length of hospital stay; MC council: Medical control council; MTOS: Major Trauma Outcome Study; Ps: Probability of survival; PT-INR: International normalized ratio of prothrombin time; RTS: Revised Trauma Score; SaO$_2$: Percutaneous oxygen saturation; SBP: Systolic blood pressure; TAE: Transcatheter arterial embolization; TBCT: Total-body CT scanning; TRISS: Trauma and Injury Severity Score; YCUMC: The Yokohama City University Medical Center

Acknowledgements

The authors would like to thank all staffs at YCUMC.

Funding

The study did not receive any funding.

Authors' contributions

SF and TA wrote the study protocol. SF collected data from the hospital. SF and TA analyzed the data and drafted the manuscript, with critical review from all authors. All authors contributed with critical revision of the protocol. All authors read and approved the final manuscript.

Competing interests

The authors declare that they have no competing interests.

Author details

[1]Department of Emergency Medicine, Yokohama City University, 4-57 Urafunecho, Minamiku, Yokohama City, Kanagawa Prefecture 232-0024, Japan. [2]Department of Surgery, Yokohama City University, 4-57 Urafunecho, Minamiku, Yokohama City, Kanagawa Prefecture 232-0024, Japan. [3]Department of Acute Medicine, Graduate School of Medicine, The University of Tokyo, 7-3-1 Hongo, Bunkyo-ku, Tokyo 113-0033, Japan.

References

1. World Health Organization. WHO. Injuries and violence: the facts 2014. http://www.who.int/violence_injury_prevention/en/. Accessed 18 Mar 2018.
2. Committee of the Japan Association of Traumatology. The Japan Advanced Trauma Evaluation and Care (JATEC). 4th ed. Tokyo: Herusu Shuppan Co, Inc; 2012.
3. Salim A, Sangthong B, Martin M, Brown C, Plurad D, Demetriades D. Whole body imaging in blunt multisystem trauma patients without obvious signs of injury: results of a prospective study. Arch Surg. 2006;141:468–75.
4. Deunk J, Dekker HM, Brink M, van Vugt R, Edwards MJ, van Vugt AB. The value of indicated computed tomography scan of the chest and abdomen in addition to the conventional radiologic work-up for blunt trauma patients. J Trauma. 2007;63:757–63.
5. Pfeifer R, Pape HC. Missed injuries in trauma patients: a literature review. Patient Saf Surg. 2008;2:20.
6. Weninger P, Mauritz W, Fridrich P, Spitaler R, Figl M, Kern B, et al. Emergency room management of patients with blunt major trauma: evaluation of the multislice computed tomography protocol exemplified by an urban trauma center. J Trauma. 2007;62:584–91.
7. Hilbert P, zur Nieden K, Hofmann GO, Hoeller I, Koch R, Stuttmann R. New aspects in the emergency room management of critically injured patients: a multi-slice CT-oriented care algorithm. Injury. 2007;38:552–8.
8. Bernhard M, Becker TK, Nowe T, Mohorovicic M, Sikinger M, Brenner T, et al. Introduction of a treatment algorithm can improve the early management of emergency patients in the resuscitation room. Resuscitation. 2007;73:362–73.
9. Wurmb TE, Frühwald P, Hopfner W, Roewer N, Brederlau J. Whole-body multislice computed tomography as the primary and sole diagnostic tool in patients with blunt trauma: searching for its appropriate indication. Am J Emerg Med. 2007;25:1057–62.
10. Yeguiayan JM, Yap A, Freysz M, Garrigue D, Jacquot C, Martin C, et al. Impact of whole-body computed tomography on mortality and surgical management of severe blunt trauma. Crit Care. 2012;16:R101.
11. Kanz KG, Paul AO, Lefering R, Kay MV, Kreimeier U, Linsenmaier U, et al. Trauma management incorporating focused assessment with computed tomography in trauma (FACTT) - potential effect on survival. J Trauma Manag Outcomes. 2010;4:4.
12. Schoeneberg C, Schilling M, Burggraf M, Fochtmann U, Lendemans S. Reduction in mortality in severely injured patients following the introduction of the "treatment of patients with severe and multiple injuries" guideline of the German society of trauma surgery—a retrospective analysis of a level 1 trauma center (2010-2012). Injury. 2014;45:635–8.
13. Huber-Wagner S, Kanz KG, Mutschler W, Lefering R. Primary pan-computed tomography for blunt multiple trauma: can the whole be better than its parts? Injury. 2009;40:S36–46.
14. Huber-Wagner S, Lefering R, Qvick LM, Körner M, Kay MV, Pfeifer KJ, et al. Effect of whole-body CT during trauma resuscitation on survival: a retrospective, multicentre study. Lancet. 2009;373:1455–61.
15. Hutter M, Woltmann A, Hierholzer C, Gärtner C, Bühren V, Stengel D. Association between a single-pass whole-body computed tomography policy and survival after blunt major trauma: a retrospective cohort study. Scand J Trauma Resusc Emerg Med. 2011;19:73.
16. Wurmb TE, Frühwald P, Hopfner W, Keil T, Kredel M, Brederlau J, et al. Whole-body multislice computed tomography as the first line diagnostic tool in patients with multiple injuries: the focus on time. J Trauma. 2009;66:658–65.
17. Wurmb TE, Quaisser C, Balling H, Kredel M, Muellenbach R, Kenn W, et al. Whole-body multislice computed tomography (MSCT) improves trauma care in patients requiring surgery after multiple trauma. Emerg Med J. 2011;28:300–4.
18. Lee KL, Graham CA, Lam JM, Yeung JH, Ahuja AT, Rainer TH. Impact on trauma patient management of installing a computed tomography scanner in the emergency department. Injury. 2009;40:873–5.
19. Fung Kon Jin PH, Goslings JC, Ponsen KJ, van Kuijk C, Hoogerwerf N, Luitse JS. Assessment of a new trauma workflow concept implementing a sliding CT scanner in the trauma room: the effect on workup times. J Trauma. 2008;64:1320–6.
20. Wada D, Nakamori Y, Yamakawa K, Fujimi S. First clinical experience with IVR-CT system in the emergency room: positive impact on trauma workflow. Scand J Trauma Resusc Emerg Med. 2012;20:52.
21. Saltzherr TP, Bakker FC, Beenen LF, Dijkgraaf MG, Reitsma JB, Goslings JC. Randomized clinical trial comparing the effect of computed tomography in the trauma room versus the radiology department on injury outcomes (REACT-1). Br J Surg. 2012;99:105–13.
22. Huber-Wagner S, Mand C, Ruchholtz S, Kühne CA, Holzapfel K, Kanz KG, et al. Effect of the localisation of the CT scanner during trauma resuscitation on survival—a retrospective, multicentre study. Injury. 2014;45:S76–82.
23. Mutze S, Madeja S, Paris S, Ostermann P, Ekkernkamp A. Helical CT examination of multiple trauma patients in a digitized radiology department. Emerg Radiol. 1999;6:77–80.
24. Hsiao KH, Dinh MM, McNamara KP, Bein KJ, Roncal S, Saade C, et al. Whole-body computed tomography in the initial assessment of trauma patients: is there optimal criteria for patient selection? Emerg Med Australas. 2013;25:182–91.
25. American College of Surgeons Committee on Trauma. ATLS advanced trauma life support program for doctors. Student course manual. 9th ed. Chicago, IL: American College of Surgeons; 2012.
26. Champion HR, Sacco WJ, Carnazzo AJ, Copes W, Fouty WJ. Trauma score. Crit Care Med. 1981;9:672–6.
27. Champion HR, Sacco WJ, Copes WS, Gann DS, Gennarelli TA, Flanagan ME. A revision of the trauma score. J Trauma. 1989;29:623–9.
28. Boyd CR, Tolson MA, Copes WS. Evaluating trauma care: the TRISS method. J Trauma. 1987;27:370–8.
29. Kanda Y. Investigation of the freely available easy-to-use software 'EZR' for medical statistics. Bone Marrow Transplant. 2013;48:452–8.

24

Pattern and nature of Neyshabur train explosion blast injuries

Katayoun Jahangiri, Hasan Ghodsi*, Ali Khodadadizadeh and Sadegh Yousef Nezhad

Abstract

Background: Explosions are classified as both man-made and complex accidents. Explosive events can cause serious damage to people, property, and the environment. This study aimed to investigate the pattern and nature of damage incurred to the victims of the Neyshabur Train Explosion.

Methods: The current study is a descriptive cross-sectional study that was retrospectively performed on 99 individuals using census method and documents victims hospitalized due to the Neyshabur train disaster (February 2004) in 2016. In this study, different variables such as age, sex, type of injury, treatment, etc. were examined using a questionnaire and were analyzed using SPSS16.

Results: The results showed that 50.5% of victims were males with mean age of 30.33 ± 4.27 years and most of them were in 20- to 40-year age group. A total of 98 victims were discharged after treatment, and 1 victim died due to the severity of injuries after 3 days of hospitalization. Second type of injuries caused by the explosion accounted for most of the injuries (55.6%), and most treatments (54.5%) were related to the specific field of orthopedics.

Conclusion: Handling and transportation of fuels and chemicals via rail transport system is one of the potential hazards that threatens human life. The results showed that the highest numbers of victims were in 20- to 40-year age group, which is the age of economic efficiency. The prevention and reduction of human and financial losses resulting from accidents require proper national planning.

Keywords: Accidents, Train explosion, Man-made crises

Background

Explosions are classified as both man-made and complex accidents. Regardless of the cause of the explosion, explosive events can cause serious damage to a lot of people. The severity of injuries and damages caused by explosions depend on several factors, including the explosion occurred at the closed or roofed place, the amount of explosives, victims distance from the explosion, and the presence of other wastes at the site of the explosions [1].

The explosions cause multiple injuries classified in four groups (primary, secondary, tertiary and quaternary injuries). Each of these injuries may occur individually or in combination with other groups [2, 3].

The primary injuries occur as a result of rapid propagation of blast waves and affect air-filled body organs such as the lungs, ears, and hollow viscera of the digestive system (colon) [4]. Bowel perforation, hemorrhage, and mesenteric shear injuries are some consequences of primary blast injuries [5].The most common organ that is affected by blast injury is the ears [6]. If the eardrum is intact, there is little risk of damage to other air-filled body organs [7]. The lung is the second organ affected by primary injuries [8]. The most common cause of death following explosions is the second injuries. Objects that are thrown around cause secondary injuries that are often penetrating wounds. Head, neck, chest, abdomen, and extremities injuries constitute the most common types of second injuries [9]. The most common tertiary injuries are closed fractures and injuries of the brain. The uncommon injuries include joint dislocations and in some cases, amputation [2, 4, 10, 11]. Damage of buildings and streets can cause blunt trauma and crush injuries [8]. Quaternary injuries include all injuries that are not included in three injury classifications such as

* Correspondence: hasan_ghodsi@sbmu.ac.ir
Department of Health in Disasters and Emergencies, School of Health, Safety and Environment, Shahid Beheshti University of Medical Sciences, Tehran, Iran

respiratory injuries, burns, breathing toxic gases such as carbon monoxide, and choking and crush of bodies [11]. This study aimed to investigate the pattern and nature of injuries incurred to the victims of the train explosion in Neyshabur.

Short summary of the scenario

At 4:42 a.m. February 18, 2004, 51 wagons of a train that stopped at Abu Moslem Station started moving and then collided with a locomotive stopped at Khayyam Station, which led to the disarrangement of wagons and a primary fire (Fig. 1) [12]. The local firefighters from all the neighboring towns arrived to rescue anybody who might have been trapped inside and to extinguish several minor fires which had broken out in the wreckage [13].

At the beginning, the incident was a local event and Initial Command System the in scene was created by the chief of firefighters, then border railway homes were evacuated. The initial fire was controlled at 9 a.m., and the people returned to their home.

Local authorities and people went to watch the scene and thank the aid workers for their work. Unfortunately, at 9:37, suddenly, a very loud explosion occurred. Immediately after the explosion, revolutionary guards cordoned off a wide area around the disaster site overnight due to fears of further blasts and pollution [14].

Description of hazard causing the accident

Fifty one wagons of a train carried sulfur, ammonium nitrate, cotton, and oil. In this incident, there were seven ammonium nitrate wagons with an approximate weight of 399 tons. After collision of wagons with a locomotive stopping at the wagon station, wagons collided and an initial fire occurred. Firefighters were not aware of wagons' contents because fire diamond on the body of the wagons was not installed. An ammonium nitrate wagon was placed next to the flames and decomposed after 5 h and resulted in the explosion of other wagons [15].

Total number and type of injuries

The explosion led to the death of more than 300 and injuries of more than 450 spectators, officials, and relief workers. A total of 24 of the firefighters, governor, firefighting director, and head of the city's energy department died in this incident [12]. All people and animals, due to the severity of the explosion, died up to 500 m away [16]. The deceased victims were transferred to Neyshabur Forensic Medicine. The severity of the explosion was such that most of the bodies were disintegrated, and it was difficult to identify them. The injured people were transferred to Neyshabur and Mashhad hospitals by ambulance, personal, and military vehicles [12].

Methods

The present study is a retrospective descriptive study that was conducted in 2016. The sample size was 99 subjects who with census method by reviewing the medical records of all the train explosion victims who were transferred to Neyshabur hospitals. After obtaining the necessary permits, researchers isolated medical records of train blast victims while visiting the medical records unit of hospitals. The instrument used in this study was two-part researcher-made questionnaire. The first part includes demographic information such as age, sex, marital status, place of residence, etc. The second part relates to the type of injury, type of treatment procedures, and the outcome of procedures. The

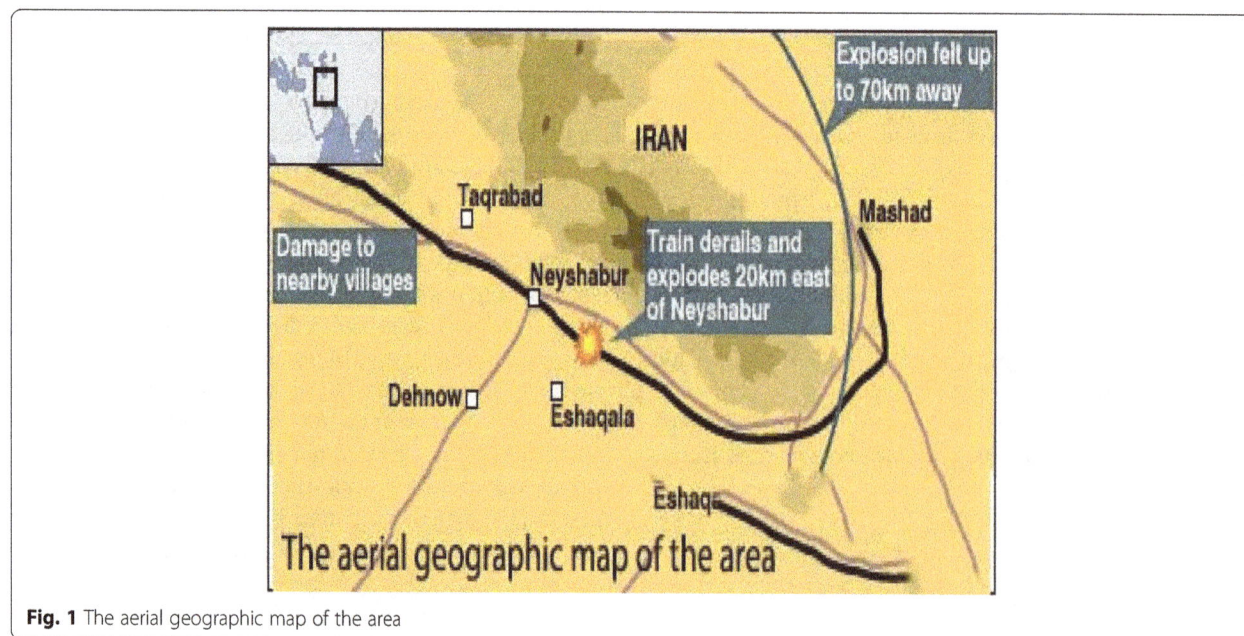

Fig. 1 The aerial geographic map of the area

data were entered into the software SPSS16 and then were described using frequency distribution tables and central and dispersion indicators.

Results

The results of investigating all medical records in medical records unit of Neyshabur hospitals (Hakim and 22 Bahman hospitals) showed that although the number of injuries was reported by executive agencies to be over 450 people, there were only a total number of 99 medical records belonging to admitted victims in these medical centers. The average age of victims was 30.33 ± 4.27 years, and most of them (36.4%) were in the 40- to 20-year age group. The youngest and oldest victims were 1.5 and 76 years old, respectively. Some demographic characteristics of the research subjects are shown in Table 1.

The majority of subjects (95%) were discharged from hospitals after the necessary treatment measures, and four patients (4%) were sent to the provincial capital after initial treatment measures for complementary therapies.

The reason stated for sending these patients was lung trauma and the absence of thoracic specialist in Neyshabur hospitals in 2003. Despite treatment procedures, one of the victims died after 3 days of hospitalization due to severe injuries (hem thorax, pneumothorax, and severe pulmonary contusion). Most treatments were performed by the departments of orthopedics (56%), neurosurgery (18%), general surgery (14%), and ENT (12%) (Fig. 2). Minimum and maximum days of hospitalization were 1 and 57 days, respectively (average 4.27 ± 6.07 days).

The second type injuries accounted for more injuries imposed on hospitalized victims (55.6%). Information on the types of injuries and the number of victims is shown in Table 2.

Discussion

The results showed that most of the victims of this accident were in 20- to 40-year age group, while most of the

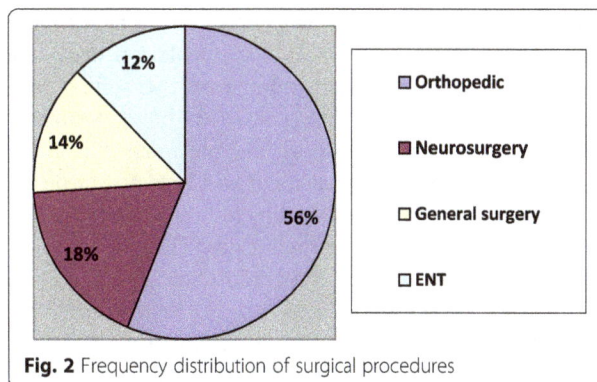

Fig. 2 Frequency distribution of surgical procedures

victims were children in Bashkir train blast [11]. The main reason for the age differences among victims is related to the type of accident in the two explosions. A freight train was exploded in Neyshabur train disaster with no passenger, while a freight train collided with a passenger train (mostly children) in the Bashkir train explosion. Many victims of Neyshabur train disaster belonged to 20- to 40-year age group because many of them who were present at the scene of the accident and had come to rescue the injured were young and middle-aged people. The results showed that the secondary injuries accounted for the most of the explosion-induced injuries imposed on hospitalized victims. Due to the severity of the blast, most people who were at 500 m away from the accident died. Also, most of those who survived and were transferred to hospitals were at a larger distance from the accident and were injured due to shrapnel hit their bodies. Furthermore, most of measures were taken by the Department of Orthopedic Surgery to remove shrapnel. This is despite the fact that most victims were hospitalized due to burns in Bashkir train explosion [11]. However, a ruptured eardrum, lungs injury, hem thorax, pneumothorax, contusion, and rupture of internal organs of the abdomen account for most of injuries in the most explosive events [17], due to the severity of the blast in Neyshabur train disaster, people with this type of injuries died at the scene of the accident; therefore, the second injuries accounted for the most of injuries. However, the results showed that there was no victim in the early hours of the accident; when officials have declared the fire was extinguished, the

Table 1 Some demographic characteristics of victims

Variable	Frequency	Percentage
Gender		
Male	50	50.5
Female	49	49.5
Marital status		
Married	61	61.6
Single	38	38.4
Hospital		
22 Bahman	72	72.7
Hakim	27	27.3

Table 2 Frequency of type of injuries incurred on Neyshabur train disaster victims

Type of injury	Frequency	Percent
Primary injuries	11	11.1
Secondary injuries	55	55.6
Tertiary injuries	29	29.3
Quaternary injuries	4	4
Total	99	100

evacuated people returned their homes and some of them also decided to watch the scene, the explosion occurred, and many people were killed and injured. In a similar incident that occurred in Baltimore in 2013, the total number of the injured was four people and the main reason for low victim number of the accident was reported to be in-time evacuation of the surrounding homes and prohibiting people to enter the scene of the incident [18].

The pattern of injury that occurs with explosions is unique. In this study, secondary injuries were higher than other injuries. And quaternary injuries were minimum in rate.

In this incident, due to the enormous blast force, most of the victims died at once at the scene of the incident.

From the above, it can be concluded that the high rate of casualty in this incident was due to the following reasons: 1—not regarding the rules of carrying hazardous materials and no installation fire diamond on the body of wagons, as a result of the lack of awareness of the firefighters and their mistake, and the decision to shut off the fire with water; 2—not protecting the perimeter of hot zone by the police and entry of unnecessary people to the scene of the incident.

Conclusion

Since the consequences of man-made and natural disasters are not predictable; therefore, to better manage events and prevent crises in the future, ordinary people should be prevented from entering the scene, until the full assurance of the safety of the scene so that we can minimize the number of affected people in case of an explosion. The blast force causes very serious injuries and often leads to the death of people. Given the extent of the injuries incurred to those present at the scene of the explosion, diagnosis and treatment of injuries are difficult.

Recommendations for the future are as follows: 1—To prevent and better response to similar incident, local authorities must supply enough resources (such as experts, equipment, information, etc.). 2—To avoid mass casualties—if needed—Incident Commander should protect the environment of incident by the police and then send EMS, fire fighters, volunteers, and other responders to hot zone. 3—The appropriate communication between the organizations involved in the incident is needed. 4—Providing executive and operational instructions for its implementation during a crisis. 5—Emergency medical technicians should learn about response to explosive events such as intentional and non-intentional incidents. They should learn how to protect themselves from dangers in the scene. They should get familiar with the type of blast injuries for better performance. In this incident, unfortunately, complete data are not available in forensic medicine, EMS department, hospitals, and other organizations involved. So, it can be said that the documentation in this incident was very weak. So, for better lesson learned from the incident, documentation is very important.

Limitation

Since this is a retrospective study, we could not get any other data such as reasons of mortality of people at the scene (cause of death and type of injuries of people who succumbed due to their injuries at scene that there were no on forensic medicine), trauma severity scores, detail about injuries frequency, and disability and the number of injured people who were treated by medical technicians on the scene.

Acknowledgements

We thank the Neyshabur University of Medical Sciences for valuable data.

Funding

The authors received no specific funding for this work.

Authors' contributions

HGH contributed to the study concept and design, acquisition and analysis of data, interpretation and making final conclusion of the results, and writing and editing the article. KJ contributed to the study supervision, interpretation and making final conclusion of the results, and editing the article. AKh and SY contributed to the study design and edition of the article and acquisition of the data. All authors read and approved the final manuscript.

Competing interests

The authors declare that they have no competing interests.

References

1. Champion HR, Holcomb JB, Young LA. Injuries from explosions: physics, biophysics, pathology, and required research focus. J Trauma. 2009;66(5): 1468–77. discussion 77
2. DePalma RG, Burris DG, Champion HR, Hodgson MJ. Blast injuries. N Engl J Med. 2005;352(13):1335–42.
3. Singh AK, Goralnick E, Velmahos G, Biddinger PD, Gates J, Sodickson A. Radiologic features of injuries from the Boston Marathon bombing at three hospitals. AJR Am J Roentgenol. 2014;203(2):235–9.
4. Sasser SM, Sattin RW, Hunt RC, Krohmer J. Blast lung injury. Prehosp Emerg Care. 2006;10(2):165–72.
5. Wani I, Parray FQ, Sheikh T, Wani RA, Amin A, Gul I, et al. Spectrum of abdominal organ injury in a primary blast type. World J Emerg Surg. 2009;4(1):46.
6. Chavko M, Prusaczyk WK, McCarron RM. Lung injury and recovery after exposure to blast overpressure. J Trauma. 2006;61(4):933–42.
7. Cho SI, Gao SS, Xia A, Wang R, Salles FT, Raphael PD, et al. Mechanisms of hearing loss after blast injury to the ear. PLoS One. 2013;8(7):e67618.
8. Mayo A, Kluger Y. Blast-induced injury of air-containing organs. ADF Health. 2006;7(1):40–4.
9. Halpern P. Bomb, blast, and crush injuries. In: Tintinalli JE, Stapczynski JS, Ma OJ, Cline DM, Cydulka RK, Meckler GD, et al., editors. Tintinalli's emergency medicine: a comprehensive study guide. New York, NY: The McGraw-Hill Companies; 2011.
10. Lemonick DM. Bombings and blast injuries: a primer for physicians. Am J Clin Med. 2011;8(3):134–40.
11. Stein M, Hirshberg A. Medical consequences of terrorism. The conventional weapon threat. Surg Clin North Am. 1999;79(6):1537–52.

12. Neyshabur train disaster: Wikipedia; 2004 [updated 9 April 2017, at 23:04].
    Available from: https://en.wikipedia.org/wiki/Nishapur_train_disaster.
13. Encyclopedia WH. Nishapur train disaster2004 [cited 2017. Available from:
    http://netlibrary.cc/articles/eng/Nishapur_train_disaster.
14. Blast danger recedes at Iran train disaster site 2004–02-19: CHINAdaily; 2004
    [updated 2004–02-19; cited 2017 June 4]. Available from: http://www.
    chinadaily.com.cn/english/doc/2004-02/19/content_307559.htm.
15. Ghanei M-h. Lessons from the explosion of the Neishabur train Shiraz: Shiraz
    fire department; 2005 [cited 2017 Oct.29]. Available from: www.shiraz.ir/
    bundles/IcmsDownloadcenter/files/.../file825.
16. Scores dead in Iranian train blast 2004 [updated Wednesday 18 February
    2004; cited 2017 Jun 9]. Available from: https://www.theguardian.com/
    world/2004/feb/18/iran.markoliver.
17. Master PB, Sekhar VC, Rangaiah YKC. Bomb blast: pattern and nature of injuries.
    Journal of Evidence based Medicine and Healthcare. 2015;2(2):165–71.
18. Winter M. Freight train derails, explodes near Baltimore. USA Today. 2013.

25

Correlation between modified LEMON score and intubation difficulty in adult trauma patients undergoing emergency surgery

Sung-Mi Ji[1], Eun-Jin Moon[2], Tae-Jun Kim[2], Jae-Woo Yi[2], Hyungseok Seo[2*] and Bong-Jae Lee[2]

Abstract

Background: Prediction of difficult airway is critical in the airway management of trauma patients. A LEMON method which consists of following assessments; Look-Evaluate-Mallampati-Obstruction-Neck mobility is a fast and easy technique to evaluate patients' airways in the emergency situation. And a modified LEMON method, which excludes the Mallampati classification from the original LEMON score, also can be used clinically. We investigated the relationship between modified LEMON score and intubation difficulty score in adult trauma patients undergoing emergency surgery.

Methods: We retrospectively reviewed electronic medical records of 114 adult trauma patients who underwent emergency surgery under general anesthesia. All patients' airways were evaluated according to the modified LEMON method before anesthesia induction and after tracheal intubation; the intubating doctor self-reported the intubation difficulty scale (IDS) score. A difficult intubation group was defined as patients who had IDS scores > 5.

Results: The modified LEMON score was significantly correlated with the IDS score ($P < 0.001$). The difficult intubation group showed higher modified LEMON score than the non-difficult intubation group (3 [2-5] vs. 2 [1-3], respectively, $P = 0.017$). Limited neck mobility was the only independent predictor of intubation difficulty (odds ratio, 6.15; $P = 0.002$).

Conclusion: The modified LEMON score is correlated with difficult intubation in adult trauma patients undergoing emergency surgery.

Keywords: Airway, Difficult intubation, Emergency surgery, LEMON score, Trauma

Background

Successful airway securement by an experienced physician is crucial in the management of trauma patient [1]. However, compared with other types of patients requiring tracheal intubation, trauma patients have a higher risk of intubation difficulty [2]. In trauma patients requiring emergency surgery, there may not have enough time to evaluate patient's airway, thereby being an increased risk of the unanticipated difficult airway. Furthermore, because of the limited number of advanced

airway securing devices or experienced staffs, such a situation that some devices or staffs are unavailable temporarily can be possible. Thus, prediction of the difficult airway and preparing appropriate device or staffs is critical in the airway management of trauma patients.

Conventional tools for predicting difficult airway, such as the Mallampati score, have a limited application in trauma patients [3]. The LEMON method, which consists of following assessments: Look-Evaluate-Mallampati-Obstruction-Neck mobility, can be used to predict difficult intubation in the emergency setting [4], and the modified LEMON score (also called "LEON" score), which excludes the Mallampati classification from the original LEMON score, has been developed for the identification of difficult airways [5].

* Correspondence: seohyungseok@gmail.com
[2]Department of Anesthesiology and Pain Medicine, Kyung Hee University Hospital at Gangdong, College of Medicine, Kyung Hee University, Seoul 05278, South Korea
Full list of author information is available at the end of the article

In the present study, we retrospectively investigated the ability of the LEON score to predict intubation difficulty by assessing the correlation between the LEON score and intubation difficulty score in adult trauma patients undergoing emergency surgery.

Methods

Patients

After the approval of the institutional review board (approval number: 2016-11-014), electronic medical records of adult trauma patients who underwent emergency surgery under general anesthesia in an operating theater between March 2016 and August 2016 were reviewed retrospectively. Patients who were already intubated before anesthesia induction or underwent surgical procedures under regional anesthesia were excluded.

Data collection

All patients' airways were evaluated by the well-trained residents or attending members of staff of the anesthesia department before anesthesia induction. Patient's airway assessment was performed according to the LEON method (Fig. 1, left) as follows: (1) Look, look at the patient externally for characteristics that are known to cause difficult laryngoscopy, intubation, or ventilation—in the LEON method, "Look" criteria assesses for presence of four features (facial trauma, large incisors, beard or mustaches, and large tongue); (2) evaluate the 3-3-2 rule—assess the alignment of the pharyngeal, laryngeal, and oral axes; (3) obstruction—presence of any conditions that can cause airway obstruction; and (4) neck mobility—assess for the presence of limited neck mobility or use of a hard neck collar immobilizer. General anesthesia was performed according to the institution's routine clinical practice. Anesthesia was induced with propofol (1 to 2 mg/kg) and maintained with volatile anesthetics, such as sevoflurane or desflurane. Target-controlled infusions of propofol and remifentanil were used. A neuromuscular blocking agent (NMBA), rocuronium bromide (0.6 mg/kg), was administered to facilitate tracheal intubation. Initially, tracheal intubation was performed by using a direct laryngoscope or video laryngoscope based on the intubating doctor's choice; however, a lightwand device or fiberoptic bronchoscopy was also used in cases of failed first attempt or difficult intubation. After tracheal intubation, the intubating doctor self-reported in the electronic medical records using the intubation difficulty scale (IDS; Fig. 1, right) as follows: N_1, the number of supplementary intubation attempts; N_2, the number of supplementary operators; N_3, the number of alternative intubation techniques used; N_4, glottic exposure as defined by the Cormack and Lehane grade (grade 1, $N_4 = 0$; grade 2, $N_4 = 1$; grade 3, $N_4 = 2$; grade 4, $N_4 = 3$); N_5, the lifting force applied during laryngoscopy ($N_5 = 1$ if a subjectively increased lifting force was required); N_6, external laryngeal pressure to improve glottic exposure ($N_6 = 1$ if external laryngeal pressure was required); and N_7, position of the vocal cords at intubation ($N_7 = 0$ if vocal cords in abduction or were not visualized; $N_7 = 1$ if vocal cords in adduction or blocking the tube passage). The IDS score is the sum of N_1 through N_7. An IDS score between 1 and 5 represents slight difficulty, and IDS score > 5 represents moderate to major difficulty. In the present study, patients were divided into the difficult intubation group (group D) and non-difficult intubation group (group ND) according to whether their IDS score was > 5 or ≤ 5.

Modified LEMON score	
Evaluation criteria	**Points**
Look externally	
Facial trauma	1
Larger incisors	1
Beard or moustache	1
Large tongue	1
Evaluate the 3-3-2 rule:	
Inter-incisor distance < 3 finger breadths	1
Hyoid-to-mental distance < 3 finger breadths	1
Thyroid-to-hyoid distance < 2 finger breadths	1
Obstruction:	
Any conditions causing airway obstruction	1
Neck mobility:	
Limited neck mobility or applying neck immobilizer.	1
Total score	9

Intubation difficulty scale		
Parameter	**Score**	**Calculation**
Number of intubation attempts > 1	N_1	Every additional attempt adds 1 point.
Number of involved anesthesiologist >1	N_2	Each additional anesthesiologist adds 1 point.
Number of alternative techniques	N_3	Each techniques adds 1 point.
Cormack-Lehane grade	N_4	N_4=grade at 1st attempt -1, if successful blind intubation N_4=0
Required lifting force	N_5	Normal; N_5=0, Required; N_5=1
Required laryngeal pressure	N_6	No; N_6=0, Required; N_6=1
Vocal cord mobility	N_7	Abduction; N_7=0, Adduction; N_7=1

Fig. 1 Modified LEMON (LEON) score and intubation difficulty scale score

Statistical analysis

All analyses were performed using MedCalc® 16.2 (MedCalc Software, Ostend, Belgium). Continuous variables were compared using the Student's t test or Mann-Whitney U test. Categorical variables were analyzed using a chi-square test, and the Cochran-Armitage test was used for trend analysis. Correlation between the LEON score and IDS was calculated using the Spearman's rank correlation. To determine the relationship between one dependent factor and one or more independent factors, a logistic regression analysis was performed. Data are expressed as means ± standard deviations, medians [interquartile ranges], or number (%). $P < 0.05$ was considered to be statistically significant.

Results

During study period, a total of 114 cases were reviewed. Patients' characteristics are shown in Table 1. There were no differences with respect to the demographic data and type of injury between group D and group ND. There was no patient who had unsuccessful intubation. Direct laryngoscope, video laryngoscope, lightwand device, and fiberoptic bronchoscope were used in 96, 17, 5, and 5 patients (84, 15, 4, and 4%, respectively).

The LEON score was significantly correlated with the IDS score (Spearman's correlation coefficient: 0.333, $P < 0.001$). The IDS score was 6 [6, 7] in group D, and it was 1 [0–3] in group ND ($P < 0.001$). The Cormack-Lehane grade was significantly higher in group D than in group ND (3 [3, 4] vs. 1 [1, 2], $P < 0.001$). The number of intubation attempts was higher in group D than in group ND (2 [1, 2] vs. 1 [1], $P < 0.001$). The median intubation

time was also longer in group D than in group ND (50 [27–80] vs. 17 [13–25] seconds, $P < 0.001$).

The LEON score was higher in group D than in group ND (3 [2–5] vs. 2 [1–3], $P = 0.017$) (Fig. 2). The incidence of difficult intubation tended to increase as the LEON score increased ($P = 0.005$). The logistic regression analysis showed that the LEON score showed a significant correlation with intubation difficulty (odds ratio, 1.55; 95% confidence interval, 1.12–2.14, $P = 0.008$). Among the variables in the LEON score, limited neck mobility was the only independent predictor of intubation difficulty (odds ratio, 6.15: 95% confidence interval, 1.909–19.819; $P = 0.002$) (Table 2).

Discussion

In the present study, we found that the LEON score correlated with the intubation difficulty and a LEON score of ≥3 could predict intubation difficulty in trauma patients.

Airway management is a challenging issue in adult trauma patients. Trauma patients may present with a variety of airway difficulties, ranging from promptly recognized to unanticipated difficult airways [6]. Moreover, most of trauma patients requiring emergency surgery do not have adequate time to undergo full preoperative airway evaluation; thus, they can be at an increased risk of unanticipated difficult airway. [4, 7] Therefore, it is crucial to be able to conduct a prompt assessment of the airway and predict difficult intubation. The LEMON score has been effectively used in emergency departments to predict difficult intubation because it can be determined based on the patient's appearance and observer's fingerbreadth, and it does not

Table 1 Patients' characteristics

Variables	Overall	Group ND ($n = 96$)	Group D ($n = 18$)	P
Age (year)	53 [38–61]	52 [18–83]	56 [19–84]	0.492
Sex (male %)	87 (76.3%)	73 (76.0%)	14 (77.8%)	0.874
Height (cm)	168.0 [162.8–175.0]	168.5 [163.0–175.0]	168.0 [159.5–174.3]	0.969
Weight (kg)	68.5 [57.0–75.0]	68.0 [57.0–75.0]	70.0 [57.3–75.8]	0.676
BMI (kg/m^2)	23.4 [21.1–25.1]	23.3 [21.0–25.1]	24.0 [22.3–25.7]	0.616
Type of injury				
Head and neck	34 (29.8%)	28 (29.2%)	6 (33.3%)	0.728
Chest	7 (6.1%)	6 (6.2%)	1 (5.6%)	0.923
Abdomen	7 (6.1%)	5 (5.2%)	2 (11.1%)	0.341
Spine	10 (8.8%)	8 (8.3%)	2 (11.1%)	0.701
Pelvis	4 (3.5%)	4 (4.2%)	0 (0%)	0.378
Extremities	52 (45.6%)	45 (46.9%)	7 (38.9%)	0.534

Data are expressed as medians [IQRs] or numbers (%)
Group ND: patients show intubation difficulty score ≤ 4
Group D: patients show intubation difficulty score > 5
Head and neck injury includes trauma to the head, facial area, and cervical spine
Spine injury indicates injury of thoracic and lumbar vertebra with/without neurologic complication
BMI body mass index

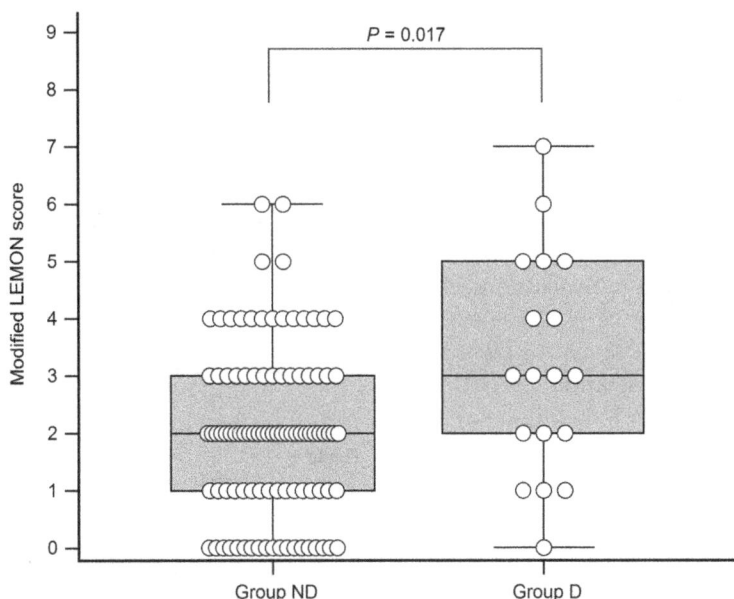

Fig. 2 Comparison of the modified LEMON (LEON) scores between group ND and group D. Patients in group ND shows intubation difficulty score ≤ 4 and patients in group D shows > 5. The modified LEMON score was 2 [1–3] in group ND and 3 [2–5] in group D (P = 0.017)

require special cut-off values or additional measurement tools [5, 8]. The Mallampati score component in the LEMON score is difficult to assess in trauma patient [7]; therefore, the LEON score, which excludes the Mallampati score, has been used effectively in clinical situations [5, 9]. Although the LEON score has been validated and widely used in emergency departments, the definitions of difficult intubation in previous studies were ambiguous (i.e., difficult tracheal intubation: tracheal intubation that requires multiple attempts in the presence or absence of tracheal pathology). In the present study, we used the IDS and defined a difficult

intubation as IDS score > 5 [2, 10]. By using the IDS, the severity of difficult intubation could be quantified; this enabled an analysis of the correlation between LEON score and intubation difficulty, which can suggest a cut-off value of LEON score in predicting difficult intubation.

It has been previously well-validated that the LEON score can effectively predict difficult intubation in the emergency department [9]. However, comparing with previous report that showed the median value of the LEON score was 1 in both the easy and difficult intubation group [5], our results showed that the median

Table 2 The incidence of each variables of modified LEMON (LEON) score and the correlation of each variables with the intubation difficulty

Variables	Overall	Group ND (n = 96)	Group D (n = 18)	Odds ratio	95% Confidence interval	P
Facial trauma, n (%)	32 (28.1%)	27 (281%)	5 (27.8%)	0.983	0.320–3.022	0.976
Large incisors, n (%)	9 (7.9%)	6 (6.2%)	3 (16.7%)	3.000	0.676–13.309	0.148
Beard or mustache, n (%)	17 (14.9%)	12 (12.5%)	5 (27.8%)	2.692	0.814–8.900	0.105
Large tongue, n (%)	16 (14.0%)	11 (11.5%)	5 (27.8%)	2.972	0.888–9.943	0.077
Inter-incisor distance < 3 FBs, n (%)	49 (43.0%)	39 (40.6%)	10 (55.6%)	1.827	0.662–5.041	0.245
Hyoid-to-mental distance < 3 FBs, n (%)	33 (28.9%)	28 (29.2%)	5 (27.8%)	0.934	0.304–2.867	0.905
Thyroid-to-hyoid distance < 2 FBs, n (%)	48 (42.1%)	39 (40.6%)	9 (50.0%)	1.462	0.533–4.012	0.461
Obstruction signs, n (%)	30 (26.3%)	22 (22.9%)	8 (44.4%)	2.691	0.917–7.617	0.063
Limited neck mobility, n (%)	16 (14.0%)	9 (9.4%)	7 (38.9%)[a]	6.152	1.909–19.821	0.002

[a] P = 0.001 compared with group ND

Group ND indicates patients show intubation difficulty score ≤ 4 and group D indicates patients show intubation difficulty score > 5

P value indicates the significance of univariable logistic regression between each variables and intubation difficulty

Obstruction signs indicate the presence of any conditions such as epiglottitis, peritonsillar abscess, sleep apnea, or upper airway trauma

FB finger breadth

value of the LEON score was 3 in the difficult intubation group and 2 in the non-difficult intubation group. Moreover, our results showed that limited neck mobility is an independent predictor of difficult intubation; this is in contrast with the results of a previous study that showed the thyroid-to-hyoid distance was not an independent predictor of difficult intubation. We thought that this difference may be because of our study population, particularly the high proportion of patients with head and neck injury. Head and neck injury is frequently associated with cervical spine injury [11, 12], and neck immobilization should be considered even without a definite cervical spine injury [13]. The point in the criteria of limited neck mobility may have contributed to a higher LEON score in this study than that reported in the previous study. Moreover, limited neck mobility, which was found to be an independent predictor of difficult intubation in the present study, may also provide evidence supporting the importance of neck mobility in the airway management of trauma patients. The thyroid-to-hyoid distance, despite its clinical significance in a previous study [5], did not significantly contribute the difficult intubation in this study, and the use of video laryngoscope may have affected this observation. Compared with direct laryngoscope, a video laryngoscope can provide an extended view in the vertical plane, which offers an advantage in cases of an anteriorly placed larynx [14]. A video laryngoscope was used for the initial intubation attempt in 15% of the subjects, which may be large enough to attenuate the influence of the thyroid-to-hyoid distance in tracheal intubation.

This study has several limitations. First, the study was conducted with a retrospective design via analysis of electronic medical records. Although the intubating doctor recorded the intubation information right after the induction of anesthesia, the data may have been unreliable because they were self-reported data. Moreover, because the initial intubation device can be selected by intubator's choice, a selection bias may affect the result. A relatively small population for a retrospective study also contributes to the result. Second, the results of the present study do not reflect patients with very severe and complex traumatic injuries that require immediate airway access. Because we evaluated patients undergoing emergency surgery in the operating theater, patients who underwent immediate tracheal intubation in the emergency department were not included. Third, we used NMBA to facilitate tracheal intubation in the present study. Since NMBA can provide the relaxation of soft tissues and comfortable condition without patient movements, the IDS score can be differed in clinical situations of tracheal intubation without NMBA.

Conclusion

The LEON score may be used as one of the evidence predicting difficult airway, thereby being helpful to increase safety in the airway management of adult trauma patients undergoing emergency surgery. A patient with LEON score ≥ 3 may have the possibility of difficult intubation, and even in using video laryngoscopy, the limited neck mobility may contribute to the intubation difficulty.

Abbreviation
IDS: Intubation difficulty scale; NMBA: Neuromuscular blocking agent

Funding
There are no funding sources for the present case report.

Authors' contributions
SMJ contributed in the interpretation of the data and drafting of the manuscript. EJM took part in the data analysis and critical revision. TJK had a hand in the data interpretation and statistical analysis. HS played a part in the study concept and design, interpretation of the data, statistical analysis, critical revision of the manuscript, and study supervision. JWY and BJL helped in the study concept, critical revision, and study supervision. All authors read and approved the final manuscript.

Competing interests
The authors declare that they have no competing interests.

Author details
[1]Department of Anesthesiology and Pain Medicine, College of Medicine, Dankook University, Cheonan, South Korea. [2]Department of Anesthesiology and Pain Medicine, Kyung Hee University Hospital at Gangdong, College of Medicine, Kyung Hee University, Seoul 05278, South Korea.

References
1. Langeron O, Birenbaum A, Amour J. Airway management in trauma. Minerva Anestesiol. 2009;75:307–11.
2. Adnet F, Racine SX, Borron SW, Clemessy JL, Fournier JL, Lapostolle F, Cupa M. A survey of tracheal intubation difficulty in the operating room: a prospective observational study. Acta Anaesthesiol Scand. 2001;45:327–32.
3. Levitan RM, Everett WW, Ochroch EA. Limitations of difficult airway prediction in patients intubated in the emergency department. Ann Emerg Med. 2004;44:307–13.
4. Reed MJ, Dunn MJ, McKeown DW. Can an airway assessment score predict difficulty at intubation in the emergency department? Emerg Med J. 2005; 22:99–102.
5. Soyuncu S, Eken C, Cete Y, Bektas F, Akcimen M. Determination of difficult intubation in the ED. Am J Emerg Med. 2009;27:905–10.
6. Walls RM. Management of the difficult airway in the trauma patient. Emerg Med Clin North Am. 1998;16:45–61.
7. Bair AE, Caravelli R, Tyler K, Laurin EG. Feasibility of the preoperative Mallampati airway assessment in emergency department patients. J Emerg Med. 2010;38:677–80.
8. Mayglothling J, Duane TM, Gibbs M, McCunn M, Legome E, Eastman AL, Whelan J, Shah KH. Eastern Association for the Surgery of T. Emergency tracheal intubation immediately following traumatic injury: an Eastern Association for the Surgery of Trauma practice management guideline. J Trauma Acute Care Surg. 2012;73:S333–40.

9.   Hagiwara Y, Watase H, Okamoto H, Goto T, Hasegawa K. Japanese
     emergency medicine network I. Prospective validation of the modified
     LEMON criteria to predict difficult intubation in the ED. Am J Emerg Med.
     2015;33:1492–6.
10. Adnet F, Borron SW, Racine SX, Clemessy JL, Fournier JL, Plaisance P,
     Lapandry C. The intubation difficulty scale (IDS): proposal and evaluation of
     a new score characterizing the complexity of endotracheal intubation.
     Anesthesiology. 1997;87:1290–7.
11. Hackl W, Hausberger K, Sailer R, Ulmer H, Gassner R. Prevalence of cervical
     spine injuries in patients with facial trauma. Oral Surg Oral Med Oral Pathol
     Oral Radiol Endod. 2001;92:370–6.
12. Mukherjee S, Abhinav K, Revington PJ. A review of cervical spine injury
     associated with maxillofacial trauma at a UK tertiary referral centre. Ann R
     Coll Surg Engl. 2015;97:66–72.
13. Austin N, Krishnamoorthy V, Dagal A. Airway management in cervical spine
     injury. Int J Crit Illn Inj Sci. 2014;4:50–6.
14. Sulser S, Ubmann D, Schlaepfer M, Brueesch M, Goliasch G, Seifert B, Spahn
     DR, Ruetzler K. C-MAC videolaryngoscope compared with direct
     laryngoscopy for rapid sequence intubation in an emergency department: a
     randomised clinical trial. Eur J Anaesthesiol. 2016;33:943–8.

26

Penetrating cardiac trauma: analysis of 240 cases from a hospital

Andres Isaza-Restrepo[1,2]* (iD), Dínimo José Bolívar-Sáenz[3], Marcos Tarazona-Lara[2] and José Rafael Tovar[4]

Abstract

Background: Trauma characteristics and its management is influenced by socioeconomic context. Cardiac trauma constitutes a challenge for surgeons, and outcomes depend on multiple factors including initial care, characteristics of the wounds, and surgical management.

Methods: This is a retrospective cross-sectional case series of patients with penetrating cardiac injuries (PCI) from January 1999 to October 2009 who underwent surgery in a trauma referral center in Bogotá, Colombia. Demographic variables, trauma characteristics, treatment, and outcomes were analyzed.

Results: The study included 240 cases: 96.2% males, mean age of 27.8 years. Overall mortality was 14.6%: 11.7% from stab wounds and 41.2% from gunshot wounds. Upon admission, 44% had a normal hemodynamic status and 67% had cardiac tamponade. About 32% had Grade II injuries and 29% Grade IV injuries. In 85% of the cases, there were ventricular compromise and 55% of patients had associated lesions. In 150 cases, a pericardial window was performed. Highest mortality occurred in wounds to the right atrium. In tamponade patients, mortality was 20% being higher for gunshot wounds (54.5%) than for stab wounds (18%) ($p = 0.0120$).

Conclusions: The study evidenced predominance of stab wounds. Based on characteristics of the trauma, patients, and survival rate, there is most likely a high pre-hospitalization mortality rate. The difference in mortality due to stab wounds and those produced by gunshots was more related to technical difficulties of the surgical repair than with the type of injury established by the Injury Grading Scale. Mortality was higher in patients with cardiac tamponade. Surgical management was satisfactory using pericardial window as the diagnostic method and sternotomy as the surgical approach.

Keywords: Cardiac trauma, Penetrating chest wounds, Heart injury, Penetrating wounds, Cardiac tamponade, Pericardial window, Sternotomy, Case series

Background

Due to high mortality rates, cardiac trauma management is a challenge for trauma teams. Based on the National Trauma Data Bank of the American College of Surgeons (ACS), Asensio et al. [1] calculated a 0.16% incidence of penetrating cardiac injury (PCI) admissions to trauma centers. Mandal and Sanusi [2] found that PCI occurred in 6.4% of the penetrating chest injuries, one of the most frequently injured body segments.

Historically, heart injuries had fatal outcomes and were considered untreatable [3]; even today, about 90% of the patients die before reaching the hospital [4–6]. Different case series have reported survival rates ranging from 3 to 84% [6–9]. Some authors have found associations between mortality and patient's hemodynamic status upon admission, kind of weapon used, wound characteristics, surgical findings, and complexity of the repair [10, 11].

Trauma characteristics may change according to social context, for example in blunt chest trauma, which is more frequent in developed countries, 30% of cardiac compromise has been reported. Survival rate for patients admitted to emergency departments in a shock state after PCI is about 35%, while for blunt chest trauma this

* Correspondence: andres.isaza@urosario.edu.co
[1]Escuela de Medicina y Ciencias de la Salud, Universidad del Rosario, Carrera 24 No 63C - 69 Barrio Siete de Agosto, Bogotá, DC, Colombia
[2]Méderi Hospital Universitario Mayor, Carrera 24 No 63C - 69 Barrio Siete de Agosto, Bogotá, DC, Colombia
Full list of author information is available at the end of the article

rate is about 2% [3]. In the USA, the ratio between PCIs from gunshots (PCI-GSW) and from stabbing (PCI-SW) is 2:1 but in developing countries the latter is more frequent [1, 6]. These differences may influence the results of reported series.

Armed conflict and urban violence in Colombia generate a high incidence of traumatic injuries, but there are few reports in the literature about experiences in their management. The series from Hospital San Juan de Dios in Bogotá in the 1980s [12] and from Hospital San Vicente de Paul in Medellín in the 1990s are the two main studies of cardiac trauma in our country [13]. Our study reports 10 years of experience in managing PCI patients on a Level III institution and trauma referral center in Bogotá, with the objective to compare and analyze it against other series reported in literature and to describe particularities encountered on our experience.

Methods

A cross-sectional retrospective case series of penetrating cardiac injury patients was done. Clinical charts of the patients with penetrating cardiac trauma that arrived to Hospital Occidente Kennedy (HOK) and underwent surgery from January 1999 to October 2009 were reviewed. Trauma team of HOK emergency service evaluated the patients, and upon admission, they were classified according to their hemodynamic status as proposed by Ivatury et al. [14]. Resuscitation was done according to the Advanced Trauma Life Support (ATLS) protocols of the ACS [15]. Patients dead upon arrival to the institution and those with Grade I cardiac wounds were excluded. Agonic patients and those with cardiac arrest were transferred immediately to an operating room for a

resuscitative thoracotomy. Patients that arrived in deep shock (SBP ≤80 mmHg after reanimation with 2000 cc crystalloids) or with signs of cardiac tamponade [16] were submitted to a closed tube thoracostomy, median sternotomy, or thoracotomy (left or right), depending on the location of the wound and clinical and in some cases post-thoracostomy findings. In the initial years of the case series, the hospital did not have a permanent echocardiography service, and later on, the echocardiogram was introduced with academic purposes but was not used for the assessment of trauma patients in the emergency department protocols; therefore, none of the patients in this study received echocardiographic evaluation. Subxiphoid pericardial window was performed for all hemodynamically stable patients with injuries in the precordial region [9, 11] to rule out cardiac compromise. The Organ Injury Scaling of the American Association for the Surgery of Trauma (OIS-AAST) classification system [17] was used for cardiac injury grading (see Table 1). Repair method was selected according to hemodynamic status, associated lesions, and surgeon preference. The following additional data was obtained: age, sex, injury characteristics, injury-surgery time, and intensive care unit (ICU) and hospitalization time stay.

Data from clinical records was collected manually using an instrument designed for that purpose, and then an EXCEL® database was created. The data was analyzed statistically using the IBM SPSS Desktop 20.0 for Windows. For quantitative variables, the mean, median, standard deviation, or range were used depending on the symmetry of data distribution. Qualitative variables, expressed in categories, were described as proportions,

Table 1 Cardiac injury grading according to OIS-ASST system (see reference [17])

Grade	Injury description
I	Blunt cardiac injury with minor ECG abnormality (non-specific ST or T wave changes, premature atrial and ventricular contraction, or persistent sinus tachycardia). Blunt or penetrating pericardial wound without cardiac injury, cardiac tamponade or cardiac herniation.
II	Blunt cardiac injury with heart block (right or left bundle branch, left anterior fasicular or atrioventricular) or ischemic changes (ST depression or T wave inversion) without cardiac failure. Penetrating tangential myocardial wound up to but not extending through the endocardium, without tamponade.
III	Blunt cardiac injury with sustained (≥5 beats/min) or multifocal ventricular contractions. Blunt or penetrating cardiac injury with septal rupture, pulmonary or tricuspid valvular incompetence, papillary muscle dysfunction, or distal coronary arterial occlusion without cardiac failure. Blunt pericardial laceration with cardiac herniation. Blunt cardiac injury with cardiac failure. Penetrating tangential myocardial wound up to but not extending through the endocardium, with tamponade.
IV	Blunt or penetrating cardiac injury with septal rupture, pulmonary or tricuspid valvular incompetence, papillary muscle dysfunction, or distal coronary arterial occlusion producing cardiac failure. Blunt or penetrating cardiac injury with aortic or mitral valve incompetence Blunt or penetrating cardiac injury of the right ventricle, right atrium, or left atrium
V	Blunt or penetrating cardiac injury with proximal coronary arterial occlusion Blunt or penetrating left ventricular perforation Stellate injuries <50% tissue loss of the right ventricle, right atrium, or left atrium
VI	Blunt avulsion of the heart: penetrating wound producing >50% tissue loss of a chamber

and to establish comparisons between proportions, the *z* test and Fisher exact test were used. A Type I error of less than 5% was accepted as being statistically significant.

Results

Diagnosis of PCI was done in 308 cases according to the manual registration of the surgical unit. After reviewing the clinical charts, a total of 68 cases were excluded: 22 were Grade I cardiac injuries (exclusive of pericardial compromise), 13 cases had insufficient information in the medical records, and 33 had the clinical information which did not coincide with the PCI diagnosis. A final sample of 240 cases was reached.

The mean age was 27.8 years (SD = 9.1); most of the patients were males (*n* = 231; 96.2%). Overall mortality was 14.6% (*n* = 35). There was a total of 223 PCI-SW cases (93%) with a mortality of 11.7%. Among the 17 PCI-GSW cases, mortality was 41.2%. In 150 cases (62.3%), a pericardial window was performed for diagnosis (11 of the PCI-GSW and 139 of the PCI-SW). According to the hemodynamic classification from Ivatury et al. [14], 44% (*n* = 106) of the patients were on a normal hemodynamic status upon admission, 34% (*n* = 82) were in profound shock, 18% (*n* = 44) were in extremis or agonic, and 3% (*n* = 8) were dead on arrival. Signs of cardiac tamponade was found in 67% (*n* = 161) of the cases, and a similar distribution was found for both injury mechanisms (67% of the PCI-SW and 65% of the PCI-GSW cases). The mean time interval between the injury and surgical procedure was 60 min. In 73.6% of the cases, that time was less than 120 min. The median stay in the ICU was 5 days (range 1–30), and the median hospital stay was 6 days (range 1–58).

Based on the OIS-AAST system [17], 33% (*n* = 79) of the patients had Grade II injuries on arrival and a mortality of 2.5% (*n* = 2 of 79); 13.3% (*n* = 32) Grade III with a mortality of 12.5% (*n* = 4 of 32); 29.2% (*n* = 70) Grade IV and a mortality of 20% (*n* = 14 of 70); and 24.5% (*n* = 59) Grade V and mortality of 25.4% (*n* = 15 of 59). There was compromise of the right ventricle in 53% of the cases, the left ventricle in 32%, the right atrium in 10%; and the left atrium in 5%. There was simultaneous injury of two chambers in 4 cases (1.6%) and two or more injuries in one cavity in 12 patients (5%). Of the 106 patients admitted with a normal hemodynamic status, 71 (67%) had Grade II cardiac injuries; 15 (14%) had Grade IV; and 13 patients (12.5%) had Grade V. In 45% (*n* = 108) of the cases, there was only cardiac lesions.

Type of weapon, surgical approach, and outcome

Mortality for PCI-SW group admitted with a normal hemodynamic status was 1% (1/99) whereas in the PCI-GSW group was 28.6% (2/7). The highest proportion of deaths occurred among individuals with Grade V injuries (12/53, 22.6%); whereas in the PCI-GSW group, 3 of the 4 patients with Grade IV wounds (75%) died (Table 2). The most frequently compromised cavities were the ventricles (*n* = 204, 85%), 127 (52.9%) cases in the right ventricle and 77 (32.1%) in the left.

Mortality

In right-ventricle injuries, mortality was 10.2% (13/127) and in left ventricle, 15.6% (12/77). Of the 18 injuries in the atriums, 7 occurred in the right atrium, of which 5 (71%) were fatal; of the 11 injuries in the left atrium, there were also 5 deaths (45.5%) (Fig. 1).

In 67.1% of the cases, there was cardiac tamponade. Mortality was 20.5% (33/161). Of the patients with tamponade, 93.2% had PCI-SW with 18% (27/150) mortality. Of the 11 PCI-GSW patients with tamponade, mortality was 54.5% (6/11). When comparing the proportions of individuals who died with tamponade injuries based on weapon type, there was a statistically significant difference (*p* = 0.0120). Of the 56 individuals remitted to the ICU, only 2 died.

Discussion

In our series, young males predominate, similar to what has been reported in the literature. In contrast, trauma characteristics, treatment, and results had some differences. The more prevalent wound mechanism was PCI-SW (93%); at admission, a total of 106 patients (44%) had a normal hemodynamic status and 161 (67%) had cardiac tamponade. The high percentage of normal hemodynamic status patients partially explains the low overall mortality in this series (14.6%) compared to what has been reported in the literature [4–6, 18–24]; nonetheless, it is similar to the reports done by Villegas (10.4%) and Duque (13%) in Colombia [25, 26]. Mortality for the PCI-SW cases was 11.7% while in other series it ranges between 13 and 78% [2, 5, 10, 23–25]. For the PCI-GSW, mortality was 41.2%, similar to what is reported in series where type of injury predominate (26–85%) [2, 5, 10, 21, 23–25].

When analyzing the differences in mortality between wound mechanism, we could not identify significant differences in the prevalence for Grades II and III injury for PCI-SW and PCI-GSW cases (46.6 and 41.2% respectively); thus, we inferred that the higher mortality in PCI-GSW was due to not receiving early hospital care rather than injury grade. Another possible explanation for the high mortality is that most of PCI-GSW cases had associated lesions: thoracoabdominal (52.9%), chest (18%), and abdominal (1 case). This observation is consistent with other experiences like those from Asensio et al. [10], Buckman et al. [27], and others who have reported that associated lesions were a poor prognosis

Table 2 Distribution of patients according to gender, hemodynamic status on admission, wound classification, surgical intervention, and post-discharge conditions related to the mechanism

Wound type	Variables		Dead	Alive	Total
Stab wounds (n = 223)	Sex	Male	25	190	215
		Female	2	6	8
	Hemodynamic status	Fatal	2	6	8
		In extremis	8	32	40
		Deep shock	16	60	76
		Normal	1	98	99
	Wound classification	Grade II injury	0	73	73
		Grade III injury	4	27	31
		Grade IV injury	11	55	66
		Grade V injury	12	41	53
	Surgical approach	Sternotomy	9	135	144
		Thoracotomy—anterolateral	18	60	78
		Clamshell incision	–	1	1
		Thoracotomy—posterolateral	–	98	98
Gunshot wounds (n = 17)	Sex	Male	8	8	16
		Female	0	1	1
	Hemodynamic status	Fatal	0	0	0
		In extremis	4	0	4
		Deep shock	2	4	6
		Normal	2	5	7
	Wound classification	Grade II injury	2	4	6
		Grade III injury	0	1	1
		Grade IV injury	3	1	4
		Grade V injury	3	3	6
	Surgical approach	Sternotomy	3	5	8
		Thoracotomy—anterolateral	5	3	8
		Clamshell incision	NA	0	0
		Thoracotomy	NA	0	0

NA not applicable

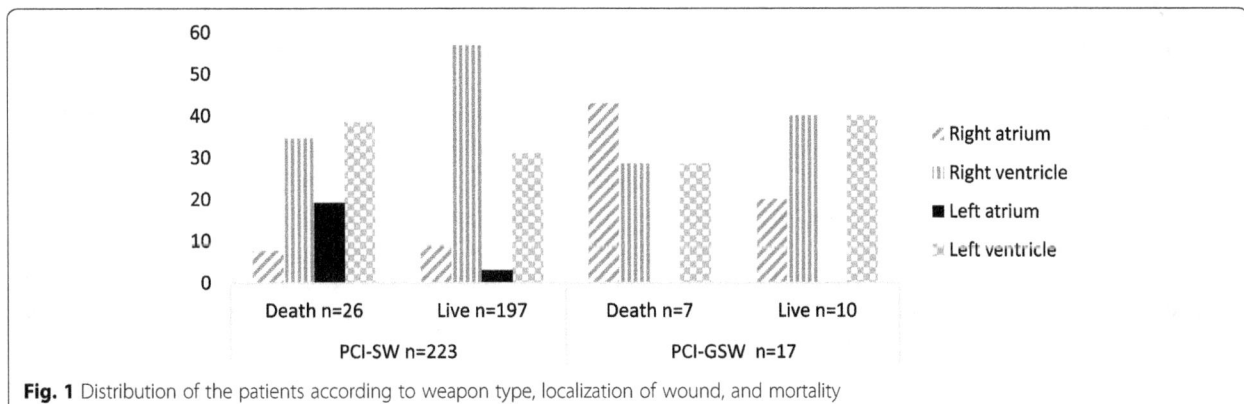

Fig. 1 Distribution of the patients according to weapon type, localization of wound, and mortality

factor for PCI patients [28–30]. It is important to remark that in our center a deep analysis was not done to stablish the final cause of death (if heart wound or associated lesions) as this process in Bogotá must be done by specialized centers in forensic medicine.

The degree of hemodynamic compromise in this series also failed to explain the difference in mortality given that 78% of the PCI-SW and 76% of the PCI-GSW were admitted with a hemodynamic status ranging from normal to profound shock. This could be explained probably due to the high prehospital mortality rate in the latter group.

Although the proportion of patients with cardiac tamponade was similar for both types of injuries, it should be noted that when there was cardiac tamponade mortality was higher than the overall mortality (20.5 vs. 14.6%). Some authors consider cardiac tamponade to be a protective factor for patient's survival [16]. Our results showed that the 2 of the 33 patients that died and had cardiac tamponade also had a normal hemodynamic status; moreover, 66% ($n = 22$ of 33) had some associated injury in the thorax or abdomen. It is important to point out that, in terms of physiopathology, filling of the pericardium space limits the stroke volume so in response cardiac frequency and right heart filling pressures are elevated through catecholamine production until right heart's distensibility limit is reached, septum is pushed to the left side, and left side's function is finally compromised [1]. For this reason, the longer the decompression of the pericardial space is delayed, a poorer prognosis should be expected which may explain our findings. As far as we know, the exact point when tamponade becomes a detrimental factor has not been stablished [27].

This series is unique in that a pericardial window was performed as the diagnostic procedure in 62.3% of the patients. As explained before, no echocardiographic assessment was done in this series, thus the protocol was to perform diagnostic pericardial windows in patients admitted with a PCI and a normal hemodynamic status. The group's experience with this procedure was satisfactory, and the results were analyzed and published [31]. In none of our cases was the pericardial sac washed to define the management as some groups propose [32], which in hindsight could have prevented the thoracotomy done in the 22 cases (8.4% of the total series) excluded from the analysis for having only the pericardium compromised.

The frequent use of pericardial window partly explains our group's preference for using sternotomy as the surgical approach and the good results obtained, similar to other series [29, 33]. In this series, a left anterolateral thoracotomy was generally used for resuscitation in patients with evident cardiac tamponade or in extremis. We concur that (i) the advantages of a sternotomy are better access to the right chambers and right pulmonary hilum, allowing cannulation for a cardiopulmonar bypass and (ii) that the left anterolateral thoracotomy facilitates access to posterior structures such as the esophagus, descending aorta, or left hilum [3]. Nevertheless, the choice of surgical approach also depends on the surgeon's experience, the expected injuries according to the probable trajectory of the wounds, and the evidence of associated lesions.

Different physiological indexes and trauma mechanism have been proposed as predictors of mortality. Among the factors that affect survival rate after a PCI are the type of weapon used, the size of myocardial injury, cardiac injured chamber, compromise of coronary arteries, initial hemodynamic status, associated lesions, and the time elapsed until reaching the hospital, factors with which our series coincide. The overall most common wound location was the ventricles ($n = 204$), and compromise of the right and left ventricle was observed in 53 and 32% respectively, with a 10–15% mortality. In contrast, of the 18 injuries to the atria, 7 occurred in the right atrium with 71% mortality and 11 in the left atrium with 5 deaths (45.5%). It was surprising that some Grade IV and V patients were admitted with a normal hemodynamic status. Despite an overall survival rate of about 85%, it is not possible to address the "benevolence" of the cardiac injuries as this and other series are based on analyses of patients that received medical attention and thus represent the cases with better prognosis.

The average time between the moment of injury and execution of the surgical procedure was 60 min, and in 73.6% of the cases, this time was less than 120 min. It can be inferred that a large number of victims die before reaching the hospital. In a previous work by Pedraza and Isaza et al. (found in the Universidad del Rosario repository under the title Caracterización de la mortalidad por trauma cardíaco penetrante en Bogotá), 127 autopsies from individuals with heart injuries were performed finding that 71% died within the first hour and that only 51% received some type of medical attention.

The clinical follow-up was done until they were discharged from the hospital. The population's socioeconomic conditions, the irregular availability of echocardiography, and the poor clinical ambulatory follow-up made it impossible for us to gather information on any residual intracardiac injuries; however, other studies have found a prevalence of valvular incompetence or septal ruptures in 19% of the cases [25, 29]. The hospital currently has stablished protocols for the clinical follow-up with electrocardiogram and strict imaging in PCI patients.

This study has limitations given that (i) it is a series of retrospective cases conducted in just one institution, where the majority of the patients come from a location with one of the highest indices of violence in Bogotá, which gives an atypical demographic profile; and (ii) the design does not permit a more in-depth statistical analysis. Nevertheless, the results permit us to generate new working hypotheses such as the need for revising the classification system of these injuries and the need of analyzing mortality from a forensic perspective.

Conclusions

Despite the study limitations, we believe the number of cases included is of great interest in the cardiac injury experience and evidence. Several interesting findings were achieved in this series. High prehospital mortality rates in PCI patients was evidenced; the difference in mortality between PCI-SW and PCI-GSW was not associated with cardiac injury grade as should be expected; an unexpected higher mortality associated to cardiac tamponade, according to what has been described in literature of PCI, was found; and that pericardial window and sternotomy were a satisfactory diagnostic and surgical approach respectively. These findings suggest that adequate and early prehospital approach is essential for reducing mortality in PCI patients. Actual cardiac injury grading requires a further revision for improving accuracy in mortality prognosis for PCI patients. Additionally, a better comprehension of cardiac tamponade pathophysiology is needed to understand when and how a factor can be a protecting or a risk factor. We also believe more autopsy studies of PCI patients could help answering lots of these questions and improving the appropriate approach and management in the future.

Acknowledgements
The authors would like to thank Juan Sebastián Martin-Saavedra for the manuscript organization and style, grammatical, and writing edition, and Omar Alejandro Gaitán for his help in data recollection during a period of the study, and to Hospital Occidente Kennedy statistics department for providing the clinical charts.

Funding
The authors declare that they have not received any kind of funding for the realization of this paper.

Authors' contributions
AIR contributed to the study design and literature research, and writing the introduction and discussion sections. DB contributed to the literature research and data collection, and writing the introduction and discussion sections. MT contributed to the data collection and critical revision. JRTC contributed to the statistical data analysis and data interpretation, and writing of the methods and results sections.

Competing interests
The authors declare that they have no competing interests.

Author details
[1]Escuela de Medicina y Ciencias de la Salud, Universidad del Rosario, Carrera 24 No 63C - 69 Barrio Siete de Agosto, Bogotá, DC, Colombia. [2]Méderi Hospital Universitario Mayor, Carrera 24 No 63C - 69 Barrio Siete de Agosto, Bogotá, DC, Colombia. [3]Hospital Occidente de Kennedy, Bogotá, D.C., Colombia. [4]Escuela de Estadística, Facultad de Ingenierías, Universidad del Valle, Santiago de Cali, Colombia.

References
1. Asensio JA, García Nuñez LM, Petrone P. Trauma to the heart. In: Feliciano DV, Mattox KL, Moore EE, editors. Trauma. 6th ed. New York, NY: McGraw Hill; 2008. p. 569–88.
2. Mandal AK, Sanusi M. Penetrating chest wounds: 24 years experience. World J Surg. 2001;25:1145–9.
3. Embrey R. Cardiac trauma. Thorac Surg Clin. 2007;17:87–93.
4. Campbell NC, Thomson SR, Muckart DJ, Meumann CM, Van Middelkoop I, Botha JB. Review of 1198 cases of penetrating cardiac trauma. Br J Surg. 1997;84:1737–40.
5. Henderson VJ, Smith RS, Fry WR, Morabito D, Peskin GW, Barkan H, Organ Jr CH. Cardiac injuries: analysis of an unselected series of 251 cases. J Trauma. 1994;36:341–8.
6. Kang N, Hsee L, Rizoli S, Alison P. Penetrating cardiac injury: overcoming the limits set by nature. Injury. 2009;40:919–27.
7. Naughton MJ, Brissie RM, Bessey PQ, McEachern MM, Donald Jr JM, Laws HL. Demography of penetrating cardiac trauma. Ann Surg. 1989;209:676–81.
8. Demetriades D, van der Veen BW. Penetrating injuries of the heart: experience over two years in South Africa. J Trauma. 1983;23:1034–41.
9. Barleben A, Huerta S, Mendoza R, Patel CV. Left ventricle injury with a normal pericardial window: case report and review of the literature. J Trauma. 2007;63:414–6.
10. Asensio JA, Murray J, Demetriades D, Berne J, Cornwell E, Velmahos G, Gomez H, Berne TV. Penetrating cardiac injuries: a prospective study of variables predicting outcomes. J Am Coll Surg. 1998;186:24–34.
11. O'Connor J, Ditillo M, Scalea T. Penetrating cardiac injury. J R Army Med Corps. 2009;155:185–90.
12. Emura F, Coral O. Injuria cardíaca penetrante: índices de trauma vs. mortalidad. Rev Col Cir. 1997;12:4–11.
13. Morales CH, Salinas CM, Henao CA, Patiño PA, Muñoz CM. Thoracoscopic pericardial window and penetrating cardiac trauma. J Trauma. 1997;42:273–5.
14. Ivatury RR, Nallathambi MN, Rohman M, Stahl WM. Penetrating cardiac trauma. Quantifying the severity of anatomic and physiologic injury. Ann Surg. 1987;205:61–6.
15. American College of Surgeons, Committee on Trauma. Advanced trauma life support manual. Chicago, IL: American College of Surgeons; 2008.
16. Moreno C, Moore EE, Majure JA, Hopeman AR. Pericardial tamponade: a critical determinant for survival following penetrating cardiac wounds. J Trauma. 1986;26:821–5.
17. Moore EE, Malangoni MA, Cogbill TH, Shackford SR, Champion HR, Jurkovich GJ, McAninch JW, Trafton PG. Organ injury scaling IV: thoracic vascular, lung, cardiac and diaphragm. J Trauma. 1994;36:299–300.
18. Ivatury RR, Rohman M, Steichen FM, Gunduz Y, Nallathambi M, Stahl WM. Penetrating cardiac injuries: twenty-year experience. Am Surg. 1987;53:310–7.
19. Sugg WL, Rea WJ, Ecker RR, Webb WR, Rose EF, Shaw RR. Penetrating wounds of the heart. An analysis of 459 cases. J Thorac Cardiovasc Surg. 1986;56:531–45.
20. Beall Jr AC, Patrick TA, Okies JE, Bricker DL, DeBakey ME. Penetrating wounds of the heart: changing patterns of surgical management. J Trauma. 1972;12:468–73.
21. Carrasquilla C, Wilson RF, Walt AJ, Arbulu A. Gunshot wounds of the heart. Ann Thorac Surg. 1972;13:208–13.
22. Asfaw I, Arbulu A. Penetrating wounds of the pericardium and heart. Surg Clin North Am. 1977;57:37–48.
23. Velmahos GC, Degiannis E, Souter I, Saadia R. Penetrating trauma to the heart: a relatively innocent injury. Surgery. 1994;115:694–7.
24. Tyburski JG, Astra L, Wilson RF, Dente C, Steffes C. Factors affecting prognosis with penetrating wounds of the heart. J Trauma. 2000;48:587–90.
25. Villegas MI, Morales CH, Rosero E, Benítez G, Restrepo FC, Fernández IM, López M, Ramírez LA. Trauma cardíaco penetrante: factores pronósticos. Rev Col Cir. 2007;22:148 56.

26. Duque HA, Florez LE, Moreno A, Jurado H, Jaramillo CJ, Restrepo MC. Penetrating cardiac trauma: follow-up study including electrocardiography, echocardiography, and functional test. World J Surg. 1999;23:1254–7.

27. Asensio JA, Berne JD, Demetriades D, Chan L, Murray J, Falabella A, Gomez H, Chahwan S, Velmahos G, Cornwell EE, et al. One hundred five penetrating cardiac injuries: a 2-year prospective evaluation. J Trauma. 1998; 44:1073–82.

28. Buckman Jr RF, Badellino MM, Mauro LH, Asensio JA, Caputo C, Gass J, Grosh JD. Penetrating cardiac wounds: prospective study of factors influencing initial resuscitation. J Trauma. 1993;34:717–25. discussion 725–727.

29. Degiannis E, Loogna P, Doll D, Bonanno F, Bowley DM, Smith MD. Penetrating cardiac injuries: recent experience in South Africa. World J Surg. 2006;30:1258–64.

30. Asensio JA, Arroyo Jr H, Veloz W, Forno W, Gambaro E, Roldan GA, Murray J, Velmahos G, Demetriades D. Penetrating thoracoabdominal injuries: ongoing dilemma-which cavity and when? World J Surg. 2002;26:539–43.

31. Ramírez MA, Rodríguez J, Roa A. Trauma precordial. Heridas penetrantes del corazón. Rev Col Cir. 1991;6:26–33.

32. Nicol AJ, Navsaria PH, Hommes M, Ball CG, Edu S, Kahn D. Sternotomy or drainage for a hemopericardium after penetrating trauma: a randomized controlled trial. Ann Surg. Epub 2013 Apr 18.

33. Mitchell ME, Muakkassa FF, Poole GV, Rhodes RS, Griswold JA. Surgical approach of choice for penetrating cardiac wounds. J Trauma. 1993;34: 17–20.

27

Laparoscopic versus open appendectomy: a retrospective cohort study assessing outcomes and cost-effectiveness

Antonio Biondi[1*], Carla Di Stefano[2], Francesco Ferrara[2], Angelo Bellia[2], Marco Vacante[3] and Luigi Piazza[2]

Abstract

Background: Appendectomy is the most common surgical procedure performed in emergency surgery. Because of lack of consensus about the most appropriate technique, appendectomy is still being performed by both open (OA) and laparoscopic (LA) methods. In this retrospective analysis, we aimed to compare the laparoscopic approach and the conventional technique in the treatment of acute appendicitis.

Methods: Retrospectively collected data from 593 consecutive patients with acute appendicitis were studied. These comprised 310 patients who underwent conventional appendectomy and 283 patients treated laparoscopically. The two groups were compared for operative time, length of hospital stay, postoperative pain, complication rate, return to normal activity and cost.

Results: Laparoscopic appendectomy was associated with a shorter hospital stay (2.7 ± 2.5 days in LA and 1.4 ± 0.6 days in OA), with a less need for analgesia and with a faster return to daily activities (11.5 ± 3.1 days in LA and 16.1 ± 3.3 in OA). Operative time was significantly shorter in the open group (31.36 ± 11.13 min in OA and 54.9 ± 14.2 in LA). Total number of complications was less in the LA group with a significantly lower incidence of wound infection (1.4 % vs 10.6 %, $P < 0.001$). The total cost of treatment was higher by 150 € in the laparoscopic group.

Conclusion: The laparoscopic approach is a safe and efficient operative procedure in appendectomy and it provides clinically beneficial advantages over open method (including shorter hospital stay, decreased need for postoperative analgesia, early food tolerance, earlier return to work, lower rate of wound infection) against only marginally higher hospital costs.

Trial registration: NCT02867072 Registered 10 August 2016. Retrospectively registered.

Keywords: Open appendectomy, Laparoscopic appendectomy, Hospital cost, Appendicitis

Abbreviations: BMI, Body mass index; CAD, Coronary artery disease; COPD, Chronic obstructive pulmonary disease; CT, Computed tomography; DM, Diabetes mellitus; LA, Laparoscopic appendectomy; OA, Open appendectomy; POD, Postoperative day; WBC, White blood cell

Background

Appendicitis is the most common cause of surgical abdomen in all age groups [1, 2]. Approximately 7–10 % of the general population develops acute appendicitis with the maximal incidence being in the second and third decades of life [3]. Open appendectomy has been the gold standard for treating patients with acute appendicitis for

more than a century, but the efficiency and superiority of laparoscopic approach compared to the open technique is the subject of much debate nowadays [3–5]. There is evidence that minimal surgical trauma through laparoscopic approach resulted in significant shorter hospital stay, less postoperative pain, faster return to daily activities in several settings related with gastrointestinal surgery [6, 7]. However, several retrospective studies [3, 8–14], several randomized trials [15–20] and meta-analyses [21, 22] comparing laparoscopic with open appendectomy have provided conflicting results.

* Correspondence: abiondi@unict.it
[1]Department of Surgery, Vittorio Emanuele Hospital, University of Catania, Via Plebiscito, 628, 95124 Catania, Italy
Full list of author information is available at the end of the article

Some of these studies have demonstrated better clinical outcomes with the laparoscopic approach [15–17, 20, 23], while other studies have shown marginal or no clinical benefits [18, 19, 24–26] and higher surgical costs [4, 19, 24, 25]. Bearing in mind that laparoscopic appendectomy, unlike other laparoscopic procedures [27], has not been found superior to open surgery for acute appendicitis, we designed the present study to determine any possible benefits of the laparoscopic approach. The aim of this study was to compare the clinical outcomes (hospital stay, operating time, postoperative complications, analgesia requirement, time to oral intake and to resume normal activity) and the hospital costs between open appendectomy and laparoscopic appendectomy.

Methods

Patients

A retrospective observational study of patients admitted to a single institution (Department of Emergency Surgery, Garibaldi Hospital-Catania) between January 2004 and July 2011 with the diagnosis of appendicitis was conducted. Pregnant women and patients with severe medical disease (hemodynamic instability, chronic medical or psychiatric illness, cirrhosis, coagulation disorders) requiring intensive care were excluded. The decision about the type of the operation was made according to the preference and experience of the surgical team on duty. We analyzed 593 patient that met the inclusion criteria and their clinical data and hospital costs. The patients were divided into two groups: open appendectomy (OA) group and laparoscopic appendectomy (LA) group. The collected clinical data included demographic data, co-morbidities, initial laboratory findings, operation time, intraoperative findings (acute, gangrenous or perforated appendix), time to soft diet, postoperative hospital stay, amount of analgesics and postoperative complications. We analyzed data on cost separately. The diagnosis was made clinically with history (right iliac fossa or periumbilical pain, nausea/vomiting), physical examination (tenderness or guarding in right iliac fossa). In patients where a clinical diagnosis could not be established, imaging studies such as abdominal ultrasound or CT were performed. Both groups of patients were given a prophylactic dose of third-generation cephalosporin and metronidazole at induction of the general anesthesia as part of the protocol. OA was performed through standard McBurney incision. After the incision, peritoneum was accessed and opened to deliver the appendix, which was removed in the usual manner. A standard 3-port technique was used for laparoscopic group. Pneumoperitoneum was produced by a continuous pressure of 12–14 mmHg of carbon dioxide *via* a Verres canula, positioned in infraumbilical site. The patient was placed in a Trendelenburg position, with a slight rotation to the left. The abdominal cavity was inspected in order to exclude other intrabdominal or pelvic pathology. After the mesoappendix was divided with bipolar forceps, the base of the appendix was secured with two legating loops, followed by dissection distal to the second loop. Then, the distal appendicular stump was closed to avoid the risk of enteric or purulent spillage. The specimen was placed in an endobag and was retrieved through a 10-mm infraumbilical port. All specimens were sent for histopathology. The patients were not given oral feed until they were fully recovered from anesthesia and had their bowel sounds returned when clear fluids were started. Soft diet was introduced when the patients tolerated the liquid diet and had passed flatus. Patients were discharged once they were able to take regular diet, afebrile, and had good pain control. The operative time (minutes) for both the procedures was counted from the skin incision to the last skin stitch applied. The length of hospital stay was determined as the number of nights spent at the hospital postoperatively. Wound infection was defined as redness or purulent or seropurulent discharge from the incision site. Seroma was defined as localized swelling without redness with ooze of clear fluid. Paralytic ileus was defined as failure of bowel sounds to return within 12 h postoperatively. The study protocol was received and approved by the Institutional Review Board and the Ethics Committee of Garibaldi Hospital. Waiver of informed consent from patients was approved because of the observational nature of the study. This study uses compliance with STROBE criteria, a checklist which has been developed to strengthen reporting standards in epidemiological research [26].

Statistical analysis

Categorical data were presented as frequencies and percentage and compared by the Chi-square test. Parametric and nonparametric continuous data were presented as mean and standard deviation and evaluated by the Student's t test and Mann–Whitney U test respectively. Comparisons between the two groups were made on an intention-to-treat basis. Thus, patients in the laparoscopic-assisted group converted to the open procedure were not excluded from the analysis. The sample size for our study was calculated based on an analysis of sample sizes required for each of the parameters (operative time, length of hospital stay, postoperative pain, complication rate, return to normal activity and cost) for an $\alpha = 0.05$ and a power of 90 %. A P-value of 0.05 was considered as significant. All calculations were performed by using the SPSS software package version 17.0 (SPSS Inc., Chicago, IL).

Results

Out of 593 patients with acute appendicitis, 310 patients underwent open appendectomy and 283 patients underwent laparoscopic appendectomy. Demographic data and preoperative clinical feature between OA group and

LA group are showed in Table 1. There were no significant differences with respect to age and associated co-morbidities. On the contrary, the difference in gender and in the white blood cell count at presentation was statistically significant. Out of the total 310 open procedures, 214 (69 %) were performed for uncomplicated appendicitis and 96 (31 %) for complicated disease including appendiceal perforation with local or widespread peritonitis. In the laparoscopic group, 241 (85 %) procedures involved uncomplicated disease and 42 (15 %) complicated appendicitis. Noteworthy, we did not observe differences between groups for all the grades of appendicitis (Table 2). In our study, the mean ± standard deviation (SD) operative time of 54.9 ± 14.7 min for the LA group was longer than the mean operative time of 31.36 ± 11.43 min for open appendectomy ($P < 0.0001$). The laparoscopic group required fewer doses of parenteral and oral analgesics in the operative and postoperative periods compared with the open appendectomy ($P < 0.0001$). Bowel movements in the first postoperative day were observed in 93 % patients subjected to laparoscopic appendectomy and 69 % in the open group ($P < 0.001$). As a result, 85 % patients in the laparoscopic group and 62 % in the open group were able to tolerate a liquid diet within the first 24 postoperative hours ($P < 0.001$). Hospital stay was significantly shorter in the laparoscopic group with a mean ± SD of 1.4 ± 0.6 days compared with 2.7 ± 2.5 of the open appendectomy group ($P = 0.015$). A highly significant difference existed between the 2 groups in time taken to return to routine daily activities, which was less in the laparoscopic group with a mean 11.5 ± 3.1 days compared with mean 16.1 ± 3.3 days in the open appendectomy group (Table 3). We observed a greater overall incidence of complications in open surgery than in laparoscopic surgery. A total of 29

complications occurred in the laparoscopic group, while 55 complications occurred in the open appendectomy group, as summarized in Table 4. We did not observe a significant difference between groups in vomiting, paralytic ileus, intrabdominal abscesses and hemoperitoneum. Differences in wound infection and wound dehiscence were significant ($P < 0.001$) (Table 4). Analysis of hospital costs are presented in Table 5. As regards laparoscopy, it is well known that the longer operative and anaesthesiological time are more expensive than the cost of the open approach (that uses reusable instruments and few and cheaper equipment). However, the shorter hospital stay (mean 1.4 ± 0.6 days) in the laparoscopic group kept low the ward cost in comparison to the open group. So, the total hospital cost for each patient of the LA group was only 150 € higher compared to patients in the OA group.

Discussion

Acute appendicitis is the most common intra-abdominal condition requiring emergency surgery [25]. The possibility of appendicitis must be considered in any patient presenting with an acute abdomen, and a certain preoperative diagnosis is still a challenge [28, 29]. Although more than 20 years have elapsed since the introduction of laparoscopic appendectomy (performed in 1983 by Semm, a gynaecologist), open appendectomy is still the

Table 1 Demographic and preoperative clinical data

	Open appendectomy (n = 310)	Laparoscopic appendectomy (n = 283)	P
Gender			<0.001
Male	184 (59.3)	121 (42.7)	
Female	126 (40.7)	162 (57.3)	
Mean age	29.66 ± 15.13	27.75 ± 14.24	0.57
WBC count (per mm³)	14903 ± 4686	13346 ± 5450	0.0002
Co-morbidities			0.244
CAD	6 (1.9)	5 (1.7)	
Hypertension	18 (5.8)	9 (3.1)	
COPD	9 (2.9)	6 (2.1)	
DM	12 (3.8)	5 (1.7)	

Data are number (%) or mean ± standard deviation values, as indicated.
WBC White blood cell, *CAD* Coronary artery disease, *COPD* Chronic obstructive pulmonary disease, *DM* Diabetes mellitus

Table 2 Surgical findings

	Open appendectomy (n = 310)	Laparoscopic appendectomy (n = 283)	P
Surgical findings, n (%)			0.074
Uncomplicated acute appendicitis	214 (69.0)	241 (85.2)	
Gangrenous appendicitis	24 (7.7)	12 (4.2)	
Appendiceal abscess	38 (12.3)	22 (7.8)	
Peritonitis	34 (11.0)	8 (2.8)	

Data are number (%)

Table 3 Operative and postoperative clinical data

	Open appendectomy (n = 310)	Laparoscopic appendectomy (n = 283)	P-value
Operative time (min)	31.36 ± 11.43	54.9 ± 14.7	<0.0001
Bowel movements (1st POD)	214 (69.0)	263 (92.9)	<0.001
Time until diet (1st POD)	192 (61.9)	241 (85.2)	<0.001
Parenteral analgesics (doses/day)	1.5 ± 0.6	1.0 ± 0.5	0.001
Oral analgesics (doses/day)	2.00 ± 2.26	1.86 ± 1.14	<0.0001
Hospital Stay (day)	2.7 ± 2.5	1.4 ± 0.6	0.015
Return to normal activity (day)	16.1 ± 3.3	11.5 ± 3.1	<0.001

Data are number (%) or mean ± standard deviation values, as indicated.
POD postoperative day

Table 4 Minor e major postoperative complications for open and laparoscopic appendectomy

Postoperative complications	Open appendectomy ($n = 76$)	Laparoscopic appendectomy ($n = 29$)	P
Minor			
Vomiting	17 (22.4)	13 (44.8)	0.621
Paralytic ileus	11 (14.5)	8 (27.6)	0.618
Wound infection	33 (43.4)	4 (13.8)	<0.001
Major			
Wound dehiscence	13 (17.1)	0 (0.0)	<0.001
Intra-abdominal abscess	1 (1.3)	4 (13.8)	0.147
Hemoperitoneum	1 (1.3)	0 (0.0)	0.339

Data are number (%)

conventional technique. Some authors consider emergency laparoscopy as a promising tool for the treatment of abdominal emergencies able to decrease costs and invasiveness and maximize outcomes and patients' comfort [30, 31]. Several studies [4, 10, 13, 16, 18, 32–34] have shown that laparoscopic appendectomy is safe and results in a faster return to normal activities with fewer wound complications. These findings have been challenged by other authors who observed no significant difference in the outcome between the two procedures, and moreover noted higher costs with laparoscopic appendectomy [3, 19, 20, 33, 35]. Anyway, a recent systematic review of meta-analyses of randomised controlled trials comparing laparoscopic versus open appendectomy concluded that both procedures are safe and effective for the treatment of acute appendicitis [36]. Total operative time in our series was significantly longer in the laparoscopic group than in open group (P <0.0001). Generally, the lack of experience of surgeons in the laparoscopic approach may contribute to a longer duration of the operation. By contrast, in the present study the learning curve effect was minimal as the surgeons performing the procedures were highly experienced in laparoscopic procedures, including laparoscopic bariatric surgery and colectomy surgery. So, in our series the longer operation time in laparoscopic appendectomy may

Table 5 Analysis of hospital cost

	Laparoscopic appendectomy	Open appendectomy
Equipment cost	1245 €	50 €
Theatre cost	300 €	300 €
Ward cost	800 €/night	800 €/night
Anesthesia cost of mean operative time	350 €	280 €
Total cost of mean in-patient hospital stay	2965 €	2810 €

be due to additional steps like setup of instruments, insufflation, making ports under vision and a phase of diagnostic laparoscopy. Length of hospital stay represents a critical factor that directly influences the economy and the well-being of the patient. We found that hospital stay was significantly shorter in laparoscopic group ($P = 0.015$) with a concomitant earlier bowel movements in patient managed laparoscopically, leading to earlier feeding and discharge from hospital. Our findings are in agreement with several studies that demonstrated a significantly short hospital stay for the laparoscopic approach [8, 22, 32, 33, 37]. In our Surgery Department, post-operative pain is assessed both subjectively *via* a visual analogue scale and objectively by the tabulation of analgesic use. In the present study, to prevent that the perception of pain may have been influenced by the patient's enthusiasm for a novel technique, we used only the number of analgesics doses (oral and parenteral) required by individual patient to compare the 2 groups. In this series, parenteral and oral analgesic requirements were less in the laparoscopic group [parenteral 1 (mean); oral 1.86 (mean)] than in the open group [parenteral 1.5 (mean); oral 2 (mean)] and we found a statistically significant difference (P <0.001) in agreement with many other studies [15, 38, 39] that reported less pain in the laparoscopic group. Several studies showed no difference between open and laparoscopic appendectomy with respect to early return to activity and performance of daily activities. However, this issue is still debated because of the different definitions and classifications of "activity" in such studies [20, 40–43]. In this study we used the return to work as an endpoint with a mean time of 11.5 ± 3.1 days in the laparoscopic group and 16.1 ± 3.3 in the open group (P <0.001). Our results are in agreement with a study by Hellberg et al. [44] and other randomized clinical trials and meta-analysis.[4, 39] The mortality rate was nil in our study. The low mortality rates reported in previous research (0.05 % and 0.3 % rate in laparoscopic and open groups [4]) indicated that appendectomy, especially in absence of complicated disease, is a safe procedure regardless of the technique used [33]. In the present study, the overall complication rates were 24.5 % and 6.7 % for open and laparoscopic appendectomy respectively, with a rate of wound infection and dehiscence significantly higher in the open group (P <0.001). Wound infection is more common in complicated appendicitis and may not represent a serious complication *per se* but has a strong impact for convalescence time and quality of life of patients. In our study no statistically difference was observed in the intraoperative findings between the two groups (Table 2), so the lower rate of wound infection in laparoscopic group may be due to placement of the detached appendix into an endobag before its removal from the abdominal cavity, reducing contact with the fascial surfaces and minimizing contamination. Conversely, intra-abdominal abscess is a serious and life-threatening complication. We observed intra-abdominal abscess formation in 4 patients in laparoscopic group (4.1 %) and in 1 patient in the open group (0.32 %). These findings are consistent with other studies that showed an increased risk of intra-abdominal abscess after laparoscopic appendectomy compared with open surgery [32, 33]. Several hypotheses have been suggested to find possible explanations: mechanical spread of bacteria in the peritoneal cavity promoted by carbon dioxide insufflation, especially in case of ruptured appendix [25, 44–47], inadequate learning curve [32], the meticulous irrigation, instead of simple suctioning, of the infected area in severe peritonitis, that leads to contamination of the entire abdominal cavity, which is difficult to aspirate latter [35]. However, in our study this finding was not statistically significant ($P = 0.147$). The management of intrabdominal abscesses included percutaneous drainage as first-line therapy, and surgical procedures. Antibiotics were given before and after percutaneous drainage or surgery. Other observed postoperative complications included vomiting, paralytic ileus and hemoperitoneum (Table 4). The higher cost of laparoscopic instruments (1245 € in our Department) compared to the conventional technique (50 € in our Department) represents an obstacle to its greater use. However, because of the shorter hospital stay, the total cost for laparoscopic appendectomy (operating room + ward costs) was only 155 € higher than open appendectomy. In addition, Moore and al. demonstrated an economic benefit of laparoscopic appendectomy from a social perspective, since earlier return to daily activities is crucial, especially for patients who are young and lead a productive life [38]. Limitations of our study included the lack of evaluation of laparoscopic surgery in obese patients, as we did not collect data on body mass index (BMI). Moreover the follow up period was only limited to two weeks after hospital discharge.

Conclusions

Our results showed the advantages of the laparoscopic approach over open appendectomy including shorter hospital stay, decreased need for postoperative analgesia, early food tolerance, earlier return to work, lower rate of wound infection, against only marginally higher hospital costs. Furthermore we found a considerable preference (during the collection of consent) of patients and a high satisfaction after the surgery in the laparoscopic group. Although the incidence of intra-abdominal abscess formation was higher after laparoscopic appendectomy, greater experience and improvements in our technique may have eradicated this catastrophic complication. Provided that surgical experience and equipment are available, laparoscopy could be considered safe and equally

efficient compared to open technique and should be undertaken as the initial procedure of choice for most case of suspected appendicitis. However, since there is no consensus to the best approach, both procedures (open and laparoscopic appendectomy) are still being practiced actively deferring the choice to the preference of surgeon and patients. In the future, laparoscopic appendectomy could represent the standard treatment for patients with appendicitis and undiagnosed abdominal pain.

Acknowledgments
None.

Funding
None.

Authors' contributions
LP, CDS, FF, and Angelo Bellia: conceived and designed the study, collected data and data interpretation. MV and Antonio Biondi: revised critically the paper. All authors wrote, read and approved the final manuscript.

Competing interests
None. This manuscript has not been published previously and is not under consideration for publication elsewhere.

Author details
[1]Department of Surgery, Vittorio Emanuele Hospital, University of Catania, Via Plebiscito, 628, 95124 Catania, Italy. [2]General and Emergency Surgery Department, Garibaldi Hospital, 95100 Catania, Italy. [3]Department of Medical and Pediatric Sciences, University of Catania, 95125 Catania, Italy.

References
1. Addiss DG, Shaffer N, Foweler BS, Tauxe R. The epidemiology of appendicitis and appendicectomy in the United States. Am J Epidemiology. 1990;132:910–25.
2. Seem K. Endoscopic appendectomy. Endoscopy. 1983;15:59–64.
3. Kurtz RJ, Heimann TM. Comparison of open and laparoscopic treatment of acute appendicitis. Am J Surg. 2001;182:211–4.
4. Garbutt JM, Soper NJ, Shannon W, Botero A, Littenberg B. Meta-analysis of randomized controlled trials comparing laparoscopic and open appendectomy. Surg Laparosc Endosc. 1999;9:17–26.
5. Biondi A, Grosso G, Mistretta A, Marventano S, Toscano C, Drago F, Gangi S, Basile F. Laparoscopic vs. open approach for colorectal cancer: evolution over time of minimal invasive surgery. BMC Surg. 2013;13 Suppl 2:S12.
6. Grosso G, Biondi A, Marventano S, Mistretta A, Calabrese G, Basile F. Major postoperative complications and survival for colon cancer elderly patients. BMC Surg. 2012;12 Suppl 1:S20.
7. Biondi A, Grosso G, Mistretta A, Marventano S, Toscano C, Gruttadauria S, Basile F. Laparoscopic-assisted versus open surgery for colorectal cancer: short-and long-term outcomes comparison. J Laparoendosc Adv Surg Tech A. 2013;23:1–7.
8. Guller U, Hervey S, Purves H, Muhlbaier LH, Peterson ED, Eubanks S, Pietrobon R. Laparoscopic versus open appendectomy: outcomes comparison based on a large administrative database. Ann Surg. 2004;239:43–52.
9. Wullstein C, Barkhausen S, Gross E. Results of laparoscopic vs. conventional appendectomy in complicated appendicitis. Dis Colon Rectum. 2001;44:1700–5.
10. Fogli L, Brulatti M, Boschi S, Di Domenico M, Papa V, Patrizi P, Capizzi FD. Laparoscopic appendectomy for acute and recurrent appendicitis:

retrospective analysis of a single-group 5-year experience. J Laparoendosc Adv Surg Tech A. 2002;12:107–10.

11. Lin HF, Wu JM, Tseng LM, Chen KH, Huang SH, Lai IR. Laparoscopic versus open a appendectomy for perforated appendicitis. J Gastrointest Surg. 2006;10:906–10.

12. Cueto J, D'Allemagne B, Vazquez-Frias JA, Gomez S, Delgado F, Trullenque L, Fajardo R, Valencia S, Poggi L, Balli J, Diaz J, Gonzalez R, Mansur JH, Franklin ME. Morbidity of laparoscopic surgery for complicated appendicitis: an international study. Surg Endosc. 2006;20:717–20.

13. Towfigh S, Chen F, Mason R, Katkhouda N, Chan L, Berne T. Laparoscopic appendectomy significantly reduces length of stay for perforated appendicitis. Surg Endosc. 2006;20:495–9.

14. Roviaro GC, Vergani C, Varoli F, Francese M, Caminiti R, Maciocco M. Videolaparoscopic appendectomy: the current outlook. Surg Endosc. 2006;20:1526–30.

15. Ortega AE, Hunter JG, Peters JH, Swanstrom LL, Schirmer B. A prospective, randomized comparison of laparoscopic appendectomy with open appendectomy. Laparoscopic Appendectomy Study Group. Am J Surg. 1995;169:208–12.

16. Milewczyk M, Michalik M, Ciesielski M. A prospective, randomized, unicenter study comparing laparoscopic and open treatments of acute appendicitis. Surg Endosc. 2003;17:1023–8.

17. Bresciani C, Perez RO, Habr-Gama A, Jacob CE, Ozaki A, Batagello C, Proscurshim I, Gama-Rodrigues J. Laparoscopic versus standard appendectomy outcomes and cost comparisons in the private sector. J Gastrointest Surg. 2005;9:1174–80.

18. Olmi S, Magnone S, Bertolini A, Croce E. Laparoscopic versus open appendectomy in acute appendicitis: a randomized prospective study. Surg Endosc. 2005;19:1193–5.

19. Katkhouda N, Mason RJ, Towfigh S, Gevorgyan A, Essani R. Laparoscopic versus open appendectomy: a prospective randomized double-blind study. Ann Surg. 2005;242:439–48.

20. Ignacio RC, Burke R, Spencer D, Bissell C, Dorsainvil C, Lucha PA. Laparoscopic versus open appendectomy: what is the real difference? Results of a prospective randomized double-blinded trial. Surg Endosc. 2004;18:334–7.

21. Wei B, Qi CL, Chen TF, Zheng ZH, Huang JL, Hu BG, Wei HB. Laparoscopic versus open appendectomy for acute appendicitis: a metaanalysis. Surg Endosc. 2011;25:1199–208.

22. Sauerland S, Lefering R, Neugebauer EA. Laparoscopic versus open surgery for suspected appendicitis. Cochrane Database Syst Rev. 2010;10:CD001546.

23. Martin LC, Puente I, Sosa JL, Bassin A, Breslaw R, McKenney MG, Ginzburg E, Sleeman D. Open versus laparoscopic appendectomy. A prospective randomized comparison. Ann Surg. 1995;222:256–61.

24. Golub R, Siddiqui F, Pohl D. Laparoscopic versus open appendectomy: a metaanalysis. J Am Coll Surg. 1998;186:545–53.

25. Chung RS, Rowland DY, Li P, Diaz J. A meta-analysis of randomized controlled trials of laparoscopic versus conventional appendectomy. Am J Surg. 1999;177:250–6.

26. Hart R, Rajgopal C, Plewes A, Sweeney J, Davies W, Gray D, Taylor B. Laparoscopic versus open appendectomy: a prospective randomized trial of 81 patient. Can J Surg. 1996;39:457–62.

27. Biondi A, Grosso G, Mistretta A, Marventano S, Tropea A, Gruttadauria S, Basile F. Predictors of conversion in laparoscopic-assisted colectomy for colorectal cancer and clinical outcomes. Surg Laparosc Endosc Percutan Tech. 2014;24:21–6.

28. Bhangu A, Søreide K, Di Saverio S, Assarsson JH, Drake FT. Acute appendicitis: modern understanding of pathogenesis, diagnosis, and management. Lancet. 2015;386:1278–87.

29. Di Saverio S, Birindelli A, Kelly MD, Catena F, Weber DG, Sartelli M, et al. WSES Jerusalem guidelines for diagnosis and treatment of acute appendicitis. World J Emerg Surg. 2016;11:34.

30. Di Saverio S, Mandrioli M, Birindelli A, Biscardi A, Di Donato L, Gomes CA, Piccinini A, Vettoretto N, Agresta F, Tugnoli G, Jovine E. Single-Incision Laparoscopic Appendectomy with a Low-Cost Technique and Surgical-Glove Port: "How To Do It" with Comparison of the Outcomes and Costs in a Consecutive Single-Operator Series of 45 Cases. J Am Coll Surg. 2016;222:e15–30.

31. Di Saverio S. Emergency laparoscopy: a new emerging discipline for treating abdominal emergencies attempting to minimize costs and invasiveness and maximize outcomes and patients' comfort. J Trauma Acute Care Surg. 2014;77:338–50.

32. Shaikh AR, Sangrasi AK, Shaikh GA. Clinical Outcomes of laparoscopic versus open Appendectomy. JSLS. 2009;13:574–80.

33. Agresta F, De Simone P, Leone L, Arezzo A, Biondi A, Bottero L, et al. Italian Society Of Young Surgeons (SPIGC). Laparoscopic appendectomy in Italy: an appraisal of 26,863 cases. J Laparoendosc Adv Surg Tech A. 2004;14:1–8.

34. Di Saverio S, Mandrioli M, Sibilio A, Smerieri N, Lombardi M, Catena F, Ansaloni L, Tugnoli G, Masetti M, Jovine E. A cost-effective technique for laparoscopic appendectomy: outcomes and costs of a case–control prospective single-operator study of 112 unselected consecutive cases of complicated acute appendicitis. J Am Coll Surg. 2014;218:e51–65.

35. Kehagias I, Karamanakos SN, Panagiotopoulos S, Panagopoulos K, Kalfarentzos F. Laparoscopic versus open appendectomy: which way to go ? World J Gastroenterol. 2008;14:4909–14.

36. Jaschinski T, Mosch C, Eikermann M, Neugebauer EA. Laparoscopic versus open appendectomy in patients with suspected appendicitis: a systematic review of meta-analyses of randomised controlled trials. BMC Gastroenterol. 2015;15:48.

37. Merhoff AM, Merhoff GC, Franklin ME. Laparoscopic versus open appendectomy. Am J Surg. 2000;179:375–8.

38. Moore DE, Speroff T, Grogan E, Poulose B, Holzman MD. Cost perspectives of laparoscopic and open appendectomy. Surg Endosc. 2005;19:374–8.

39. Frazee RC, Roberts JW, Symmonds RE, et al. A prospective randomized trial comparing open versus laparoscopic appendectomy. Ann Surg. 1994;219:725–8.

40. Yong JL, Law WL, Lo CY, Lam CM. A comparative study of routine laparoscopic versus open appendectomy. JSLS. 2006;10:188–92.

41. Pedersen AG, Petersen OB, Wara P, Rønning H, Qvist N, Laurberg S. Randomized clinical trial of laparoscopic versus open appendectomy. Br J Surg. 2001;88:200–5.

42. Marzouk M, Khater M, Elsadek M, Abdelmoghny A. Laparoscopic versus open appendectomy: a prospective comparative study of 227 patients. Surg Endosc. 2003;17:721–4.

43. Katkhouda N, Mason RJ, Towfigh S. Laparoscopic versus open appendectomy: a prospective, randomized, double-blind study. Adv Surg. 2006;40:1–19.

44. Hellberg A, Rudberg C, Kullmann E, et al. Prospective randomized multicentre study of laparoscopic versus open appendectomy. Br J Surg. 1999;86:48–53.

45. Evasovich MR, Clark TC, Horattas MC, Holda S, Treen L. Does pneumoperitoneum during laparoscopy increase bacterial translocation? Surg Endosc. 1996;10:1176–9.

46. Gurtner GC, Robertson CS, Chung SC, Ling TK, Ip SM, Li AK. Effect of carbon dioxide pneumoperitoneum on bacteraemia and endotoxaemia in an animal model of peritonitis. Br J Surg. 1995;82:844–8.

47. Jacobi CA, Ordemann J, Bohm B, Zieren HU, Volk HD, Lorenz W, Halle E, Muller JM. Does laparoscopy increase bacteremia and endotoxemia in a peritonitis model? Surg Endosc. 1997;11:235–8.

28

LBP rs2232618 polymorphism contributes to risk of sepsis after trauma

Hong-xiang Lu, Jian-hui Sun, Da-lin Wen, Juan Du, Ling Zeng, An-qiang Zhang[*] and Jian-xin Jiang[*]

Abstract

Background: Previous study revealed that rs2232618 polymorphism (Phe436Leu) within LBP gene is a functional variant and associated with susceptibility of sepsis in traumatic patients. Our aim was to confirm the reported association by enlarging the population sample size and perform a meta-analysis to find additional evidence.

Methods: Traumatic patients from Southwest ($n = 1296$) and Southeast ($n = 445$) of China were enrolled in our study. After genotyping, the relationship between rs2232618 and the risk of sepsis was analyzed. Furthermore, we proceeded with a comprehensive literature search and meta-analysis to determine whether the rs2232618 polymorphism conferred susceptibility to sepsis.

Results: Significance correlation was observed between rs2232618 and risk of sepsis in Southwest patients ($P = 0.002$ for the dominant model, $P = 0.006$ for the recessive model). The association was confirmed in Southeast cohort ($P = 0.005$ for the dominant model) and overall combined cohorts ($P = 4.5 \times 10^{-4}$, $P = 0.041$ for the dominant and recessive model). Multiple logistical regression analyses suggested that rs2232618 polymorphism was related to higher risk of sepsis (OR = 1.77, 95% CI = 1.26–2.48, $P = 0.001$ in Southwest patients; OR = 2.11, 95% CI = 1.24–3.58, $P = 0.006$ in Southeast cohort; OR = 1.54, 95% CI = 1.34–2.08, $P = 0.006$ in overall cohort). Furthermore, meta-analysis of four studies (including the present study) confirmed that rs2232618 within LBP increased the risk of sepsis (OR = 1.75, $P < 0.001$ for the dominant model; OR = 6.08, $P = 0.003$ for the recessive model; OR = 2.72, $P < 0.001$ for the allelic model).

Conclusions: The results from our replication study and meta-analysis provided firm evidence that rs2232618T allele significantly increased the risk of sepsis.

Keywords: Trauma, Sepsis, Lipopolysaccharide-binding protein, Single nucleotide polymorphism, Meta-analysis

Backgrounds

According to WHO, 10% of deaths and 16% of disabilities around the world were due to traumatic injuries [1]. With the development of first aid and hospital treatment, the early mortality of major trauma patients declined in recent years [2]. However, the incidence of mortality caused by post-injury sepsis remained unchanged during the past decades [3, 4]. Despite the obtained increasing research progress in sepsis after trauma, current knowledge about the molecular mechanisms of the development of sepsis is still limited [5]. Therefore, early diagnosis and treatment based on the special clinical signs and laboratory results become imperative requirements [6].

Previous studies indicated that gene variants (generally single nucleotide polymorphisms, SNPs) in inflammatory response genes could contribute to different outcomes which are observed in sepsis and infectious diseases both in laboratory animal models and clinical patient cohorts [7, 8]. Candidate gene studies for traumatic patients identified several SNPs in lipopolysaccharide-binding protein (LBP), toll-like receptor 1(TLR1), and tumor necrosis factor-alpha (TNF-α) which were related to the development of sepsis [9–11]. The assessment of sepsis-specific genetic variants in these patients could explain the individual differences in susceptibility for trauma-related sepsis to some extent [7, 12]. Therefore, those SNPs could serve as beneficial biomarkers to

* Correspondence: zhanganqiang@126.com; hellojjx@126.com
State Key Laboratory of Trauma, Burns and Combined Injury, Institute of Surgery Research, Daping Hospital, Third Military Medical University, Chongqing 400042, China

evaluate and monitor infection or inflammatory responses to trauma patients.

Lipopolysaccharide-binding protein (LBP), a key gene in the host innate immune response, has been reported to play a crucial role in the pathophysiologic process of sepsis after major traumatic injury [13]. We previously found that the rs2232618 (Phe436Leu) polymorphism in LBP had a significant association with the incidence of sepsis and MOD score in two non-dependent cohorts of major traumatic patients admitted from Chongqing (Southwest of China) and Zhejiang (Southeast of China). The correlation analysis showed these patients with variant C allele had higher sepsis morbidity risk and MOD score. Other studies also showed that rs2232618 could affect the outcome of sepsis patients [14, 15]. In addition, protein activities could enhance after C allele mutated to T allele at rs2232618 [16]. Thus, the current study was designed to examine the association between rs2232618 and sepsis after trauma by enlarging the sample size. Furthermore, a meta-analysis including previously published studies was carried out to provide a more precise estimate of this association.

Materials and methods
Study populations
Two unrelated study cohorts of traumatic injury patients in Southwest (Chongqing) and Southeast (Zhejiang) of China were performed for this study. Traumatic patients in the ICU at the Department of Trauma Surgery in the Daping Hospital and the Chongqing Emergency Medical Center were recruited during the period of between January 2005 and October 2016. The traumatic injury patients in the Second Affiliated Hospital, Zhejiang University, were enrolled between January 2008 and July 2015. The including criteria and excluding criteria were described previously [16]. Trauma severity of each person was assessed using the Injury Severity Score (ISS) (The Abbreviated Injury Scale: 2005 revisions) by two independent researchers. Demographic characteristics and clinical information were taken from the electronic medical record. Consequently, the diagnosis of sepsis was according to the criteria of the American College of Chest Physicians and Society of Critical Care Medicine Consensus Committee. Definition of infection was clinically positive bacterial cultures from blood, sputum, urine tissue, catheter tips, and wounds. For those trauma patients with multiple positive cultures, the first significant culture of gram-positive or gram-negative organisms occurring after admission was selected. Multiple organ dysfunction (MOD) score was the sum of single organ score calculated during every day the patients stayed in the hospital. The patient sampling and experiments got approval from the Institutional Ethics Review Board of the Third Military Medical University.

Informed consent for all subjects was acquired from the patients or their kin.

Genotyping
Blood samples of trauma patients were obtained immediately after admission by physicians or nurses. Total DNA of every patient was extracted from whole blood according to the laboratory protocol. Samples were stored at – 80 °C with a 40 µg/ml concentration. Pyrosequencing was utilized to genotype rs2232618 similar to our previous report [16, 17]. The double-blind method was implemented. Approximately 10% of the samples was genotyped in duplicate to ensure genotyping quality.

Statistical analysis
Categorical data were shown as counts and percentages. Continuous data were given as means ± SD. Comparison of categorical data was conducted by χ^2 analysis, and continuous data were analyzed using Student's t test. Genotype frequencies were determined according to gene number. Hardy-Weinberg equilibrium (HWE) was assessed to detect whether the rs2232618 polymorphism distribution among the study population was stable by χ^2 analyses. The correlation between rs2232618 polymorphisms and the incidence of sepsis was performed by χ^2 analyses in three genetic effects (allele dose genetic model, dominant genetic model, and recessive genetic model). Furthermore, the allelic odds ratio (OR) and 95% confidence intervals (CI) were calculated by a multiple stepwise logistic regression analysis adjusted by identified confounding variables of age, sex, and ISS. Moreover, we also compared the MOD scores between different genotypes with Student's t test. The exact P values were considered significant if $P < 0.05$. All statistical analyses were performed in SPSS 17.

Meta-analysis of rs2232618 in association with sepsis risk
To confirm the involvement of rs2232618 in sepsis susceptibility, a meta-analysis combining published studies and our study was carried out. PubMed, Embase, and Web of Knowledge were searched in order to identify all published studies up to December 15, 2017, that had evaluated the associations between rs2232618 polymorphism and sepsis. Key words used for search were "rs2232618 or Leu436Pro" and "sepsis or severe sepsis or septic shock or septicemia." The inclusion criteria were as follows: (1) independent case-control or cohort study evaluating the association between rs2232618 and sepsis risk and (2) the number or frequency of genotypes was provided in detail or obtained by contacting the authors.

Information such as first author's name, publication year, country origin and the ethnicity of study population, genotype number, or allele frequency for case and control were collected from each study using a standardized data collection protocol. The odds ratio (OR) and its 95% confidence interval (CI) were used to evaluate the strength of the association between rs2232618 and sepsis susceptibility based on genotype frequencies in cases and controls. The pooled ORs were performed for dominant (TT versus CC + CT), recessive (TT + CT versus CC), and allelic (T versus C) genetic models, respectively. The significance of pooled ORs was tested by Z test ($P < 0.05$ was considered statistically significant).

Between-study heterogeneity across all eligible comparisons was estimated by the Cochran's Q statistic and the I^2 metric. Heterogeneity was considered significant at $P < 0.05$ for the Q statistic. For the I^2 metric, the following cut-off points were used: $I^2 = 0$–25%, no heterogeneity; $I^2 = 25$–50%, moderate heterogeneity; $I^2 = 50$–75%, large heterogeneity; $I^2 = 75$–100%, extreme heterogeneity. A fixed-effects model, using Mantel-Haenszel method, was applied to pool data from studies when heterogeneity was negligible based on P for Q statistic greater than 0.1; otherwise, a random-effects model, using DerSimonian and Laird method was applied. The meta-analysis was conducted using Review Manager 5.0.

Results

Overall clinical characteristics of major traumatic patients

There were1296 major traumatic patients from Southwest of China and 445 patients from Southeast of China enrolled and genotyped in our study. The demographic and clinical information of those patients was presented in Table 1. Most of the trauma patients were male. Patients were of young age (mean age 42.5 ± 12.9 and 41.4 ± 12.3). All patients in the study survived more than 48 h after admitted to the hospital. Average ISS in Southwest and Southeast are 21.2 ± 9.4 and 21.7 ± 9.3, respectively. Among them, incidence of trauma sepsis is 33.3% and 37.5% in the Southwest and Southeast of China, respectively. The main type of infection was respiratory tract infection in the two study cohorts (27.6% and 43.1%). According to infection of bacterial species, gram-negative infections occupied about 41.4% and 38.9% and gram-positive infections were about 29.6% and 9.6%. Among the trauma population, the mean of MOD score was 7.17 ± 1.02 and 6.41 ± 0.85 in Southwest and Southeast, respectively.

Clinical correlation of the rs2232618with trauma-related sepsis

The rs2232618 was successfully genotyped in 1296 Southwest of China trauma patients. The overall minor allele frequency (MAF = 5.5%) was consistent with the 86 Chinese Han Beijing in HapMap datasets (MAF = 9.1%). The genotype frequencies of rs2232618 was in line with Hardy-Weinberg equilibrium ($P = 0.06$)

Table 1 Overall clinical characteristics of patients with major trauma

Variables	Southwest ($n = 1296$)	Southeast ($n = 445$)
Age, years	42.5 ± 12.9	41.4 ± 12.3
Male/female, %	81.2/18.8	77.8/22.2
AIS max abdomen	2.6 ± 0.9	2.5 ± 0.6
AIS max extremities/pelvis	2.7 ± 0.8	2.8 ± 0.5
AIS max face	1.5 ± 0.7	1.7 ± 0.3
AIS max head/neck	2.9 ± 1.3	2.5 ± 1.1
AIS max thorax	3.1 ± 0.6	3.4 ± 0.2
ISS	21.2 ± 9.4	21.7 ± 9.3
MOD scores	7.17 ± 1.02	6.41 ± 0.85
Sepsis, n (%)	432 (33.3%)	167 (37.5%)
Source of infection, n (%)		
Respiratory tract infection, n (%)	70 (27.6)	72 (43.1)
Primary bloodstream infection, n (%)	43 (16.5)	33 (19.8)
Urinary tract infection, n (%)	24 (9.2)	20 (12.0)
Catheter associated infection, n (%)	55 (21.1)	15 (9.0)
Wound infection, n (%)	44 (16.9)	17 (10.1)
Others, n (%)	18 (6.8)	9 (6.0)
Pathogens, n (%) (positive blood cultures)		
Gram-negative, n (%)	179 (41.4)	65 (38.9)
Gram-positive, n (%)	128 (29.6)	16 (9.6)
Fungi, n (%)	4 (0.9)	0 (0)
Mixed gram-negative and gram-positive, n (%)	5 (1.2)	0 (0)
Negative blood cultures, n (%)	116 (26.9)	86 (51.5)

(Table 2). Both allele and genotype frequencies of rs2232618 remained constant in the Southwest cohort. As presented in Table 3, no statistically significant difference in age, gender, or ISS was detected among traumatic patients with different genotypes. In the Southwest cohort, we found a strong association between rs2232618 and incidence of sepsis both in the dominant model ($P = 0.002$) and in recessive effect of the allele ($P = 0.006$), so the trauma patients with more C allele would be more likely to suffer from sepsis (TT 32.0%, TC 43.9%, CC 71.4%). For multiple logistical regression analyses, data from allele dose model analyses adjusted by age, sex, and ISS also suggested that rs2232618 polymorphism had a significant correlation with higher morbidity rate of sepsis (OR = 1.77, 95% CI − 1.26–2.48, $P = 0.001$) (Table 3). In addition, when comparing the MOD score among patients with different genotypes, results indicated that C carriers had a higher MOD score than the T carrier patients ($P = 1.8 \times 10^{-6}$ in case of dominant model) (Table 3). Therefore, C carriers may be more likely to have bad outcome.

Table 2 Distribution of rs2232618 in the LBP gene among trauma patients in the two cohorts

	Patients	MAF, %		Genotypes, N			
		Databank*	Patients	Wild	Heterozygous	Variant	HWE
Southwest	1296	9.1	5.5	1166	123	7	0.06
Southeast	445	9.1	6.1	388	54	3	0.46

*Data were from HapMap database for Chinese Han Beijing (n = 139)

We further validated those results in another distinct trauma cohort (Southeast of China). The characteristics and clinical data of injury patients from Southeast of China are shown in Table 1. The overall MAF of rs2232618 (MAF = 6.1%) in the validation trauma cohort was consistent with those from Southwest of China and HapMap datasets. The genotype distribution conformed to the HWE (P = 0.46). As shown in Table 3, the risk rate of sepsis increased when the patients were with more C allele (TT 35.1%, TC 53.75%, CC 66.7%). There was a strong association between rs2232618 and development of post-traumatic sepsis in the dominant effect (P = 0.005). However, relevance of rs2232618 and sepsis morbidity in recessive genetic model was not detected again; the reason might be that there were just three TT genotype trauma patients from Southeast of China and it was not enough to validate the significant association. A multiple analysis was performed by stepwise logistic regression; the results suggested that rs2232618 polymorphism was related to higher risk of sepsis (OR = 2.11, 95% CI = 1.24–3.58, P = 0.006). Furthermore, we found that the C carriers also had higher MOD score than those patients with T allele in the dominant model (P = 0.005) (Table 3).

Due to no significant differences in the distribution of age, sex, and injury severity among patients from Southwest

and Southeast of China were identified, the two cohorts were combined to enlarge the study cohort. Just as presented in Table 3, there was a stronger relevance between rs2232618 polymorphism and incidence of sepsis or MOD scores. The results suggested that rs2232618T → C would greatly increase the risk of sepsis in dominant and recessive model (P = 4.5 × 10^{-4} and P = 0.041). Similar with previous results, allele dose effect analyses also confirmed the relevance for rs2232618 polymorphism and morbidity of sepsis (OR = 1.54, 95% CI = 1.34–2.08, P = 0.005). Furthermore, a significant difference in MOD score was observed among traumatic patients with different genotypes (P = 1.4×10^{-9} in dominant genetic model).

Results of meta-analysis

Finally, three relevant articles were included in final meta-analysis [14–16]. There were 4 studies with 917 cases, and 1291 controls determined the association between rs2232618 polymorphism and sepsis risk (Table 4). However, Jabandziev's study [15] just provided genotype number for TT vs. TT + TC, so this study was just included in the dominant genetic model. Because Zeng et al.'s Chongqing and Zhejiang cohorts were included in our study, they were presented in study 1 and study 2 [16]. As shown in Figs. 1, 2, and 3, no significant

Table 3 Clinical relevance of rs2232618 among trauma patients in the two cohorts

	Genotypes	N	Age (years)	Sex (M/F, %)	ISS	Sepsis, n (%)	MOD score
Southwest	TT	1166	42.6 ± 12.8	81.4/18.6	20.8 ± 9.3	373 (32.0)	6.11 ± 2.24
	TC	123	41.7 ± 13.9	77.2/22.8	25.0 ± 9.7	54 (43.9)	7.20 ± 2.23
	CC	7	43.0 ± 10.7	100/0	24.1 ± 13.2	5 (71.4)	8.17 ± 3.19
						a1, b1, c1	a2
Southeast	TT	388	41.3 ± 12.2	78.1/21.9	21.5 ± 9.3	136 (35.1)	5.88 ± 2.32
	TC	54	42.1 ± 12.9	79.6/20.4	23.4 ± 9.3	29 (53.7)	7.39 ± 3.73
	CC	3	32.7 ± 8.1	33.3/66.7	21.3 ± 7.2	2 (66.7)	6.00 ± 1.41
						a3, c2	a4
Total	TT	1554	42.3 ± 12.6	80.6/19.4	21.0 ± 9.3	509 (33.0)	6.07 ± 2.24
	TC	177	41.2 ± 13.7	92.1/7.9	22.5 ± 10.3	83 (46.9)	7.27 ± 2.87
	CC	10	43.4 ± 12.1	80.0/20.0	23.8 ± 11.9	7 (70.0)	8.00 ± 2.94
						a5, b2, c3	a6

Dominant effect (variant homozygotes + heterozygotes vs. wild homozygotes) as analyzed by ANCOVA: [a1]P = 0.002, [a2]P = 1.8E–6, [a3]P = 0.002, [a4]P = 0.005, [a5]P = 4.5 × 10^{-4}, [a6]P = 1.4E–9
Recessive effect (variant homozygotes vs. heterozygotes + wild homozygotes) as analyzed by ANCOVA: [b1]P = 0.032, [b2]P = 0.041
Allele dose association by logistic regression: [c1]P = 0.001(OR = 1.77, 95% CI = 1.26–2.48), [c2]P = 0.006(OR = 2.11, 95% CI = 1.24–3.58), [c3]P = 0.005(OR = 1.54, 95% CI = 1.34–2.08)

Table 4 Characteristics of the studies included in the meta-analysis

Author	Country	Ethnicity	Case/control	Case			Control		
				TT	TC	CC	TT	TC	CC
Study1[#1]	China	Han	432/864	373	54	5	793	69	2
Study2[#2]	China	Han	167/278	136	29	2	252	25	1
Jabandziev 2014*	Czech	NA	114/529	85	29		432	97	
Hubacek 2001	Germany	NA	204/250	157	42	5	212	38	0

Zeng's Chongqing and Zhejiang cohorts were included in our study, so they were not presented independently

[#1]Study1 represented the Southwest cohorts in our study

[#2]Study2 represented Southeast cohorts in our study

*Jabandziev's study just provided genotype number for TT vs. TT + TC. The number of TT and CC was not shown separately. 29 and 97 represented the TT + TC in case and control, respectively

evidence of heterogeneity was observed in all genetic models (dominant model, $I^2 = 0$, $P = 0.79$; recessive model $I^2 = 0$, $P = 0.74$; allelic model $I^2 = 0$, $P = 0.71$), so a fix-effects model was to pool the OR. In the dominant genetic model (TT VS. TC + CC), overall pooled OR for four studies combined was 1.75 (95% CI = 1.40–2.19) ($P < 0.001$) (Fig. 1). Similarly, the recessive and allelic models were all significantly associated with sepsis risk (recessive genetic model OR = 6.08, 95% CI = 1.82–20.37, $P = 0.003$ (Fig. 2); allelic genetic model OR = 2.72, 95% CI = 2.13–3.47, $P < 0.001$) (Fig. 3).

Discussion

Patients after major traumatic injury were at high risk of sepsis and sepsis-associated multiple organ dysfunction syndrome [18, 19]. Therefore, increasing interest in identifying sepsis early in clinical management and providing timely and accurate therapies shorten hospital stays and improve overall outcomes [19]. Recently, researchers paid great attention to the potential action for genetic variation in sepsis susceptibility after traumatic injury. Various investigators had detected potential relevance between immune-related gene polymorphisms and risk of septic episodes [9]. SNPs could regulate the expression of innate immune system components, inflammatory cytokines, and coagulation cascade, so illuminating the influence of variation on immune inflammatory response from a cellular and molecular level might contribute to enhance management in the later stage of trauma [15, 20]. Our study indicated that rs2232618 in LBP gene was associated with the morbidity of trauma-related sepsis and C allele carriers had higher sepsis rate in Southwest and Southwest of China trauma patients. Moreover, meta-analysis also revealed that rs2232618 was related with risk of sepsis under all genetic models.

LBP as a class I acute-phase protein of hepatic origin could mediate innate immune responses after recognizing lipopolysaccharides (LPS) originating from different gram-negative bacteria [21, 22]. LBP could form a high-affinity complex with LPS, then LPS was delivered to cell through CD14 or TLR4-MD2 and triggered a cascade of cytokines and pro-inflammatory mediators [23]. During sepsis, previous studies suggested that levels of serum LBP elevated almost seven times higher than normal levels [24]. Therefore, LBP might be a promising tool for the early clinical diagnosis of sepsis and appropriated in differentiating sepsis and systemic inflammatory response syndrome (SIRS) [25]. It was reasonable to suppose the SNP affecting the expression or activities of LBP might also have influence on individual susceptibility for sepsis. Flores et al. [26] have reported a common SNP risk haplotype of LBP gene that was strongly related to susceptibility to severe sepsis and mutant

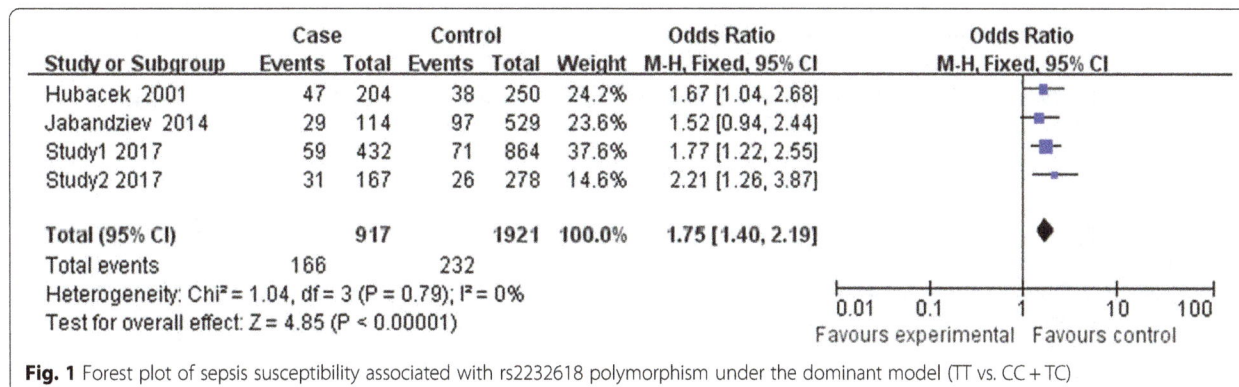

Fig. 1 Forest plot of sepsis susceptibility associated with rs2232618 polymorphism under the dominant model (TT vs. CC + TC)

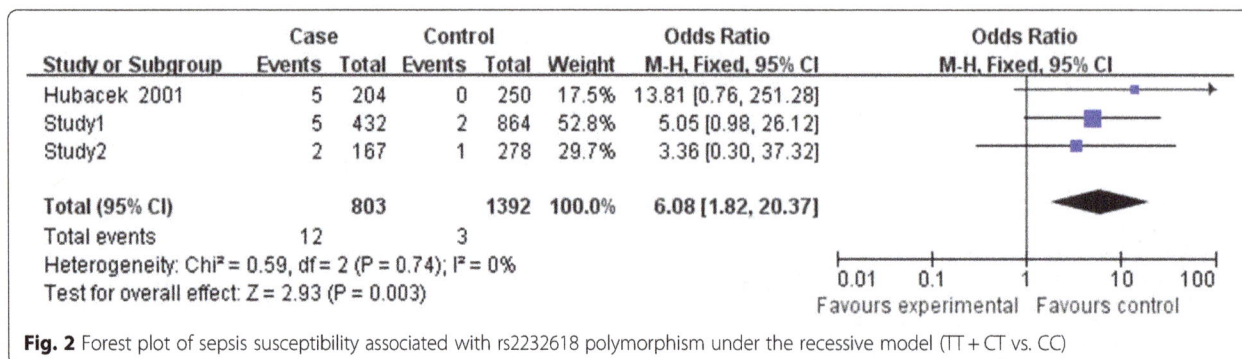

Fig. 2 Forest plot of sepsis susceptibility associated with rs2232618 polymorphism under the recessive model (TT + CT vs. CC)

homozygous individuals had increased risk of severe sepsis. Previous studies also reported that a frequent human LBP SNP (minor allelic frequency = 0.08) affecting an amino acid led to a dysfunctional LBP and had a reduced binding capacity for LPS and lipopeptides. Decreased cytokine response after LPS exposure was also identified in variant carriers. Furthermore, retrospective trial evidence suggested that this LBP SNP was correlated with increased mortality rate during sepsis and pneumonia [27]. Therefore, LBP gene polymorphisms might have an association with sepsis susceptibility.

The T → C variant in rs2232618 polymorphism leaded phenylalanine transformation leucine at amino acid 436 (Phe436Leu) in the LBP protein [28]. Therefore, rs2232618 may influence interaction for LPS and CD14. Our previous investigation reported that rs2232618C allele carriers had higher sepsis morbidity and MOD score. Mechanism research suggested rs2232618 was also related to LPS-induced activation of peripheral blood leukocytes in patients with major traumatic injury, and the rs2232618 polymorphism had impact on activities of LBP protein, but not the production of LBP protein [16]. Furthermore, Hubacek et al. showed patients which were homozygote for Phe436Leu alleles exclusively had higher mortality after sepsis [14]. Jabandziev et al. reported combing rs2232618 in LBP with additional four SNPs could be used as a predictor of sepsis outcome in children [15]. Therefore, we concluded the

rs2232618 was a functional variation and might play an important role in the pathophysiologic process of sepsis and MODS. In order to further investigate the clinical association between rs2232618 and risk of sepsis in larger major traumatic patient cohorts, we enlarged the sample size in the Southwest and Southeast of China. Similar to our previous findings, individuals with more C genotype for rs2232618 polymorphism had higher incidence of sepsis in both study populations. The following meta-analysis further confirmed the association. Thus, the results presented here indicated the rs2232618 polymorphism might be a functional risk variant for sepsis in patients with major traumatic injury.

However, our study had several limitations. Firstly, owing to the lower incidence of gram-positive or mixed-infected sepsis, sub-group analysis between rs2232618 polymorphism and trauma-related sepsis was not completed. Secondly, the diagnosis criterion of sepsis had been revised as sepsis-3 for patients who had a daily SOFA score ≥ 2 with suspected infection in 2016 [29]. However, majority of our sepsis patients were diagnosed based on the sepsis-2 for patients who met ≥ 2 SIRS criteria with suspected infection, so whether the association would exist in patients identified by new sepsis criteria was unsure. Finally, we only recruited trauma patients in Chinese Han population, which is different from other ethnic populations in some aspects; further studies in other ethnic populations should be included to fully explore the association.

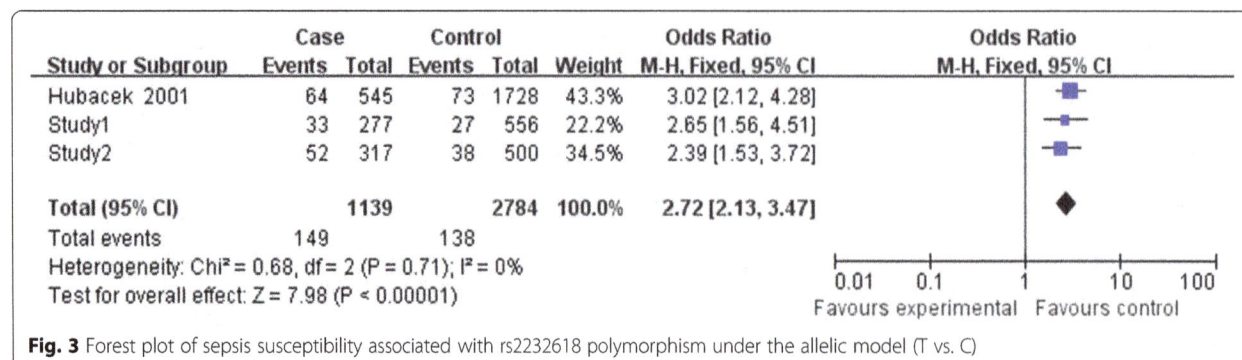

Fig. 3 Forest plot of sepsis susceptibility associated with rs2232618 polymorphism under the allelic model (T vs. C)

Conclusions

In summary, our study enlarged the sample size to further define the clinical relation between rs2232618 and the incidence of sepsis after severe traumatic injury. The follow-up meta-analysis strongly clarified the significant association between rs2232618 and sepsis. Future studies would explore whether rs2232618 could improve early clinical therapeutic interventions in patients with sepsis.

Abbreviations

CI: Confidence intervals; HWE: Hardy-Weinberg equilibrium; ISS: Injury Severity Score; LBP: Lipopolysaccharide-binding protein; LPS: Lipopolysaccharides; MAF: Minor allele frequency; MOD: Multiple organ dysfunction; OR: Odds ratio; SIRS: Systemic inflammatory response syndrome; SNP: Single nucleotide polymorphisms; TLR1: Toll-like receptor 1; TNF-α: Tumor necrosis factor-alpha

Acknowledgements

The authors thank PhD Kan Zhu (University of California, Davis, USA) for the language correction throughout the manuscript. We also thank all the participants who participated in this study.

Funding

This work is supported by National Natural Science Foundation of China (81601677 and 81571892) and Medical Research Funding of PLA of China (AWS14C003 and 17QNP005).

Authors' contributions

D-LW curated the data. LZ carried out the investigation. J-XJ administered the project and visualization. D-LW and JD contributed to the resources. J-HS contributed to the software. H-XL and A-QZ wrote the original draft. A-QZ wrote, reviewed, and edited the manuscript. All authors read and approved the final manuscript.

Competing interests

All authors declare that they have no competing interests.

References

1. Lord JM, Midwinter MJ, Chen YF, Belli A, Brohi K, Kovacs EJ, Koenderman L, Kubes P, Lilford RJ. The systemic immune response to trauma: an overview of pathophysiology and treatment. Lancet. 2014;384(9952):1455–65.
2. Park JH, Choi SH, Yoon YH, Park SJ, Kim JY, Cho HJ. Risk factors for sepsis in Korean trauma patients. Eur J Trauma Emerg Surg. 2016;42(4):453–8.
3. Raju R. Immune and metabolic alterations following trauma and sepsis - an overview. Biochim Biophys Acta. 2017;1863(10 Pt B):2523–5.
4. Cabrera CP, Manson J, Shepherd JM, Torrance HD, Watson D, Longhi MP, Hoti M, Patel MB, O'Dwyer M, Nourshargh S, et al. Signatures of inflammation and impending multiple organ dysfunction in the hyperacute phase of trauma: a prospective cohort study. PLoS Med. 2017;14(7): e1002352.
5. Xiao W, Mindrinos MN, Seok J, Cuschieri J, Cuenca AG, Gao H, Hayden DL, Hennessy L, Moore EE, Minei JP, et al. A genomic storm in critically injured humans. J Exp Med. 2011;208(13):2581–90.
6. Eriksson J, Gidlof A, Eriksson M, Larsson E, Brattstrom O, Oldner A. Thioredoxin a novel biomarker of post-injury sepsis. Free Radic Biol Med. 2017;104:138–43.
7. Rautanen A, Mills TC, Gordon AC, Hutton P, Steffens M, Nuamah R, Chiche JD, Parks T, Chapman SJ, Davenport EE, et al. Genome-wide association study of survival from sepsis due to pneumonia: an observational cohort study. Lancet Respir Med. 2015;3(1):53–60.
8. Wurfel MM. Genetic insights into sepsis: what have we learned and how will it help? Curr Pharm Des. 2008;14(19):1900–11.
9. David VL, Ercisli MF, Rogobete AF, Boia ES, Horhat R, Nitu R, Diaconu MM, Pirtea L, Ciuca I, Horhat D, et al. Early prediction of sepsis incidence in critically ill patients using specific genetic polymorphisms. Biochem Genet. 2016;55(3):193–203.
10. Teuffel O, Ethier MC, Beyene J, Sung L. Association between tumor necrosis factor-alpha promoter -308 A/G polymorphism and susceptibility to sepsis and sepsis mortality: a systematic review and meta-analysis. Crit Care Med. 2010;38(1):276–82.
11. Thompson CM, Holden TD, Rona G, Laxmanan B, Black RA, O'Keefe GE, Wurfel MM. Toll-like receptor 1 polymorphisms and associated outcomes in sepsis after traumatic injury: a candidate gene association study. Ann Surg. 2014;259(1):179–85.
12. Bronkhorst MW, Patka P, Van Lieshout EM. Effects of sequence variations in innate immune response genes on infectious outcome in trauma patients: a comprehensive review. Shock. 2015;44(5):390–6.
13. Cunningham SC, Malone DL, Bochicchio GV, Genuit T, Keledjian K, Tracy JK, Napolitano LM. Serum lipopolysaccharide-binding protein concentrations in trauma victims. Surg Infect. 2006;7(3):251–61.
14. Hubacek JA, Stuber F, Frohlich D, Book M, Wetegrove S, Ritter M, Rothe G, Schmitz G. Gene variants of the bactericidal/permeability increasing protein and lipopolysaccharide binding protein in sepsis patients: gender-specific genetic predisposition to sepsis. Crit Care Med. 2001;29(3):557–61.
15. Jabandziev P, Smerek M, Michalek J, Fedora M, Kosinova L, Hubacek JA, Michalek J. Multiple gene-to-gene interactions in children with sepsis: a combination of five gene variants predicts outcome of life-threatening sepsis. Crit Care. 2014;18(1):R1.
16. Zeng L, Gu W, Zhang AQ, Zhang M, Zhang LY, Du DY, Huang SN, Jiang JX. A functional variant of lipopolysaccharide binding protein predisposes to sepsis and organ dysfunction in patients with major trauma. Ann Surg. 2012;255(1):147–57.
17. Alderborn A, Kristofferson A, Hammerling U. Determination of single-nucleotide polymorphisms by real-time pyrophosphate DNA sequencing. Genome Res. 2000;10(8):1249–58.
18. Rittirsch D, Schoenborn V, Lindig S, Wanner E, Sprengel K, Gunkel S, Blaess M, Schaarschmidt B, Sailer P, Marsmann S, et al. An integrated clinico-transcriptomic approach identifies a central role of the Heme degradation pathway for septic complications after trauma. Ann Surg. 2016;264(6):1125–34.
19. Ciriello V, Gudipati S, Stavrou PZ, Kanakaris NK, Bellamy MC, Giannoudis PV. Biomarkers predicting sepsis in polytrauma patients: current evidence. Injury. 2013;44(12):1680–92.
20. Cornell TT, Wynn J, Shanley TP, Wheeler DS, Wong HR. Mechanisms and regulation of the gene-expression response to sepsis. Pediatrics. 2010;125(6): 1248–58.
21. Rietschel ET, Brade H, Holst O, Brade L, Muller-Loennies S, Mamat U, Zahringer U, Beckmann F, Seydel U, Brandenburg K, et al. Bacterial endotoxin: chemical constitution, biological recognition, host response, and immunological detoxification. Curr Top Microbiol Immunol. 1996;216:39–81.
22. Schumann RR, Kirschning CJ, Unbehaun A, Aberle HP, Knope HP, Lamping N, Ulevitch RJ, Herrmann F. The lipopolysaccharide-binding protein is a secretory class 1 acute-phase protein whose gene is transcriptionally activated by APRF/STAT/3 and other cytokine-inducible nuclear proteins. Mol Cell Biol. 1996;16(7):3490–503.
23. Ryu JK, Kim SJ, Rah SH, Kang JI, Jung HE, Lee D, Lee HK, Lee JO, Park BS, Yoon TY, et al. Reconstruction of LPS transfer cascade reveals structural determinants within LBP, CD14, and TLR4-MD2 for efficient LPS recognition and transfer. Immunity. 2017;46(1):38–50.
24. Chen KF, Chou CH, Jiang JY, Yu HW, Meng YH, Tang WC, Wu CC. Diagnostic accuracy of lipopolysaccharide-binding protein as biomarker for sepsis in adult patients: a systematic review and meta-analysis. PLoS One. 2016;11(4):e0153188.
25. Garcia de Guadiana Romualdo L, Albaladejo Oton MD, Rebollo Acebes S, Esteban Torrella P, Hernando Holgado A, Jimenez Santos E, Jimenez Sanchez R, Orton Freire A. Diagnostic accuracy of lipopolysaccharide-binding protein for sepsis in patients with suspected infection in the

emergency department. Ann Clin Biochem. 2017;55(1):143–8. https://doi.org/10.1177/0004563217694378.

26. Flores C, Perez-Mendez L, Maca-Meyer N, Muriel A, Espinosa E, Blanco J, Sanguesa R, Muros M, Garcia JG, Villar J, et al. A common haplotype of the LBP gene predisposes to severe sepsis. Crit Care Med. 2009;37(10):2759–66.

27. Eckert JK, Kim YJ, Kim JI, Gurtler K, Oh DY, Sur S, Lundvall L, Hamann L, van der Ploeg A, Pickkers P, et al. The crystal structure of lipopolysaccharide binding protein reveals the location of a frequent mutation that impairs innate immunity. Immunity. 2013;39(4):647–60.

28. Iovine N, Eastvold J, Elsbach P, Weiss JP, Gioannini TL. The carboxyl-terminal domain of closely related endotoxin-binding proteins determines the target of protein-lipopolysaccharide complexes. J Biol Chem. 2002;277(10):7970–8.

29. Singer M, Deutschman CS, Seymour CW, Shankar-Hari M, Annane D, Bauer M, Bellomo R, Bernard GR, Chiche JD, Coopersmith CM, et al. The third international consensus definitions for sepsis and septic shock (sepsis-3). Jama. 2016;315(8):801–10.

Non-operative management for penetrating splenic trauma: how far can we go to save splenic function?

Roy Spijkerman[1][*] [iD], Michel Paul Johan Teuben[1], Fatima Hoosain[2], Liezel Phyllis Taylor[2], Timothy Craig Hardcastle[3], Taco Johan Blokhuis[1], Brian Leigh Warren[2] and Luke Petrus Hendrikus Leenen[1]

Abstract

Background: Selective non-operative management (NOM) for the treatment of blunt splenic trauma is safe. Currently, the feasibility of selective NOM for penetrating splenic injury (PSI) is unclear. Unfortunately, little is known about the success rate of spleen-preserving surgical procedures. The aim of this study was to investigate the outcome of selective NOM for penetrating splenic injuries.

Methods: A dual-centre study is performed in two level-one trauma centres. All identified patients treated for PSI were identified. Patients were grouped based on the treatment they received. Group one consisted of splenectomised patients, the second group included patients treated by a spleen-preserving surgical intervention, and group three included those patients who were treated by NOM.

Results: A total of 118 patients with a median age of 27 and a median ISS of 25 (interquartile range (IQR) 16–34) were included. Ninety-six patients required operative intervention, of whom 45 underwent a total splenectomy and 51 underwent spleen-preserving surgical procedures. Furthermore, 22 patients (12 stab wounds and 10 gunshot wounds) were treated by NOM. There were several anticipated significant differences in the baseline encountered. The median hospitalization time was 8 (5–12) days, with no significant differences between the groups. The splenectomy group had significantly more intensive care unit (ICU) days (2(0–6) vs. 0(0–1)) and ventilation days (1(0–3) vs. 0(0–0)) compared to the NOM group. Mortality was only noted in the splenectomy group.

Conclusions: Spleen-preserving surgical therapy for PSI is a feasible treatment modality and is not associated with increased mortality. Moreover, a select group of patients can be treated without any surgical intervention at all.

Keywords: Spleen, Penetrating, Non-operative, Trauma, Gunshot wound, Stab wound, Mortality

Background

The spleen plays an important role in the immune system, and asplenia is associated with a lifelong increased risk of severe infectious diseases [1, 2]. Currently, splenic injuries are therefore preferably treated in a way that splenic function can be preserved [3, 4]. It has been shown that over 80% of blunt injuries to the spleen can be treated by non-operative management (NOM) [3, 5]. Moreover, when laparotomy is indicated, there are several surgical options to treat splenic injuries besides a total splenectomy [6, 7].

These spleen-saving procedures have been shown to be safe and effective in saving the immunologic function of the spleen in blunt splenic trauma [8].

It is unclear, however, whether selective NOM and spleen-preserving surgery is suitable for the treatment of penetrating splenic injuries as well. Non-operative and spleen-preserving surgery for the treatment of penetrating solid intra-abdominal organs is becoming more common in large trauma centres that frequently deal with penetrating trauma [9–11]. Most studies that address the feasibility of NOM focus on the injured liver or kidney [12, 13]. As splenic injuries are relatively rare, most other studies only analyse pooled data from all intra-abdominal organs (including the spleen) [9–11]. In

* Correspondence: spijkermanroy@gmail.com
[1]Department of Trauma, University Medical Centre Utrecht, Heidelberglaan 100, 3584CX Utrecht, The Netherlands
Full list of author information is available at the end of the article

order to investigate the feasibility of selective NOM and spleen-preserving surgery for the spleen, it is essential not to consider the injured spleen comparable to liver and kidney injuries. The clinical course of splenic injuries is considerably different from other solid intra-abdominal organs as splenic injuries are notorious for the risk of delayed bleeding [14]. When the spleen is injured, there is a high chance of concurrent intra-abdominal solid and hollow organ injuries as well as thoracic and diaphragmatic injuries [15].

Little is known about the feasibility and safety of NOM and spleen-preserving surgery for the treatment of PSI (penetrating splenic injury). One recent single-centre study from Berg et al. indicated that NOM can be utilized in a select group of patients with penetrating splenic trauma [15]. In our institutions, more liberal inclusion criteria for selective non-operative management are used; therefore, we aimed to explore the safety of our protocols, in which we push spleen-saving therapy to the limits.

Methods

We performed a dual-centre study in two level-one trauma centres in South-Africa to investigate the feasibility of selective NOM in PSI. We received approval from the Health Research Ethics Committee (HREC) in Cape Town and the Biomedical Research Ethics Committee (BREC) in Durban. From the prospectively composed trauma database in Tygerberg Hospital in Cape Town as well as the Inkosi Albert Luthuli Central Hospital (IALCH) in Durban, we retrospectively identified patients that presented to either institution for the treatment of penetrating splenic injury. The study period in Tygerberg Hospital was between September 1, 2010, and September 1, 2014, while we included all patients presented to IALCH between April 1, 2007, and April 1, 2014. All patients with a splenic injury presenting to the IALCH were identified from the institutional trauma registry (UKZN BREC BE207–09). We identified the patients at Tygerberg Hospital by reviewing a maintained operation logbook as well as the radiology database (HREC S14/02/046). All patients above the age of 14 were included. For the purpose of the study, we excluded patients who died in the emergency department before diagnostic work-up was completed.

Study group characteristics

Documented data included patient demographics: age in years, gender, systolic blood pressure (SBP) in millimetre of mercury, pulse rate (PR) in beats per minute, Glasgow Coma Score (GCS), serum haemoglobin (Hb) in grams per decilitre, serum haematocrit (Ht) in L/L, thrombocyte count in $\times 10^9$/L, Abbreviated Injury Scale (AIS) [16] and Injury Severity Score (ISS) [17]. We further documented the specific underlying mechanism of injury,

thereby distinguishing stab wounds (SW) from gunshot wounds (GSW).

Imaging

Computed tomography (CT)-scan reports were documented and used for this study. All patients that were haemodynamically stable enough were preoperatively scanned by CT. Also, all patients that were selected for NOM underwent a CT-scan.

Treatment modalities

Patients were categorized by the type of treatment that they received. Group I consisted of patients treated by a total splenectomy, patients that underwent a spleen-preserving surgical procedure were included in group II, and patients treated by NOM were analysed as group III. Spleen-preserving surgery is a procedure where the bleeding from the spleen was either stopped by the use of sutures or by the use of haemostatic techniques, such as the application of Surgicel® (Ethicon, Johannesburg). Patients that were treated by NOM underwent a successful trial of NOM. In order to make a trial of NOM successful, we created new treatment guidelines (Fig. 1). Not all the patients included in our study period followed this protocol, but we have started using it currently.

We suggest a trial of NOM in patients with penetrating splenic injury without a strict indication (such as HVI) for operative management (OM). We utilize the following other exclusion criteria for NOM: decreased level of consciousness, spinal cord injuries, blood in nasogastric tube, and blood on rectal examination. All patients have to undergo CT scanning to identify concurrent HVI and to grade concurrent intra-abdominal injuries. A trial of NOM includes a strict observation period of 24 h with serial clinical examination and temperature every 4 h, no oral intake, no antibiotics, one hourly blood pressure and pulse/respiratory rate measurements for the first 6 h and thereafter every 4 h. If the first 24 h are uneventful, it is recommended to give a trial of feeding and perform clinical examination every 4 h during the next 12 h without antibiotics. If there are signs of neurological problems, signs that indicate HVI or signs of haemodynamic instability consider operative management (OM). It is recommended to discharge patients no earlier than 36 h after admission.

Outcomes

The primary outcome was mortality. The secondary outcomes were post-operative complications, mechanical ventilation days, length of hospital stay (LOS) and length of intensive care unit (ICU) stay. We also compared the outcome of patients sustaining gunshot wounds with those that sustained stab wounds. Splenic-AIS and AIS

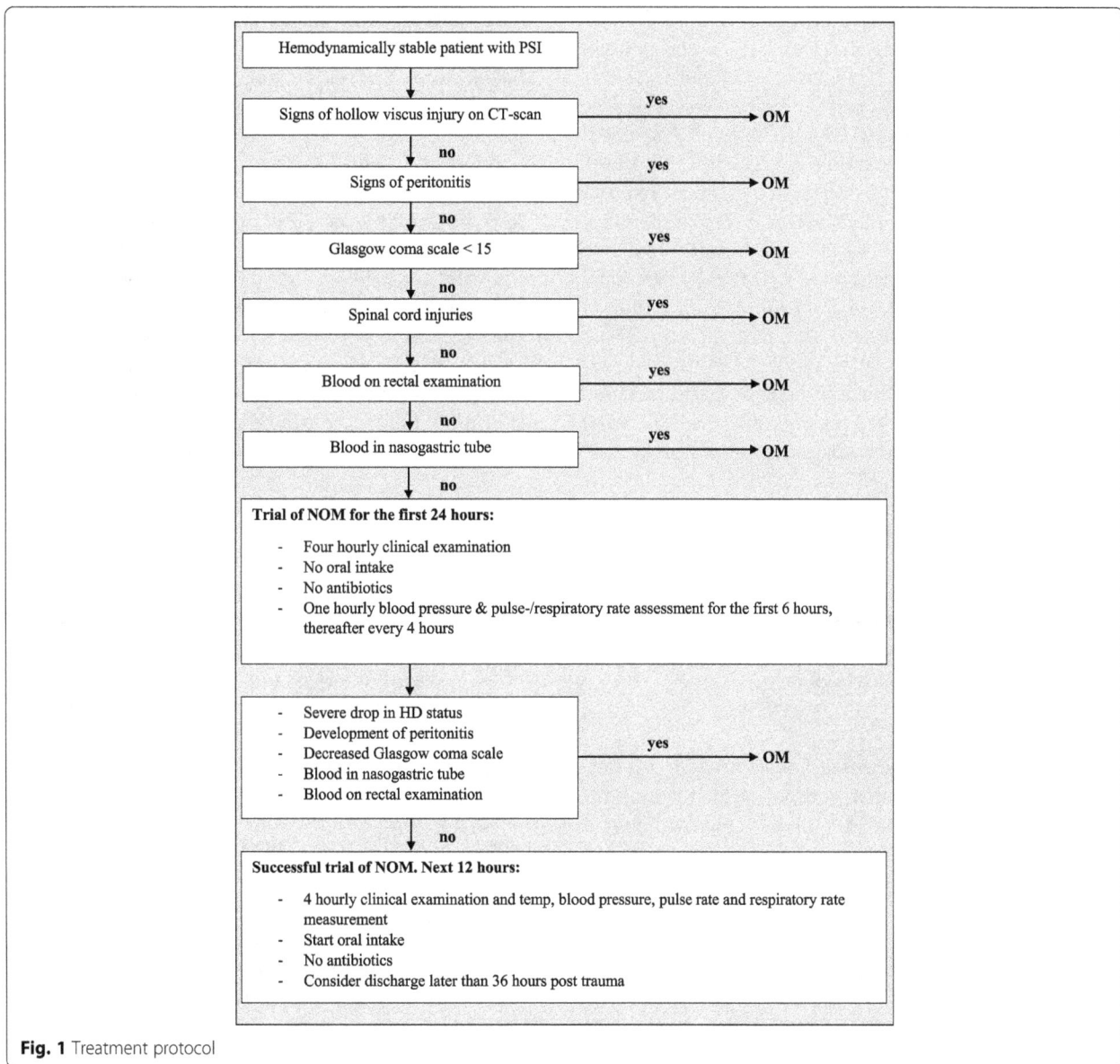

Fig. 1 Treatment protocol

of associated injuries were determined by using the 1998 version of the Abbreviated Injury Scale.

Statistical analysis

Statistical analysis was performed using SPSS for Windows 20.0 (IBM, Chicago, Illinois). Differences between groups were calculated with Fisher's exact test and chi-square test for ordinal data and two-tailed t test and Mann-Whitney U test for continuous data. P values less than 0.05 were considered significant.

Results

For the purpose of this study, we identified, during a 4-year period at the Tygerberg Hospital and a 6-year period at the Inkosi Albert Luthuli Central Hospital, all patients with penetrating splenic injuries.

Study group characteristics

A total of 118 patients (109 (92%) male and 9 (8%) female) with a median (interquartile range (IQR)) age of 27 (20–32) presented to the emergency departments. On admission, they had a median (IQR) systolic blood pressure of 122 (105–136), a pulse rate of 94 (80–113) beats per minute and a Glasgow Coma Scale-score of 15 (15–15). Nineteen patients (16%) had an altered mental state (GCS < 15). Fifty-three patients (45%) were admitted for the treatment of stab wound injuries, whereas 65 patients (55%) sustained gunshot injuries. The median (IQR) Abbreviated Injury Scale of the encountered splenic lesions was 3 (3–4). Seventy-eight individuals (66%) had a splenic AIS <4, while 40 patients (33%) were diagnosed with a grade 4 or 5 splenic injury. The patients had a median total Injury Severity Score of 25 (16–34).

Comparison of baseline characteristics

A comparison of baseline characteristics of the populations is shown in Table 1. As expected, there were significant differences in age, systolic blood pressure, pulse rate, GCS and thrombocyte count between the splenectomy and the spleen-preserving surgical therapy group. Furthermore, median (IQR) Abbreviated Injury Score (4 (3–5) vs. 2 (2–3)) and Injury Severity Score (25 (19–16) vs. 18 (13–25)) were both significantly higher in patients who underwent a splenectomy. In the splenectomy group, 20 patients (44%) had a splenic-AIS <3, a total of six patients (13%) had a splenic-AIS of 4 and 19 patients (43%) were found with an AIS of 5. In the spleen-preserving surgical treatment group, 43 patients (84%) had a splenic-AIS <4, three patients (6%) had AIS of 4, and five patients (10%) were diagnosed with an AIS of 5.

Non-operatively managed patients had a significantly lower systolic blood pressure (117 (105–124) vs. 129 (115–141)) and a significantly higher splenic-AIS (3 (2–4) vs. 2 (2–3)) compared to patients selected for spleen-preserving surgical therapy. Fifteen out of 22 patients (68%) that were selected for non-operative management had an AIS <3, two patients (9%) had an AIS of 4, and five patients (23%) had an AIS of 5.

Mechanism of injury

We compared the characteristics, management and outcome of patients with either gunshot or stab wound injuries. As anticipated, the AIS of the splenic injury (3 (2–5) vs. 2 (2–3)) as well as total ISS (25 (18–41) vs. 18 (13–25)) were significantly higher in patients suffering from gunshot wounds.

A comparison between the management and outcome of stab wounds and gunshot wounds is shown in Table 2. Splenectomy was relatively more frequently performed in the patients suffering from gunshot wounds (SW = 10/53 (19%) vs. GSW = 35/65 (54%)). The amount of patients managed non-operatively does not significantly differ between stab wounds and gunshot wounds (SW = 12/53 (23%) vs. GSW = 10/65 (15%)). The total number of complications is significantly higher in patients with gunshot wounds (50 vs. 6). The number of ventilation days (1 (0–3) vs. 0 (0–0)), the number of days in the ICU (3 (1–8) vs. 0 (0–0)) and hospitalization days (9 (6–18) vs. 6 (5–9)) are significantly higher in patients suffering from gunshot wounds then those treated for stab wound injuries. Furthermore, fatalities were only seen in the patients with gunshot injuries (N = 7).

Associated injuries

The associated injuries found in our distinct study groups are shown in Table 3. Concomitant solid intra-abdominal organ injuries were encountered in all groups. Left kidney injuries are the most frequently associated abdominal injuries, a total of 48 out of 118 patients (41%) were diagnosed with this injury. Stomach and colon injury are the two most frequently seen hollow viscus injuries (HVIs). There were no HVIs found in the patients managed non-operatively. Thirty-two out of 45 patients (71%) from the splenectomy group had a concurrent diaphragm injury, while 35 out of 51 patients (69%) from the patients treated by a spleen-preserving surgical intervention had a diaphragmatic lesion. The most common injured extra abdominal organ is the lung (93 out of 118 patients (79%)), most frequently due to a pneumothorax. Furthermore, two of the splenectomised patients (4%) had a concurrent cardiac injury.

Table 1 Comparison of baseline characteristics

	Group 1: Splenectomy (n = 45)	Group 2: Spleen-preserving surgical therapy (n = 51)	Group 3: Non-operative management (n = 22)
Age (years)	29 (22–34)[a]	26 (19–30)[a]	26 (20–32)
Gender (M/F)	42/3	47/4	20/2
SBP (mmHg)	117 (94–137)[a]	129 (115–141)[a,Φ]	117 (105–124)[Φ]
Pulse rate (bpm)	103 (82–124)[a]	89 (74–108)[a]	98 (83–106)
GCS	15 (14–15)[†]	15 (15–15)[†]	15 (15–15)
Serum Hb (g/dL)	11 (9.2–12.7)	11.5 (9.7–13.4)	11.8 (10–12.8)
Thrombocytes count (×10⁹/L)	212 (124–290)[a,‡]	274 (208–319)[a]	281 (208–391)[‡]
AIS spleen	4 (3–5)[†]	2 (2–3)[†,∞]	3 (2–4)[∞]
ISS	25 (19–36)[a]	18 (13–25)[a]	27 (18–41)

All variables are in median (IQR)
SBP systolic blood pressure, *bpm* beats per minute, *GCS* Glasgow Coma Score, *Hb* haemoglobin, *Ht* haematocrit, *ISS* Injury Severity Score, *AIS* Abbreviated Injury Score
Group 1 vs. group 2 with $p < 0.05$ by [a]t test and [†]Mann-Whitney U test
Group 2 vs. group 3 with $p < 0.05$ by [∞]t test and [Φ]Mann-Whitney U test
Group 1 vs. group 3 with $p < 0.05$ by [‡]t test

Table 2 Mechanism of injury

	Stab wounds n = 53	Gunshot wounds n = 65
Total splenectomy	10	35
Spleen-preserving therapy	31	20
Non-operative management	12	10
Total number of complications	6[a]	50[a]
No. of patients with complications	5	27
Ventilation days	0 (0–0)[∞]	1 (0–3)[∞]
ICU stay (days)	0 (0–0)[∞]	3 (1–8)[∞]
Length of hospital stay (days)	6 (5–9)[∞]	9 (6–18)[∞]
Mortality	0[†]	7[†]

All variables are in median (IQR). All frequencies are in absolute number
ICU intensive care unit
$p < 0.05$ by [a]chi-square test, [†]Fisher's exact test and [∞]Mann-Whitney U test

Table 3 Associated injuries

	Group 1: Splenectomy (n = 45)	Group 2: Spleen-preserving surgical therapy (n = 51)	Group 3: Non-operative management (n = 22)
Abdominal solid organ injuries			
Kidney	29	20	10
Liver	18	10	3
Pancreas	16	7	1
Abdominal hollow organ injuries			
Stomach	22	15	0
Colon	16	12	0
Small bowel	6	7	0
Duodenum	1	0	0
Extra-abdominal injuries			
Lung	32	43	18
Diaphragm	33	35	5
Spine	7	6	7
Craniocerebral	2	1	4
Heart	2	0	0
Neck	2	1	0
Maxillofacial	1	0	1
Ureter	1	0	0

Treatment modalities

A total of 96 out of 118 patients (81%) required immediate surgical intervention, of whom 91 patients (77%) underwent a laparotomy and five patients (4%) underwent a diagnostic laparoscopy. Forty-five of the 118 patients (38%) were splenectomised. One of the splenectomised patients was initially selected for non-operative management; however, during an electively executed diaphragmatic repair procedure, the spleen started bleeding again after manipulation. As haemostatic techniques were unable to stop the blood loss, a splenectomy was inevitable. A total of 51 of the 118 patients (43%) were treated by spleen-preserving surgical treatment. There were several indications for an operative intervention without the need for splenectomy. We can divide into two big groups. The first group included patients that needed emergency surgery for haemodynamic instability, but where the main source of bleeding was mostly a different organ/vessel. In 17 of these 51 patients (33%), the spleen was bleeding, but the bleeding could be stopped by haemostatic agents. The second big group included patients that received an operative intervention for delayed peritonitis or where the patient was operated upon for the evaluation of diaphragm injuries. Thirty-four out of 51 patients (66%) underwent an operative intervention for the treatment of their abdominal injuries without the need to actively treat the splenic injury. Of this group, 29 of the 34 patients

(85%) underwent a laparotomy and five patients (15%) underwent a laparoscopy for repair of their diaphragm injury. Furthermore, 22 of the 118 patients (19%) with splenic injuries were treated by non-operative management. The treatment modalities that were used in our patients are illustrated in Fig. 2.

Morbidity and mortality

A comparison of outcome measurements in patients treated by different treatment modalities is demonstrated in Table 4. The number of complications did not differ in terms of statistical significance between groups. Nevertheless, the splenectomy group had a significantly higher number of people suffering from complications than the spleen-preserving group (19/45 (42%) vs. 9/51 (18%)). Mechanical ventilation days (1 (0–3) vs. 0 (0–0)) and duration of ICU stay (2 (0–6) vs. 0 (0–1)) were significantly longer in splenectomised patients compared to non-operated patients. All the complications are listed in Table 5. The majority of our complications were found in the splenectomy group. The most prevalent complications in our study were intra-abdominal collections which complicated the clinical course of patients 16 times (14%). Six patients (5%) had pneumonia, and 10 patients (8%) were diagnosed with sepsis. A total of three patients (3%) developed multi-organ dysfunction syndrome (MODS). There was a statistically significant difference in mortality between the splenectomy group and the spleen-preserving surgical treatment group. There was no mortality in patients selected for spleen-preserving surgical procedures and in the non-operative group, while

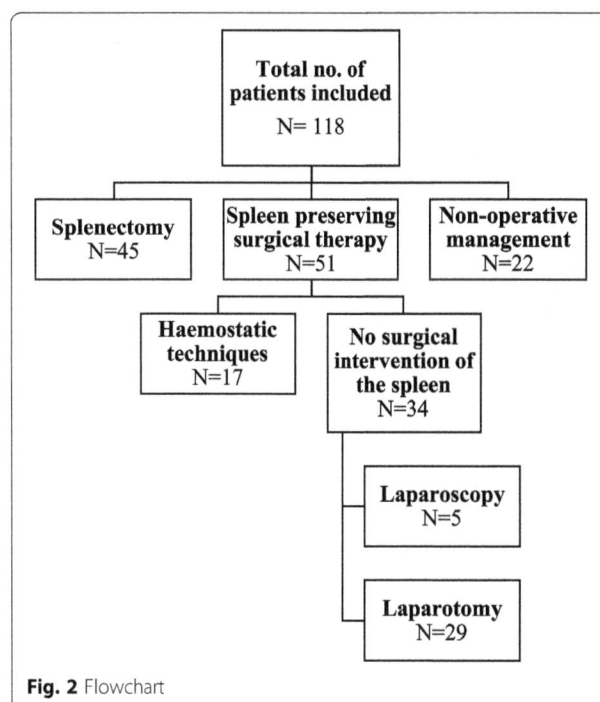

Fig. 2 Flowchart

Table 4 Comparison of outcome between treatment groups

	Group 1: Splenectomy (n = 45)	Group 2: Spleen-preserving surgical therapy (n = 51)	Group 3: Non-operative management (n = 22)
Total number of complications	30	21	5
No. of patients with complications	19[a]	9[a]	4
Ventilation days	1 (0–3)[∞]	0 (0–1)	0 (0–0)[∞]
ICU stay (days)	2 (0–6)[∞]	0 (0–3)	0 (0–1)[∞]
Length of hospital stay (days)	8 (7–12)	7 (5–12)	8 (5–15)
Mortality	7[†]	0[†]	0

All variables are in median (IQR). All frequencies are in absolute number
ICU intensive care unit
Group 1 vs. group 2 with *p* < 0.05 by [a]chi-square test and [†]Fisher's exact test
Group 1 vs. group 3 with *p* < 0.05 by [∞]Mann-Whitney *U* test

Table 5 Post-operative complications

	Group 1: Splenectomy (n = 45)	Group 2: Spleen-preserving surgical therapy (n = 51)	Group 3: Non-operative management (n = 22)
Intra-abdominal collections	7	7	2
Perisplenic	5	1	1
Other location	3	6	1
Sepsis	6	3	1
Pneumonia	2	2	2
Ileus	3	–	–
MODS	3	–	–
Wound infection	1	2	–
Ongoing bleeding	2	–	–
Re-bleed	2	–	–
Subglottic stenosis	–	2	–
Renal pseudo aneurysm	1	–	–
Lung empyema	1	1	–
Upper GI bleed	1	–	–
Enterocutaneous fistula	1	–	–
Exudative pleural adhesions	–	1	–
Extra-abdominal collections	–	1	–
Infected urinoma	–	1	–
Urinoma	–	1	–

All frequencies are in absolute number
MODS multi-organ dysfunction syndrome, *GI* gastrointestinal

seven of the 45 patients (16%) from the splenectomy group died during hospitalization. Three of the 45 patients (7%) died several hours after operative intervention due to massive and ongoing blood loss, while four other patients (9%) died later mainly due to MODS.

Discussion

In our study, 22 out of 118 patients (19%) with penetrating splenic injuries were successfully treated by non-operative management; therefore, we can conclude that NOM is feasible in a selected group of patients. More than half of the patients (51/98) with PSI that required emergency laparotomy were successfully treated by spleen-preserving surgical procedures, and therefore, we conclude that spleen-saving surgery is a safe alternative to total splenectomy, even for penetrating trauma. This study also noted that both NOM and spleen-saving surgery can be applied in both stab and gunshot injuries. Thus, based on our findings, we recommend considering non-operative therapy in all haemodynamically stable patients with penetrating splenic injuries, without concurrent injuries that need an operation, as a feasible alternative to routine operative exploration in appropriate high-level trauma care facilities.

Stab wounds

We found that splenic stab wound injuries in patients, without concurrent intra-abdominal hollow viscus organ injuries and haemodynamic instability, can be successfully treated by non-operative management. Complication rates are low, and delayed re-bleeds are rare as only one non-operatively treated patient required splenectomy for the treatment of secondary bleeding. Furthermore, it cannot be excluded that this single case of delayed splenic bleeding was not a result of iatrogenic injury, as it occurred during an elective diaphragm repair operation. Hence, we would recommend consideration of non-operative management in all haemodynamically stable patients with splenic injury caused by stabbing. Nevertheless, due to the high number of associated concurrent hollow organ injuries (57 out of 118 had at least one concurrent HVI), we strongly advise to routinely perform computed tomography scanning and good clinical review in all patients with splenic stab wounds selected for non-operative management.

Gunshot wounds

Given the high complication rates in patients with gunshot injuries, we believe that our study does not provide sufficient evidence to recommend selective NOM for patients with splenic gunshot injuries. According to our univariate analysis, it appears that the mechanism of injury has to be considered as a key predictive factor for morbidity. Patients non-operatively treated for gunshot injuries had significantly more complications than those treated for stab wound injuries. This difference can be explained by the increased number of associated hollow and solid intra-abdominal, as well as thoracic, injuries. Additionally, both ICU stay and hospitalization time were statistically significantly prolonged in patients treated for gunshot injuries. We do not recommend the routine use of NOM for patients suffering from gunshot injuries. These findings are in line with a systematic review performed by Singh and Hardcastle, where they concluded that NOM is feasible for GSW, but it can not be used routinely [18]. More studies should be performed in order to define specific criteria for adequate patient selection. Until these studies are executed, we feel safe to select stable patients with minor gunshot injuries to the spleen and normal mental status for a trial of non-operative management. In our study, a total of 10 patients with gunshot injuries to the spleen were successfully treated without surgical intervention. A key pre-requisite for these guidelines is the availability of decent monitoring facilities and adequately trained staff.

Haemodynamically unstable patients

When a haemodynamically unstable patient with penetrating splenic injury presents to the emergency department, a trial of NOM is not possible. Emergency laparotomy is indicated. However, in contrast to haemodynamically unstable patients with blunt splenic trauma, patients with penetrating injuries have frequently less concomitant foci of blood loss. This diminishes the necessity of a fast splenectomy aimed to reduce crucial operation time in the damage control setting. We opt to utilize an alternative surgical strategy in which the spleen is not routinely and directly taken out, but packed or treated by local haemostatic techniques and then left untouched during the rest of the inspection of the abdomen. In accordance with our treatment guidelines, attempts to preserve splenic function are the preferred treatment for penetrating splenic injuries. In more than half of our patients, we managed to preserve the spleen by this approach.

Reflection of the literature

Our results of stab and gunshot injuries are in line with the literature. A retrospective study performed by Berg et al. concluded that a select group of patients without haemodynamic instability, peritonitis and radiologic evidence of hollow organ injuries might be adequate candidates for a trial of NOM [15]. They further suggested the need to gather multi-centre data in order to define more precisely the selection criteria for NOM. Their study was executed in a level one trauma centre in the USA and investigated 238 cases of PSI of whom eventually less than 10% (24 patients) were successfully treated by non-operative treatment. In fact, 10 of these

24 patients cannot, however, be considered as proper cases of NOM, since those patients underwent minimally invasive surgery for the evaluation of their abdominal injuries. According to our more strictly defined definitions of NOM in their study, only 2.4% of patients were successfully treated by non-operative therapy. We treated approximately 20% of patients with PSI successfully by NOM. The fraction of patients that is suitable for NOM seems to be almost 10 times larger than that suggested by Berg et al. [15].

In a study from Clancy et al., 57 out of 197 patients with penetrating splenic injuries were initially selected for non-operative therapy; however, the failure rate of NOM is not documented [19]. In other series from Pachter et al. [20], Demetriades et al. [11] and Kaseje et al. [21], relatively less patients with PSI were selected for NOM (respectively 6/43, 3/28 and 5/25). In the study from Demetriades et al., NOM failed in two out of three patients while there was no failure documented in the other studies [11]. Despite the absence of failure rates of NOM, our study is the first to describe successful non-operative treatment of about 20% of patients admitted to level one trauma centres for the treatment of PSI.

Key points and limitations

The key points of this study are that we were able to combine data from two large South African trauma centres and that patients in both institutions were treated according to the same treatment guidelines. Furthermore, this study is unique in enabling us to describe the natural course of penetrating splenic injuries without immediate treatment. We were (unwillingly) forced to push non-operative management to its limits. Hence, given our results, we have probably not reached these limits yet, at least not for stab wound injuries of the spleen.

The main limitation of this study is the retrospective design. However, due to a strictly maintained trauma and radiology data registry, we were able to identify a large number of patients and we had unlimited excess to all patient charts and laboratory results. So the chance of under registration of findings is considered to be very low. Another disadvantage of the study is the fact that we had to exclude several patients as they were transferred from referring hospitals to our level one trauma centres. Also due to the retrospective design, the baseline characteristics show some significant differences between the treatment groups. Most of the differences can be attributed to the fact that patients that need surgical intervention are in a different clinical state than patients that can be selected for NOM. However, there might be some part of selection bias due to these baseline differences. There also is a risk of selection bias due to the situation in the hospitals in South Africa; it is different to the situation in hospitals in the western world. Doctors have to deal with limited resources, and different decisions are made regarding treatment modalities.

Conclusions

In conclusion, our study is the first to show that non-operative management for penetrating splenic trauma is a feasible alternative in selected patients. Given the large number of complications in patients with gunshot wounds to the spleen, we recommend to be reluctant with applying NOM in this group. However, patients with stab wounds seem to be feasible candidates for non-operative therapy. Due to the high prevalence of concurrent hollow viscus organ injuries in patients with PSI, we consider adequate computed tomography imaging as a key pre-requisite for NOM. Furthermore, we believe that spleen-saving techniques must have an important place in treatment algorithms of emergency surgery.

Abbreviations

AIS: Abbreviated Injury Score; BPM: Beats per minute); CT: Computed tomography; GCS: Glasgow coma scale; GWS: Gunshot wound; Hb: Haemoglobin; Ht: Haematocrit; HVI: Hollow viscus unjury; IALCH: Inkosi Albert Luthuli Central Hospital; ICU: Intensive care unit; IQR: Interquartile range; ISS: Injury Severity Score; LOS: Length of hospital stay; MODS: Multi-organ dysfunction syndrome; NOM: Non-operative management; OM: Operative management; PR: Pulse rate; PSI: Penetrating splenic injury; SBP: Systolic blood pressure; SW: Stab wound

Acknowledgements

Not applicable.

Funding

Parts of this study have been presented at international meetings, and funding was obtained from the Alexandre Suerman Fund and Utrecht University Visiting Fellowship Fund.

Authors' contributions

All authors contributed equally to this study. All authors read and approved the final manuscript.

Competing interests

The authors declare that they have no competing interests.

Author details

[1]Department of Trauma, University Medical Centre Utrecht, Heidelberglaan 100, 3584CX Utrecht, The Netherlands. [2]Department of Trauma, Tygerberg Hospital (University of Stellenbosch), Francie van Zijl Avenue, Cape Town 7505, South Africa. [3]Department of Trauma, Inkosi Albert Luthuli Central Hospital (University of Kwazulu-Natal), 800 Bellair Road, Durban 4091, South Africa.

References

1. Shumacker HB, King H. Splenic studies. AMA Arch Surg. 1952;65:499–510.
2. Mebius RE, Kraal G. Structure and function of the spleen. Nat Rev Immunol. 2005;5:606–16.
3. Richardson JD. Changes in the management of injuries to the liver and spleen. J Am Coll Surg. 2005;200:648–69.
4. Hsieh T-M, Cheng Tsai T, Liang J-L, Che LC. Non-operative management attempted for selective high grade blunt hepatosplenic trauma is a feasible strategy. World J Emerg Surg. 2014;9:51.
5. Peitzman AB, Heil B, Rivera L, Federle MB, Harbrecht BG, Clancy KD, et al. Blunt splenic injury in adults: multi-institutional study of the Eastern Association for the Surgery of Trauma. J. Trauma. 2000;49:177–87-9.
6. Büyükünal C, Danişmend N, Yeker D. Spleen-saving procedures in paediatric splenic trauma. Br J Surg. 1987;74:350–2.
7. Resende V, Petroianu A. Subtotal splenectomy for treatment of severe splenic injuries. J Trauma. 1998;44:933–5.
8. Resende V, Petroianu A. Functions of the splenic remnant after subtotal splenectomy for treatment of severe splenic injuries. Am J Surg. 2003;185:311–5.
9. Navsaria PH, Nicol AJ, Edu S, Gandhi R, Ball CG. Selective nonoperative management in 1106 patients with abdominal gunshot wounds: conclusions on safety, efficacy, and the role of selective CT imaging in a prospective single-center study. Ann Surg. 2015;261:760–4.
10. Kong V, Oosthuizen G, Sartorius B, Clarke D. Selective non-operative management of stab wounds to the posterior abdomen is safe: the Pietermaritzburg experience. Injury. 2015;46:1753–8.
11. Demetriades D, Hadjizacharia P, Constantinou C, Brown C, Inaba K, Rhee P, et al. Selective nonoperative management of penetrating abdominal solid organ injuries. Trans Meet Am Surg Assoc. 2006;124:285–93.
12. Moolman C, Navsaria PH, Lazarus J, Pontin A, Nicol AJ. Nonoperative management of penetrating kidney injuries: a prospective audit. J Urol. 2012;188:169–73.
13. MacGoey P, Navarro A, Beckingham IJ, Cameron IC, Brooks AJ. Selective non-operative management of penetrating liver injuries at a UK tertiary referral centre. Ann R Coll Surg Engl. 2014;96:423–6.
14. Kluger Y, Paul DB, Raves JJ, Fonda M, Young JC, Townsend RN, et al. Delayed rupture of the spleen—myths, facts, and their importance: case reports and literature review. J Trauma. 1994;36:568–71.
15. Berg RJ, Inaba K, Okoye O, Pasley J, Teixeira PG, Esparza M, et al. The contemporary management of penetrating splenic injury. Injury. 2014;45:1394–400.
16. Moore EE, Cogbill TH, Jurkovich GJ, Shackford SR, Malangoni MA, Champion HR. Organ injury scaling: spleen and liver (1994 revision). J Trauma. 1995;38:323–4.
17. Baker SP, O'Neill B, Haddon W, Long WB. The injury severity score: a method for describing patients with multiple injuries and evaluating emergency care. J Trauma. 1974;14:187–96.
18. Singh N, Hardcastle TC. Selective non operative management of gunshot wounds to the abdomen: a collective review. Int Emerg Nurs. 2015;23:22–31.
19. Clancy TV, Ramshaw DG, Maxwell JG, Covington DL, Churchill MP, Rutledge R, et al. Management outcomes in splenic injury: a statewide trauma center review. Ann Surg. 1997;226:17–24.
20. Pachter HL, Guth AA, Hofstetter SR, Spencer FC. Changing patterns in the management of splenic trauma: the impact of nonoperative management. Ann. Surg.. 1998 ;227:708–17-9.
21. Kaseje N, Agarwal S, Burch M, Glantz A, Emhoff T, Burke P, et al. Short-term outcomes of splenectomy avoidance in trauma patients. Am J Surg. 2008;196:213–7.

30

Lower gastrointestinal bleeding—Computed Tomographic Angiography, Colonoscopy or both?

Daniel Clerc[1], Fabian Grass[1], Markus Schäfer[1], Alban Denys[2], Nicolas Demartines[1*] and Martin Hübner[1]

Abstract

Background: Lower endoscopy (LE) is the standard diagnostic modality for lower gastrointestinal bleeding (LGIB). Conversely, computed tomographic angiography (CTA) offers an immediate non-invasive diagnosis visualizing the entire gastrointestinal tract. The aim of this study was to compare these 2 modalities with regards to diagnostic value and bleeding control.

Methods: Tertiary center retrospective analysis of consecutive patients admitted for LGIB between 2006 and 2012. Comparison of patients with LE *vs.* CTA as first exam, respectively, with emphasis on diagnostic accuracy and bleeding control.

Results: Final analysis included 183 patients; 122 (66.7%) had LE first, while 32 (17.5%) had CTA; 29 (15.8%) had neither of both exams. Median time to CTA was shorter compared to LE (3 (IQR = 8.2) *vs.* 22 (IQR = 36.9) hours, $P < 0.001$). Active bleeding was identified in 31% with CTA *vs.* 15% with LE ($P = 0.031$); a non-actively bleeding source was found by CTA and LE in 22 *vs.* 31%, respectively ($P = 0.305$). Bleeding control required endoscopy in 19%, surgery in 14% and embolization in 1.6%, while 66% were treated conservatively. Post-interventional bleeding was mostly controlled by endoscopic therapy (57%). 80% of patients with active bleeding on CTA required surgery.

Conclusions: Post-interventional LGIB was effectively addressed by LE. For other causes of LGIB, CTA was efficient, and more available than colonoscopy. Treatment was conservative for most patients. In case of active bleeding, CTA could localize the bleeding source and predict the need for surgery.

Keywords: Gastrointestinal hemorrhage, Colonoscopy, Computed tomographic angiography, Endoscopy

Background

Lower gastrointestinal bleeding (LGIB) is a common clinical problem, representing 20 to 30% of patients presenting with gastrointestinal bleeding [1, 2]. LGIB incidence is increasing over time, as it is associated with older age and pre-existing comorbidities [3]. Very distal bleeding, e.g. due to hemorrhoids and low rectal cancer, is rather easy to diagnose, but bleeding from the colon and small bowel remains a diagnostic challenge. According to recent guidelines, hemodynamic stabilization and resuscitation must be performed prior to search any bleeding source. While

nasogastric lavage and/or esophagogastroduodenoscopy can be considered to rule out upper gastrointestinal bleeding for patients presenting severe hematochezia, lower endoscopy (LE) is the preferred diagnostic approach for LGIB [1, 4]. Nevertheless, computed tomographic angiography (CTA) for evaluation of GI bleeding is increasingly used and may challenges lower endoscopy as most appropriate tool. This non-invasive diagnostic modality is readily available in most hospitals and can be rapidly performed without any bowel preparation. Reported sensitivity and specificity rates are 86 and 95%, respectively and bleeding as low as 0.4ml/min can be detected [5, 6].

So far, there is only limited evidence on the routine use of CTA in the initial management of LGIB. Its accuracy compared to LE remains unclear; and subsequently, its

* Correspondence: demartines@chuv.ch
This study was presented at the Annual Swiss Surgical Meeting 2015, May 20–22, Bern, Switzerland
[1]Department of Visceral Surgery, University Hospital of Lausanne (CHUV), Lausanne, Switzerland
Full list of author information is available at the end of the article

use as a first-line diagnostic modality is not considered in current management algorithms [1, 4].

This current study aimed to compare the accuracy of CTA and colonoscopy in the diagnosis of LGIB and their influence on bleeding control.

Methods

Retrospective cohort study conducted at a tertiary care academic center. The study was approved by the local ethics committee (protocol 389/12) performed according the STROBE recommendations, and registered under www.researchregistry.com (# 726).

Patients and data collection

All consecutive patients admitted for LGIB to the department of visceral surgery between January 2006 and December 2012 were potentially eligible. The following patients were excluded from analysis: (I) proctological bleeding, (II) LGIB not being the primary cause of admission, and (III) patients with LGIB admitted for elective surgery. Patients underwent primary evaluation at the emergency department by emergency physicians and by a gastrointestinal consultant surgeon before admission to the visceral surgery department. The initial diagnostic modality (LE or CTA) was defined by the physician in charge of the patient.

LE was defined as a flexible lower endoscopy performed by a gastroenterologist. Procedures were performed by an attending, junior staff or resident gastroenterologist according to the policy of a Swiss university hospital. Resident procedures were supervised by a board-certified gastro-enterologist. Gastroenterology consultant is available 24/7 in our institution, with in-hospital presence during daytime, and available within 30 min during the nightshift. Type of bowel preparation, if any, was upon the choice of the gastroenterologist performing the procedure. A standard flexible colonoscope was used for all procedures. Conscious sedation or general anesthesia was used depending upon patient's general condition. Whenever possible, examination was performed up to the ileo-caecal valve. Exam findings were classified as positive with actively bleeding lesion, positive with non-actively bleeding lesion or inconclusive. LE was defined inconclusive when no lesion was detected regardless of the quality of preparation and the amount of blood clots present in the endoscopic view.

For actively bleeding lesions or non-actively bleeding lesions with high risk of re-bleeding, endoscopic therapy was directly applied with clips, adrenaline infusion or thermal probe depending on the gastroenterologist's preference.

CTA was defined as a contrast-enhanced abdominal and pelvic CT scan performed in a triphasic acquisition. First, a native acquisition was followed by contrast-enhanced arterial phase after a bolus injection of 100ml contrast media (300mg iodine/ml, 4ml/s) with automatic triggering (collimation 16 × 0.625mm; pitch 1.75; table speed 35mm/s). The venous acquisition was performed 70–80 s later. Exam findings were classified as positive with active bleeding when CTA showed intraluminal contrast material extravasation. CTA were defined positive without active bleeding when the cause of bleeding was spotted without contrast material extravasation. CTA were defined inconclusive when no cause of bleeding was found.

The time spent from the admission to the emergency room to the execution of the diagnostic exams was recorded. First hemodynamic parameters (heart rate (HR), blood pressure) and hemoglobin (Hb) values recorded upon admission were retrieved. The shock index (SI), defined as the ratio of heart rate to systolic blood pressure, and the mean arterial pressure (MAP), were calculated.

The cause of bleeding was classified in six categories: small bowel, diverticular, colorectal neoplasia, colorectal lesion, post-interventional, and unknown location. Small bowel bleeding was defined as the source of bleeding arising from the ligament of Treitz to the ileo-caecal valve. Diverticular bleeding was defined as the source of bleeding being related to a colonic diverticular disease. A colorectal neoplasia was defined as benign or malignant lesion being the cause of bleeding. Non-neoplastic, non-diverticular colorectal lesions being the source of bleeding (colitis, colonic ulcers or angiodysplasias) were grouped in the colorectal lesion category. Post-interventional bleeding was defined as a bleeding occurring following endoscopic or surgical procedure. Bleeding of unknown location was defined when the cause of bleeding was not found during hospital stay. The control of bleeding was recorded according to the last therapeutic intervention performed (surgery, angio-embolization, endoscopic intervention or conservative).

Patient's characteristics, information on the performed diagnostic procedures and clinical outcomes were defined a priori. All eligible patients were collected by ICD codes. Data was retrieved by retrospective chart review and entered in a coded computerized database. Patients were stratified according to the first diagnostic exam performed at hospital admission, i.e. LE, CTA or none of both exams.

Statistical analysis

Descriptive statistics for categorical variables were reported as frequency (%), while continuous variables were reported as median (interquartile range). Chi-square and Student's t-test were used for comparison of categorical and continuous variables, respectively. All statistical tests were two-sided and a level of 0.05 was used to indicate statistical significance. Data analysis was performed with the Statistical Software for the Social Sciences SPSS

Advanced Statistics 22 (IBM Software Group, 200 W. Madison St., Chicago, IL; 60606 USA).

Results

Patients and clinical outcome

Within the study period, 301 patients were hospitalized in the visceral surgery department with diagnostic of GIB. 118 patients were excluded according to the *a priori* defined rules. Final analysis included 183 patients, with 109 male and 74 female patients with a median age of 75 years (Fig. 1). One hundred and twenty-two patients (66.7%) had LE as first diagnostic intervention, 32 (17.5%) had CTA. The remaining 29 patients (15.8%) had neither of the two exams during their hospital stay. Patient characteristics are presented in Table 1. Median length of hospital stay (LOS) was 5 (IQR = 7) days. In the CTA group, LOS was longer compared to the LE group with 9 (IQR = 12.7) versus 5 (IQR = 6.6) days, respectively (P = 0.026). In-hospital mortality rate was 2.7% and concerned 5 patients. 3 patients died of postoperative complications (septic shock, intravascular disseminated coagulopathy, cardiac failure), one patient of multi-organ failure following hemorrhagic shock and one patient presented sudden cardiac arrest. Four out of these 5 deceased patients were examined with CTA first. Twenty-eight patients (15.3%) were referred after initial evaluation in a regional center. The CTA group had the higher proportion of referred patients (34.4%) compared with the LE group (9.8%). Patients' hemodynamics are detailed in

Table 1 Patient characteristics

	All patients (n = 183)	CTA (n = 32)	LE (n = 122)	P
Age, median (range)	75 (21–99)	68 (21–94)	77 (33–99)	**0.004**
Male, n (%)	109 (59.6)	19 (59.4)	71 (58.2)	*0.909*
Hb (g/L), Mean ± SD	110 ± 27	102 ± 30	112 ± 24	*0.090*
MAP (mmHg), Mean ± SD	93 ± 18	85 ± 18	95 ± 16	**0.006**
HR, Mean ± SD	83 ± 16	82 ± 15	83 ± 16	*0.881*
SI, Mean ± SD	0.66 ± 0.22	0.72 ± 0.27	0.63 ± 0.18	*0.082*
Diagnostic, n (%)				
Diverticular	48 (26.2)	9 (28.1)	38 (31.1)	*0.741*
Unknown location	41 (22.4)	5 (15.6)	21 (17.2)	*0.831*
Colo-rectal lesion	34 (18.6)	5 (15.6)	27 (22.1)	*0.419*
Post-interventional	23 (12.6)	2 (6.2)	17 (13.9)	*0.239*
Small bowel	20 (10.9)	11 (34.4)	4 (3.3)	**<0.001**
Colo-rectal neoplasia	17 (9.3)	0 (0)	15 (12.3)	**0.037**

Comparison of baseline characteristics of patients who had CTA and patients who had LE. Significant P-values (<0.05) are indicated in bold characters. SI is defined as HR/Systolic blood pressure

CTA Computed tomographic angiography, *LE* Lower endoscopy, *Hb* Hemoglobin level, *MAP* Mean arterial pressure, *HR* Heart rate, *SI* Shock index

Table 1. MAP was significantly lower in the CTA group, compared with the LE group with 85 ± 18 versus 95 ± 16 mmHg, respectively (P = 0.006). Patients in the CTA group had similar Hb levels at admission compared with the LE group (102 ± 30 versus 112 ± 24 g/L, respectively; P = 0.09). SI was also similar in patients in the CTA group,

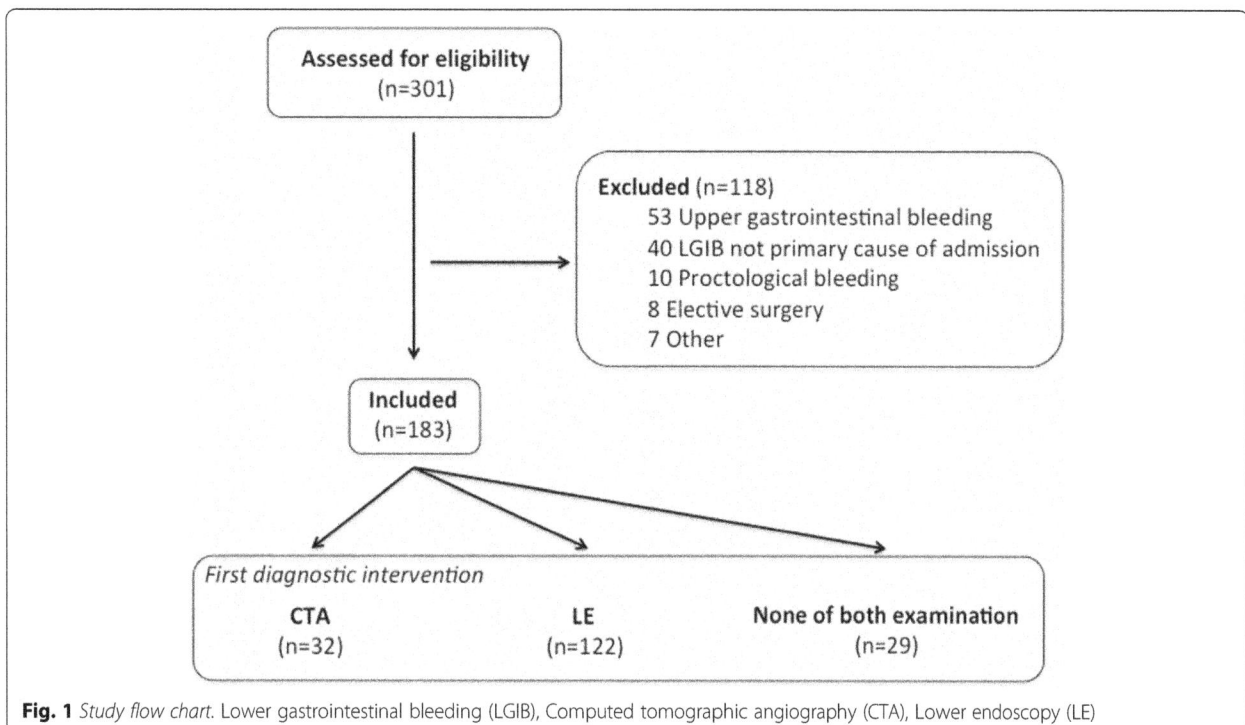

Fig. 1 *Study flow chart.* Lower gastrointestinal bleeding (LGIB), Computed tomographic angiography (CTA), Lower endoscopy (LE)

with 0.72 ± 0.27 versus 0.63 ± 0.18 in those of LE group ($P = 0.082$). No significant difference was observed in the comparison of HR at admission in both groups (Table 1).

Radiological and endoscopic findings

In the first 3 years of the study period, LE was the predominating diagnostic tool, while CTA gained of importance in the second part of the study period only (Fig. 2).

Following hospital admission, CTA was performed significantly earlier than colonoscopy, after a median of 3 (IQR = 8.2) versus 22 (IQR = 36.9) hours ($P < 0.001$).

Active bleeding was found significantly more frequently with CTA compared to LE (31.3 vs. 14.8%, $P = 0.031$). A non-active bleeding source was identified in 21.8 vs. 31.1% by CTA and LE, respectively ($P = 0.305$). The rate of inconclusive exams was similar in both groups (46,9 vs. 54.1%, $P = 0.396$).

Patients presenting post-interventional bleeding were mostly evaluated by LE first, and rarely by CTA first (73.9 vs. 8.7%, respectively). Patients with small bowel bleeding underwent predominantly CTA first (55%) compared to LE first (20%), this difference was statistically significant ($P < 0.001$).

Bleeding control

The control of bleeding was achieved by conservative measures in 120 (65.6%) patients, by endoscopic intervention in 34 (18.6%), by surgery in 26 (14.2%) and by embolization in 3 patients (1.6%), respectively. There were no differences in the rate of conservatively managed patients in the CTA group compared to the LE group (56.3 vs. 61.5%, $P = 0.591$). A summary of the final bleeding control according to the first exam used is

shown in Fig. 3. Active bleeding on CTA was found in 10 patients and surgery was needed for the final control of the bleeding in 80% of cases, whereas the remaining 20% of patients were treated conservatively. After positive CTA for these 10 patients, 4 underwent surgery directly, 3 LE and 3 angiography. All 3 LE were inconclusive because of impaired vision due to blood clots, and only 1 out of 3 angiographies was positive allowing embolization in one single patient who eventually needed surgery for re-bleeding. In all these cases except for one, the bleeding localization was confirmed by the pathology report. Patients presenting post-interventional bleeding were primarily controlled by LE in 57%. Patients with small bowel bleeding needed more often surgery (35%) compared with other pathologies (Fig. 4). Of the 29 patients with no exam during hospital stay, 27 patients had conservative treatment and 2 underwent immediate invasive treatment due to hemodynamic instability. Embolization was performed for 1 patient and 1 patient underwent surgery directly. The remaining 27 patients were not further examined because of clinically minor bleeding, with spontaneous resolution.

Discussion

The results of this study suggest that CTA may be a good choice in most patients with LGIB despite the fact that LE was the most used modality in our series and remains best choice for post-interventional bleeding. CTA was quickly available, reliable to indentify the bleeding source and helpful to guide further management.

In the group of patients assessed by CTA first, a significantly greater rate of active bleeding was observed compared to patients examined with LE first (31.3 vs. 14.8%, respectively, $P = 0.031$). While the shorter waiting

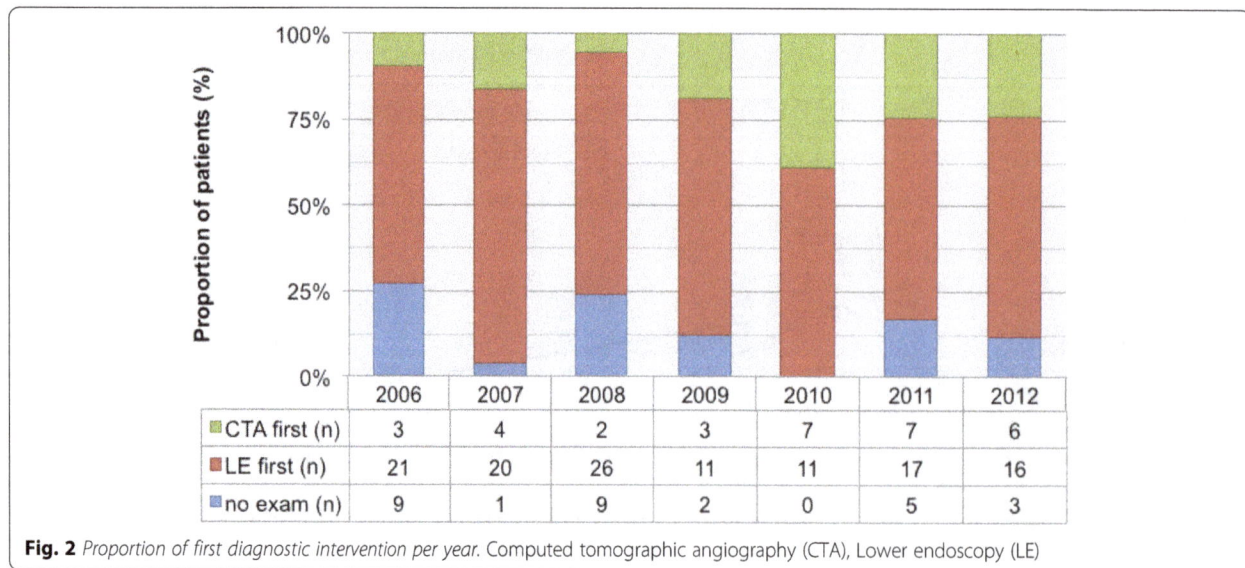

	2006	2007	2008	2009	2010	2011	2012
CTA first (n)	3	4	2	3	7	7	6
LE first (n)	21	20	26	11	11	17	16
no exam (n)	9	1	9	2	0	5	3

Fig. 2 *Proportion of first diagnostic intervention per year.* Computed tomographic angiography (CTA), Lower endoscopy (LE)

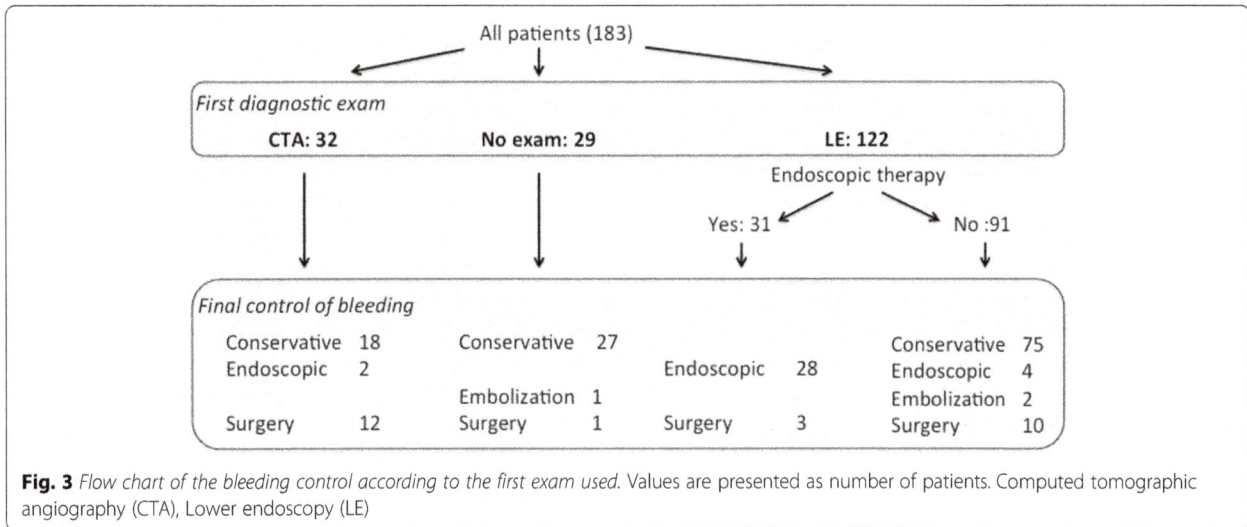

Fig. 3 *Flow chart of the bleeding control according to the first exam used.* Values are presented as number of patients. Computed tomographic angiography (CTA), Lower endoscopy (LE)

time in the CTA group very likely increased the chance to identify actively bleeding lesions, the delay taken to perform LE increased the chance for spontaneous bleeding cessation. Delay in performing LE is explained by prior bowel preparation and limited gastroenterology consultant availability out of office hours. Nonetheless, about half of the exams were inconclusive in both groups, without significant difference. In a study including 115 patients with LGIB who underwent CTA, Chan & al. found that 77% of patients with negative studies did not need further intervention. In 68% of cases the exam did not show features of active bleeding, which is consistent with the present findings [7].

In the literature, the optimal time point of colonoscopy for LGIB remains controversial. In a retrospective analysis, Strate & al. revealed that shorter time to colonoscopy was an independent predictor of shorter LOS, particularly if colonoscopies were performed within 12–24 h [8]. A further trial confirmed that the source of bleeding was more frequently found with urgent colonoscopy (within 8 h) compared to elective colonoscopy (within 4 days) [9]. On the other hand, in a randomized trial comparing colonoscopies performed within 12 h of presentation to those executed within 36–60 h, the authors did not show differences in clinical outcomes. However non-diagnostic colonoscopies were more common in the elective group [10].

In this series, 65.6% of patients had spontaneous cessation of bleeding regardless of the first diagnostic exam chosen. This suggests that most patients presenting with LGIB can be managed conservatively. In the literature, self-limiting LGIB rates of up to 80% have been reported, especially in case of diverticular bleeding [4, 11, 12].

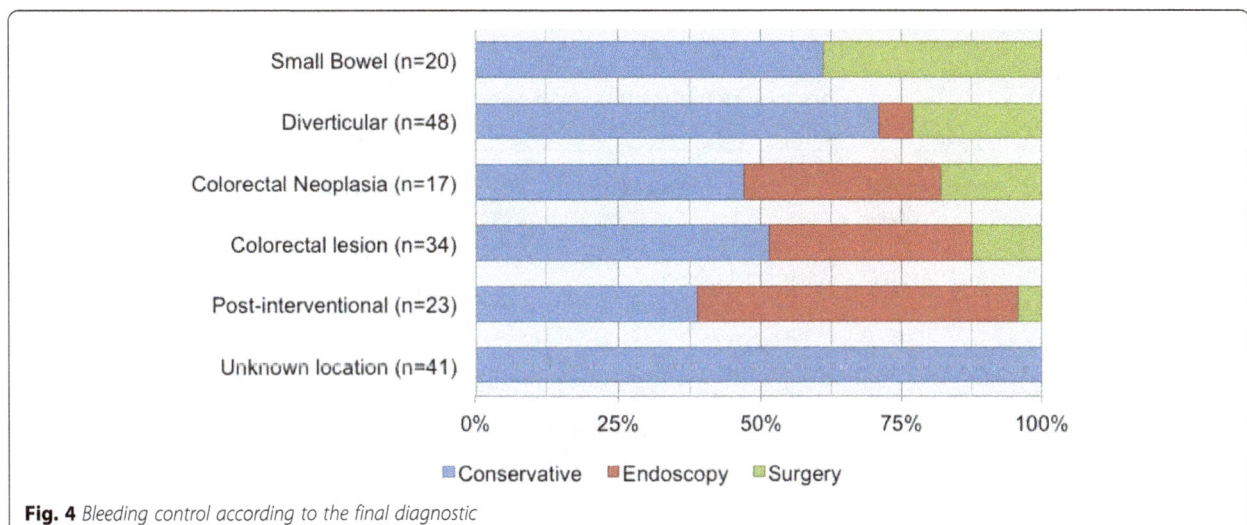

Fig. 4 *Bleeding control according to the final diagnostic*

Surgery was required in 14% of patients in this serie which is similar to the published range of 2.6 to 18% [8, 9, 13, 14]. In-hospital mortality was 2.7% in the present study. Previously published mortality rates ranged from 2.4 to 8.8%, [3, 8, 13, 15].

The present results suggest that most patients with post-interventional bleeding were effectively treated with colonoscopy. In this sub-group of patients, examination with CTA was not necessary, and patients should directly undergo early colonoscopy to confirm diagnosis and deliver treatment at the same time. In the literature, several authors reported successful endoscopic management of post-polypectomy bleeding for most patients [16–18]. In the present series, 80% of patients with active bleeding on CTA required surgery for bleeding control. This is in line with Chan & al. reporting about 90% of patients with LGIB and positive CTA needing intervention for bleeding control. However, surgery was performed in 24% of cases whereas embolization was successful in 64% of patients [7]. In a study from Nagata & al., early colonoscopy following CTA resulted in a higher detection rate of colonic vascular lesions than colonoscopy alone [19]. These results contrast the present findings were all 3 LE performed after positive CTA were negative due to impaired visualization. Koh & al. suggested that angiography should be performed as soon as possible after positive CTA to allow embolization [20]. In their series, angiography was performed only after CTA with signs of active bleeding and about half of them were negative. In the present study, only 3 patients underwent angiography after positive CTA, 2 of them were negative and one patient underwent embolization first, followed by salvage surgery because of early re-bleeding.

Based on these findings, our own institutional algorithm for the management of LGIB was adapted (Fig. 5). For post-interventional bleeding, urgent LE is advocated.

Patients presenting with minor bleeding can be observed and prepared for elective colonoscopy within 24 h. Patients presenting with more significant bleeding should undergo CTA as first-line procedure. It is hypothesized that this algorithm may help to decrease time to diagnosis and guide successful treatment. In published practice guidelines algorithms, radionuclide red blood cell scan followed by mesenteric angiography is indicated for patients unfit for colonoscopy or those with failed endoscopic therapy, but use of CTA is not included [1, 4]. Other authors have integrated CTA in their management algorithm. Copland & al. proposed, for clinically active bleeding, CTA as first-line procedure after exclusion of UGIB with nasogastric lavage. Colonoscopy is then performed if CTA localized the bleeding [21]. Another report proposed an algorithm including CTA for all patients with LGIB [22]. Chan & al. proposed a management pathway including CTA after negative endoscopic evaluation [7]. The fact that so much various algorithms are proposed suggests that further research is needed.

This study has several limitations besides its retrospective design and a limited number of patients. Within the study period, there was a change in care providers and hence in practice. Furthermore, the choice of the first diagnostic exam was decided by the treating physician. Significant lower MAP and trends to lower Hb level and higher SI indicate a selection bias as the severely affected patients were more likely to undergo CTA first. Longer LOS in the CTA group also probably reflects the greater severity of the bleeding. Patients' comorbidites, medication, medical or surgical history also probably led to a selection bias in the choice of the first exam. The retrospective nature of the study precluded us to ensure a valid comparison. We could not account for the delay in performing LE during the night, as the gastroenterology consultant's availability was lower outside office hours.

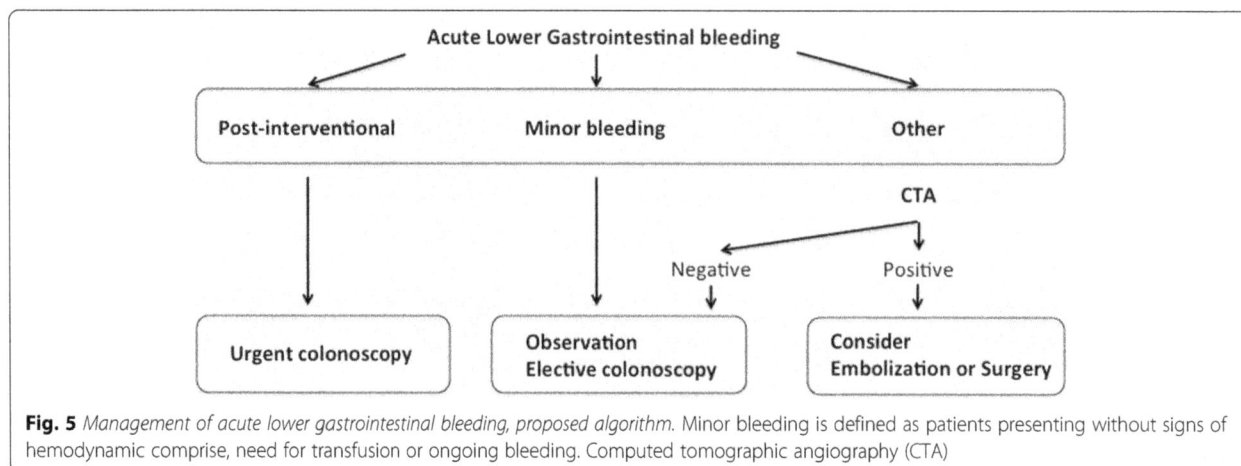

Fig. 5 *Management of acute lower gastrointestinal bleeding, proposed algorithm.* Minor bleeding is defined as patients presenting without signs of hemodynamic comprise, need for transfusion or ongoing bleeding. Computed tomographic angiography (CTA)

Conclusion

In conclusion, our analysis describes current practice of management for LGIB in a "real-world" setting in order to propose a new treatment algorithm that needs to be evaluated prospectively. The present study suggests that CTA is an efficient and readily available tool to manage patients with LGIB. CTA could be considered a suitable first diagnostic option for acute LGIB except for post-interventional bleeding which should entail immediate LE. However, most patients with LGIB can be treated conservatively.

Acknowledgements
Not applicable.

Funding
Not applicable.

Authors' contributions
DC: design, analysis and interpretation, drafting/FG: analysis and interpretation, critical revision/MS: design, interpretation, critical revision/AD: design, interpretation, critical revision/ND: conception, interpretation, critical revision/ MH: conception and design, analysis and interpretation, drafting/All authors approved the final version.

Competing interests
The authors declare that they have no competing interests.

Author details
[1]Department of Visceral Surgery, University Hospital of Lausanne (CHUV), Lausanne, Switzerland. [2]Department of Interventional Radiology, University Hospital of Lausanne (CHUV), Lausanne, Switzerland.

References
1. ASGE Standards of Practice Committee, Pasha SF, Shergill A, Acosta RD, Chandrasekhara V, Chathadi KV, Early D, Evans JA, Fisher D, Fonkalsrud L, Hwang JH, Khashab MA, Lightdale JR, Muthusamy VR, Saltzman JR, Cash BD. The role of endoscopy in the patient with lower GI bleeding. Gastrointest Endosc. 2014;79(6):875–85. doi:10.1016/j.gie.2013.10.039. Epub 2014 Apr 2.
2. Strate LL. Lower GI, bleeding: epidemiology and diagnosis. Gastroenterol Clin North Am. 2005;34(4):643–64. Review.
3. Lanas A, García-Rodríguez LA, Polo-Tomás M, Ponce M, Alonso-Abreu I, Perez-Aisa MA, Perez-Gisbert J, Bujanda L, Castro M, Muñoz M, Rodrigo L, Calvet X, Del-Pino D, Garcia S. Time trends and impact of upper and lower gastrointestinal bleeding and perforation in clinical practice. Am J Gastroenterol. 2009;104(7):1633–41. doi:10.1038/ajg.2009.164. Epub 2009 May 5.
4. Zuccaro Jr G. Management of the adult patient with acute lower gastrointestinal bleeding. American College of Gastroenterology. Practice Parameters Committee. Am J Gastroenterol. 1998;93(8):1202–8.
5. Chua AE, Ridley LJ. Diagnostic accuracy of CT angiography in acute gastrointestinal bleeding. J Med Imaging Radiat Oncol. 2008;52(4):333–8. doi:10.1111/j.1440-1673.2008.01964.x.
6. Geffroy Y, Rodallec MH, Boulay-Coletta I, Jullès MC, Ridereau-Zins C, Zins M. Multidetector CT angiography in acute gastrointestinal bleeding: why, when, and how. Radiographics. 2011;31(3):E35–46. Review. Erratum in: Radiographics. 2011 Sep-Oct;31(5):1496. Radiographics. 2011 Nov-Dec;31(7): 2114. Fullès, Marie-Christine [corrected to Jullès, Marie-Christine].
7. Chan V, Tse D, Dixon S, Shrivastava V, Bratby M, Anthony S, Patel R, Tapping C, Uberoi R. Outcome following a negative CT Angiogram for gastrointestinal hemorrhage. Cardiovasc Intervent Radiol. 2015;38(2):329–35. doi:10.1007/s00270-014-0928-8. Epub 2014 Jul 15.
8. Strate LL, Syngal S. Timing of colonoscopy: impact on length of hospital stay in patients with acute lower intestinal bleeding. Am J Gastroenterol. 2003;98(2):317–22.
9. Green BT, Rockey DC, Portwood G, Tarnasky PR, Guarisco S, Branch MS, Leung J, Jowell P. Urgent colonoscopy for evaluation and management of acute lower gastrointestinal hemorrhage: a randomized controlled trial. Am J Gastroenterol. 2005;100(11):2395–402.
10. Laine L, Shah A. Randomized trial of urgent vs. elective colonoscopy in patients hospitalized with lower GI bleeding. Am J Gastroenterol. 2010; 105(12):2636–41. doi:10.1038/ajg.2010.277. quiz 2642. Epub 2010 Jul 20.
11. Barnert J, Messmann H. Diagnosis and management of lower gastrointestinal bleeding. Nat Rev Gastroenterol Hepatol. 2009;6(11):637–46. doi:10.1038/nrgastro.2009.167. Review.
12. Farrell JJ, Friedman LS. Review article: the management of lower gastrointestinal bleeding. Aliment Pharmacol Ther. 2005;21(11):1281–98. Review.
13. Strate LL, Saltzman JR, Ookubo R, Mutinga ML, Syngal S. Validation of a clinical prediction rule for severe acute lower intestinal bleeding. Am J Gastroenterol. 2005;100(8):1821–7.
14. Jacovides CL, Nadolski G, Allen SR, Martin ND, Holena DN, Reilly PM, Trerotola S, Braslow BM, Kaplan LJ, Pascual JL. Arteriography for lower gastrointestinal hemorrhage: role of preceding abdominal computed tomographic angiogram in diagnosis and localization. JAMA Surg. 2015; 150(7):650–6. doi:10.1001/jamasurg.2015.97.
15. Strate LL, Ayanian JZ, Kotler G, Syngal S. Risk factors for mortality in lower intestinal bleeding. Clin Gastroenterol Hepatol. 2008 Sep;6(9):1004–10; quiz 955-. doi: 10.1016/j.cgh.2008.03.021. Epub 2008 Jun 16.
16. Parra-Blanco A, Kaminaga N, Kojima T, Endo Y, Uragami N, Okawa N, Hattori T, Takahashi H, Fujita R. Hemoclipping for postpolypectomy and postbiopsy colonic bleeding. Gastrointest Endosc. 2000;51(1):37–41.
17. Sorbi D, Norton I, Conio M, Balm R, Zinsmeister A, Gostout CJ. Postpolypectomy lower GI bleeding: descriptive analysis. Gastrointest Endosc. 2000;51(6):690–6.
18. ASGE Standards of Practice Committee, Fisher DA, Maple JT, Ben-Menachem T, Cash BD, Decker GA, Early DS, Evans JA, Fanelli RD, Fukami N, Hwang JH, Jain R, Jue TL, Khan KM, Malpas PM, Sharaf RN, Shergill AK, Dominitz JA. Complications of colonoscopy. Gastrointest Endosc. 2011;74(4): 745–52. doi:10.1016/j.gie.2011.07.025.
19. Nagata N, Niikura R, Aoki T, Moriyasu S, Sakurai T, Shimbo T, Shinozaki M, Sekine K, Okubo H, Watanabe K, Yokoi C, Yanase M, Akiyama J, Uemura N. Role of urgent contrast-enhanced multidetector computed tomography for acute lower gastrointestinal bleeding in patients undergoing early colonoscopy. J Gastroenterol. 2015;50(12):1162–72. doi:10.1007/s00535-015-1069-9. Epub 2015 Mar 27.
20. Koh FH, Soong J, Lieske B, Cheong WK, Tan KK. Does the timing of an invasive mesenteric angiography following a positive CT mesenteric angiography make a difference? Int J Colorectal Dis. 2015;30(1):57–61. doi:10.1007/s00384-014-2055-z. Epub 2014 Nov 4.
21. Copland A, Munroe CA, Friedland S, Triadafilopoulos G. Integrating urgent multidetector CT scanning in the diagnostic algorithm of active lower GI bleeding. Gastrointest Endosc. 2010;72(2):402–5. doi:10.1016/j.gie.2010.04. 014. Review.
22. Sabharwal R, Vladica P, Chou R, Law WP. Helical CT in the diagnosis of acute lower gastrointestinal haemorrhage. Eur J Radiol. 2006;58(2):273–9. Epub 2006 Jan 18.

31

Nonoperative management of appendiceal phlegmon or abscess in children less than 3 years of age

Hailan Zhang*, Yuzuo Bai and Weilin Wang

Abstract

Background: In children less than 3 years of age, there is little experience in the nonoperative management of appendiceal phlegmon or abscess (APA), especially in APA with an appendicolith. The purposes of this study were to evaluate the effects of an appendicolith and the success rate of nonoperative management for APA in these young children.

Methods: Children younger than 3 years of age with APA who underwent attempted initial nonoperative treatment between January 2008 and December 2016 were reviewed. Based on the presence or absence of an appendicolith on admission ultrasonography examination or computed tomography scan, children were divided into two groups: appendicolith group and no appendicolith group.

Results: There were 50 children who met the study criteria. Among 50 children, three children failed to respond to nonoperative treatment because of aggravated intestinal obstruction or recurrent appendicitis within 30 days of admission. The overall success rate for nonoperative management of APA was 94% (47/50) in children younger than 3 years old. The rate of diarrhea and CRP levels were higher in the appendicolith group than that of the no appendicolith group ($P < 0.05$). However, the success rate and the hospital length of stay for nonoperative treatment in the appendicolith group and the no appendicolith group were similar without statistical significance.

Conclusion: APA with or without an appendicolith can have nonoperative management without immediate appendectomy in children less than 3 years old.

Keywords: Appendiceal phlegmon, Appendiceal abscess, Nonoperative treatment, Children, Appendicolith

Background

Acute appendicitis is the most common surgical emergency in children [1]. In young children less than 3 years of age, however, the incidence of appendicitis is low (approximately 2.3% of all children with acute appendicitis); thus, appendicitis in this age group is easily missed by pediatricians [2]. Furthermore, in young children, the clinical symptoms and physical signs of appendicitis are atypical and frequently overlap with other common gastrointestinal diseases. Therefore, delayed diagnosis and a higher perforation rate occur more often [3–5]. The appendiceal phlegmon or abscess (APA) at presentation occurs in

about 33 to 50% in this young age group [6, 7]. The optimal management of APA is controversial, especially in APA with an appendicolith. The debates predominantly focus on the effects of an appendicolith and the success rate of nonoperative treatment. Some surgeons preferred immediate operation for APA [8], whereas some researches supported nonsurgical management with antibiotics because appendectomy could be technically difficult and complication rates rose [9–12]. The presence of an appendicolith might predict failure of nonoperative treatment of APA, and immediate appendectomy may be a better choice [13]. Some studies found no correlation between clinical outcomes and the presence of an appendicolith [14]. Current studies mainly focused on adults and older children; however, little experience exists with the

* Correspondence: hailanzhang2008@sina.com
Department of Pediatric Surgery, Shengjing Hospital of China Medical University, No. 36 SanHao St., Heping District, Shenyang 110004, China

nonoperative treatment of APA during the first 3 years of life. The purposes of this retrospective study were to evaluate the appendicolith effects and the success rate of nonoperative management for APA in children under 3 years old.

Methods

Patients

The medical records of all pediatric patients (< 3 years of age) with APA who underwent attempted initial nonoperative treatment between January 2008 and December 2016 were reviewed. There were no signs of generalized peritonitis or apparent intestinal obstruction among the patients. The data collected included the patient's characteristics, duration of symptoms, common symptoms (e.g., pain, fever, vomiting, and diarrhea), physical examinations (e.g., mass, tenderness, rebound, and rigidity), white blood cell (WBC) counts, C-reactive protein (CRP) levels, antibiotics administered, length of stay (LOS), ultrasonography (US) findings, and computed tomography (CT) scan findings.

Treatment failure with nonoperative management was defined as unsuccessful in case of an appendectomy during the initial hospitalization or a subsequent readmission within 30 days of admission. Periappendiceal abscesses were not generally drained unless the condition of children did not improve or abscesses gradually increased. The non-surgically treated children were given intravenous, broad-spectrum antibiotics such as cefoperazone and sulbactam sodium and ceftriaxone and tazobactam sodium. The therapy was continued for at least 5 days. When the patients improved, US or CT was repeated. If regression of appendiceal inflammation was noted on US or CT and the children remained afebrile, physical signs improved, and the WBC counts and CRP levels decreased; the children were discharged home with oral broad-spectrum antibiotics such as cefdinir and cefaclor.

Statistical analysis

Data were presented as mean ± standard deviation. Statistical evaluation of data was performed by independent-samples t test and chi-square test (Fisher's exact test was used when $T < 5$) depending on data (SPSS 17.0, SPSS, Chicago, IL). A P value of < 0.05 was considered as significant.

Results

Fifty children less than 3 years old underwent attempted initial nonoperative management during the study period. There were 29 boys and 21 girls, with an average age of 24.60 ± 8.49 months (range 5–35 months). The mean duration of symptoms was 8.58 ± 5.49 days. The most common symptoms were fever in 48 patients (96%), abdominal pain in 42 (84%), vomiting in 25 (50%), and diarrhea in 24 (48%). Tenderness was found

in all children; 30 of them (60%) also presented localized peritonitis. The WBC counts and CRP levels were 19.20 ± 6.37 × 10⁹/L and 100.27 ± 74.73 mg/L, respectively. Mean inflammatory areas of APA were 20.08 ± 14.77 cm². Two children underwent US-guided percutaneous drainage. One child with an appendicolith underwent early appendectomy because of aggravated intestinal obstruction, while two children without an appendicolith required subsequent readmission because of recurrent pain within 30 days of admission. They responded to antibiotics with complete resolution clinically and were discharged 5 days later. The hospital LOS was 13.24 ± 5.41 days and the overall success rate for nonoperative management of APA was 94% (47/50).

Among 50 children, 46 (92%) were performed with admission US; 45 (90%) were examined with CT scans. Based on the presence or absence of an appendicolith on admission US or CT imaging, the patients were categorized into two groups: appendicolith group [$n = 27$] and no appendicolith group [$n = 23$]. A summary of patient characteristics is displayed in Table 1. No difference existed between the appendicolith group and the no appendicolith group when comparing age, duration of symptoms, pain, fever, vomiting, localized peritonitis, WBC, and mean inflammatory areas. The rate of diarrhea (63.0 vs. 30.4%) and CRP levels (126.83 ± 83.46 vs. 69.10 ± 48.21) were higher in the appendicolith group than the no appendicolith group ($P < .05$). The overall success rates (96.3 vs. 91.3%) and LOS (14.26 ± 5.55 vs.12.04 ± 5.09) for nonoperative treatment in the appendicolith group and the no appendicolith group were similar without statistical significance.

Table 1 Clinical characteristics between the appendicolith group and no appendicolith group

	Appendicolith ($n = 27$)	No appendicolith ($n = 23$)	P value
Sex (male:female)	15:12	14:9	0.704
Age (months)	25.89 ± 7.47	23.09 ± 9.49	0.249
Duration of symptoms	8.04 ± 4.17	9.22 ± 6.77	0.472
Pain	23 (85.2%)	19 (82.6%)	0.804
Fever	26 (96.3%)	22 (95.7%)	1.000
Vomiting	12 (44.4%)	13 (56.5%)	0.395
Diarrhea	17 (63.0%)	7 (30.4%)	0.022*
Localized peritonitis	19 (70.4%)	11 (47.8%)	0.105
WBC	20.69 ± 6.79	14.44 ± 5.46	0.072
CRP	126.83 ± 83.46	69.10 ± 48.21	0.004*
Inflammatory area (cm²)	21.58 ± 15.15	18.32 ± 14.45	0.442
LOS	14.26 ± 5.55	12.04 ± 5.09	0.151
Overall success	26 (96.3%)	21 (91.3%)	0.588

*$P < 0.05$

Discussion

The peak incidence of acute appendicitis occurs in the second decade of life, while it is uncommon to face appendicitis in children younger than 3 years of age. The incidence is approximately 2.3% of all children with acute appendicitis in this young age group [2]. Inability of a young child to communicate to the parents or clinicians, atypical presentation, and other associated illness may delay the diagnosis. So, perforated appendices could be already present in 60–100% when the diagnosis is performed in young children [3, 15, 16]. Some surgeons preferred immediate operations even if intra- and postoperative complications were higher because the anatomic immaturity and an inadequate omental barrier of young children might lead to diffusion of appendiceal inflammation. However, some studies had reported that the ability to localize intraperitoneal inflammatory processes was well-developed. An appendix mass is discovered at the time of presentation in about 33 to 50% of young children under 3 years of age [6, 7].

Although some reviews report antibiotic therapy is safe and effective [17–20], first-line treatment of acute appendicitis remains to be appendectomy, especially laparoscopic appendectomy [21–23]. The best treatment strategy for APA is very controversial. Immediate appendectomy may be technically demanding because of the distorted anatomy and the difficulties to close the appendiceal stump because of the inflamed tissues. It is rare but it exists that the exploration has to end up in an ileocaecal resection or a right-sided hemicolectomy due to the technical problems or a suspicion of malignancy because of the distorted tissues [8, 24, 25]. So, nonoperative management is suggested because of a good and extensively documented success rate [10, 26]. The disadvantages of nonoperative management are that the actual pathology remains unclear and that appendicitis can "recur" after successful nonsurgical treatment. Many researches indicated the risks of recurrence and undetected serious diseases were very low and supported the nonoperative treatment [10, 26–30]. In 2015, the World Society of Emergency Surgery Jerusalem guidelines also suggested that nonoperative management was a reasonable first-line treatment for APA [12]. Weber and Di Saverio advocated for a clinical approach that is tailored to the individual patient's circumstances and reflective of the situational realities of each patients [31]. However, these researches mainly focus on adults and older children. Little experience exists with the nonoperative treatment of APA in children less than 3 years old.

The success rate for nonoperative treatment of APA was 94% during the first 3 years of life in our review. This is similar to previous researches that the success rate ranged from 84 to 98% in adults and children [10, 26, 32, 33]. The post-operative complications of immediate appendectomy

were obvious higher, and laparoscopic appendectomy occurred significantly less in children younger than 3 years [2, 34–36]. These indicated the nonoperative management of APA is superior to immediate appendectomy in children younger than 3 years of age.

Three children with APA failed to respond to nonoperative treatment. Among them, two patients returned to the hospital and required intravenous antibiotics and an admission of 5 days because of recurrent pain. One child deteriorated during antibiotic therapy and required early appendectomy. The rate of early appendectomy was only 2% during the nonoperative treatment in young children under 3 years old. Our high success rate of nonoperative management might be connected with our nonoperative strategy. Generalized peritonitis or apparent intestinal obstruction was excluded from the nonsurgical treatment of APA. Under these clinical conditions, it was difficult to succeed according to our experiences to treat APA in older children.

An appendicolith, or fecalith, is composed of inspissated fecal material, mucus with entrapped calcium phosphate, and inorganic salts. The appendicolith has long been implicated as an important cause of APA [37]. When an appendicolith was present in APA, it was believed to predict failure of nonsurgical therapy and immediate appendectomy was suggested [13]. However, some researches indicated that APA with an appendicolith can be managed nonoperatively and immediate appendectomy is not necessary in older children [14, 26]. To our knowledge, nonoperative management of APA with an appendicolith has not been systematically reported in children younger than 3 years old.

With respect to the influence of appendicoliths on nonoperative treatment of APA, the rate of diarrhea and CRP levels were higher in the appendicolith group compared to the no appendicolith group; however, these have no influence on the nonoperative treatment outcomes, including the hospital LOS and overall success rate. The nonoperative success rate of the appendicolith group was 96.3%. Hence, APA with an appendicolith can be treated nonoperatively and the presence of an appendicolith does not affect the therapeutic effect in young children less than 3 years of age.

It is allowed to diagnose children appendicitis by CT scan in our country and Simanovsky N et al. had reported non-diagnostic or equivocal US in the evaluation of acute abdominal pain in children younger than 10 years old is probably sufficient to justify the additional CT radiation burden [38]. CT scanning had been done in most young children because the ultrasonic diagnosis was uncertain, little experience existed with the nonoperative treatment of APA, and the effect of an appendicolith on clinical outcomes was unclear. The diagnostic performance of US depends on the technique of the examiners, and it is not always easy to detect the presence or absence of an appendicolith in APA. Now, the use of CT scan had been obviously decreased in our hospital because of higher success rate for nonoperative treatment and no correlation between clinical outcomes and the presence of appendicolith if APA could be diagnosed by US.

This review has some limitations. It was a single-center research. The number of patients was small because of the lower morbidity and the higher pre-operative misdiagnosis. Another limitation was that the data were retrospectively collected. These might have resulted in some degree of bias. Additional prospective trials with a larger number of subjects are needed to validate our conclusions about the optimal management of APA in young children.

Conclusions

The presence of an appendicolith does not affect the nonoperative therapeutic effect of APA in young children. In the absence of generalized peritonitis or apparent intestinal obstruction, APA can be managed nonoperatively without immediate appendectomy in children less than 3 years old.

Acknowledgements
None.

Funding
None.

Authors' contributions
ZHL and BYZ conceived and designed the study, collected data, interpreted data, and prepared for manuscript writing. WWL designed the study and interpreted data. All authors read and approved the final manuscript submission.

Competing interests
The authors declare that they have no competing interests.

References
1. Davenport M. Acute abdominal pain in children. BMJ. 1996;312:498–501.
2. Alloo J, Gerstle T, Shilyansky J, Ein SH. Appendicitis in children less than 3 years of age: a 28-year review. Pediatr Surg Int. 2004;19:777–9.
3. Mallick MS. Appendicitis in pre-school children: a continuing clinical challenge. A retrospective study. Int J Surg. 2008;6:371–3.
4. Nance ML, Adamson WT, Hedrick HL. Appendicitis in the young child: a continuing diagnostic challenge. Pediatr Emerg Care. 2000;16:160–2.
5. Cappendijk VC, Hazebroek FW. The impact of diagnostic delay on the course of acute appendicitis. Arch Dis Child. 2000;83:64–6.
6. Puri P, Boyd E, Guiney EJ, O'Donnell B. Appendix mass in the very young child. J Pediatr Surg. 1981;16:55–7.
7. Puri P, O'Donnell B. Appendicitis in infancy. J Pediatr Surg. 1978;13:173–4.
8. Mentula P, Sammalkorpi H, Leppäniemi A. Laparoscopic surgery or conservative treatment for appendiceal abscess in adults? A randomized controlled trial. Ann Surg. 2015;262:237–42.
9. Roach JP, Partrick DA, Bruny JL, Allshouse MJ, Karrer FM, Ziegler MM. Complicated appendicitis in children: a clear role for drainage and delayed appendectomy. Am J Surg. 2007;194:769–72.
10. Andersson RE, Petzold MG. Nonsurgical treatment of appendiceal abscess or phlegmon: a systematic review and meta-analysis. Ann Surg. 2007;246:741–8.
11. Simillis C, Symeonides P, Shorthouse AJ, Tekkis PP. A meta-analysis comparing conservative treatment versus acute appendectomy for complicated appendicitis (abscess or phlegmon). Surgery 2010;147:818–829.
12. Di Saverio S, Birindelli A, Kelly MD, Catena F, Weber DG, Sartelli M, et al. WSES Jerusalem guidelines for diagnosis and treatment of acute appendicitis. World J Emerg Surg. 2016;11:34.
13. Aprahamian CJ, Barnhart DC, Bledsoe SE, Vaid Y, Harmon CM. Failure in the nonoperative management of pediatric ruptured appendicitis: predictors and consequences. J Pediatr Surg. 2007;42:934–8.
14. Levin T, Whyte C, Borzykowski R, Han B, Blitman N, Harris B. Nonoperative management of perforated appendicitis in children: can CT predict outcome? Pediatr Radiol. 2007;37:251–5.
15. Bansal S, Banever GT, Karrer FM, Partrick DA. Appendicitis in children less than 5 years old: influence of age on presentation and outcome. Am J Surg. 2012;204:1031–5.
16. Nelson DS, Bateman B, Bolte RG. Appendiceal perforation in children diagnosed in a pediatric emergency department. Pediatr Emerg Care. 2000; 16:233–7.
17. Di Saverio S, Sibilio A, Giorgini E, Biscardi A, Villani S, Coccolini F, et al. The NOTA Study (Non Operative Treatment for Acute Appendicitis): prospective study on the efficacy and safety of antibiotics (amoxicillin and clavulanic acid) for treating patients with right lower quadrant abdominal pain and long-term follow-up of conservatively treated suspected appendicitis. Ann Surg. 2014;260:109–17.
18. Svensson JF, Patkova B, Almström M, Naji H, Hall NJ, Eaton S, et al. Nonoperative treatment with antibiotics versus surgery for acute nonperforated appendicitis in children: a pilot randomized controlled trial. Ann Surg. 2015;261:67–71.
19. Gorter RR, van der Lee JH, Cense HA, Kneepkens CM, Wijnen MH, In't Hof KH, et al. Initial antibiotic treatment for acute simple appendicitis in children is safe: short-term results from a multicenter, prospective cohort study. Surgery. 2015;157:916–23.
20. Hansson J, Körner U, Khorram-Manesh A, Solberg A, Lundholm K. Randomized clinical trial of antibiotic therapy versus appendicectomy as primary treatment of acute appendicitis in unselected patients. Br J Surg. 2009;96:473–81.
21. Podda M, Cillara N, Di Saverio S, Lai A, Feroci F, Luridiana G, et al. Antibiotics-first strategy for uncomplicated acute appendicitis in adults is associated with increased rates of peritonitis at surgery. A systematic review with meta-analysis of randomized controlled trials comparing appendectomy and non-operative management with antibiotics. Surgeon. 2017;15:303–14.
22. Di Saverio S, Mandrioli M, Sibilio A, Smerieri N, Lombardi R, Catena F, et al. A cost-effective technique for laparoscopic appendectomy: outcomes and costs of a case-control prospective single-operator study of 112 unselected consecutive cases of complicated acute appendicitis. J Am Coll Surg. 2014; 218:e51–65.
23. Bozkurt MA, Unsal MG, Kapan S, Gonenc M, Dogan M, Kalayci MU, et al. Is laparoscopic appendectomy going to be standard procedure for acute appendicitis; a 5-year single center experience with 1,788 patients. Eur J Trauma Emerg Surg. 2015;41:87–9.
24. Lane JS, Schmit PJ, Chandler CF, Bennion RS, Thompson JE Jr. Ileocecectomy is definitive treatment for advanced appendicitis. Am Surg 2001;67:1117–1122.
25. St Peter SD, Aquayo P, Fraser JD, Keckler SJ, Sharp SW, Leys CM, et al. Initial laparoscopic appendectomy versus initial nonoperative management and interval appendectomy for perforated appendicitis with abscess: a prospective, randomized trial. J Pediatr Surg. 2010;45:236–40.
26. Zhang HL, Bai YZ, Zhou X, Wang WL. Nonoperative management of appendiceal phlegmon or abscess with an appendicolith in children. J Gastrointest Surg. 2013;17:766–70.
27. Willemsen PJ, Hoorntje LE, Eddes EH, Ploeg RJ. The need for interval appendectomy after resolution of an appendiceal mass questioned. Dig Surg. 2002;19:216–20.
28. Tekin A, Kurtoğlu HC, Can I, Oztan S. Routine interval appendectomy is unnecessary after conservative treatment of appendiceal mass. Color Dis. 2008;10:465–8.
29. Puapong D, Lee SL, Haigh PI, Kaminski A, Liu IL, Applebaum H. Routine interval appendectomy in children is not indicated. J Pediatr Surg. 2007;42: 1500–3.

30. Lai HW, Loong CC, Chiu JH, Chau GY, Wu CW, Lui WY. Interval appendectomy after conservative treatment of an appendiceal mass. World J Surg. 2006;30:352–7.

31. Weber DG, Di Saverio S. Letter to the editor: laparoscopic surgery or conservative treatment for appendiceal abscess in adults? Ann Surg. 2017; 266:e58–9.

32. Gillick J, Velayudham M, Puri P. Conservative management of appendix mass in children. Br J Surg. 2001;88:1539–42.

33. Erdoğan D, Karaman I, Narci A, Karaman A, Cavuşoğlu YH, Aslan MK, et al. Comparison of two methods for the management of appendicular mass in children. Pediatr Surg Int. 2005;21:81–3.

34. Chang YT, Lin JY, Huang YS. Appendicitis in children younger than 3 years of age: an 18-year experience. Kaohsiung J Med Sci. 2006;22:432–6.

35. Cheong LH, Emil S. Pediatric laparoscopic appendectomy: a population-based study of trends, associations, and outcomes. J Pediatr Surg. 2014;49: 1714–8.

36. Lee SL, Stark R, Yaghoubian A, Shekherdimian S, Kaji A. Does age affect the outcomes and management of pediatric appendicitis? J Pediatr Surg. 2011; 46:2342–5.

37. Alaedeen DI, Cook M, Chwals WJ. Appendiceal fecalith is associated with early perforation in pediatric patients. J Pediatr Surg. 2008;43:889–92.

38. Simanovsky N, Dola T, Hiller N. Diagnostic value of CT compared to ultrasound in the evaluation of acute abdominal pain in children younger than 10 years old. Emerg Radiol. 2016;23:23–7.

32

Youth traffic-related injuries: a prospective study

Michal Grivna[1], Hani O. Eid[2] and Fikri M. Abu-Zidan[3*]

Abstract

Background: Traffic-related injuries are the most common cause of morbidity and mortality of the youth. Our aim was to study epidemiology, risk factors and outcome of hospitalized youth patients injured in road traffic collisions in order to give recommendations for prevention.

Methods: We prospectively studied all youth (15–24 years) patients having traffic-related injuries who were admitted to Al Ain or Tawam Hospitals, Al Ain City, or who died after arrival to these hospitals during an 18 months period. Demography, location and time of injury, injured body regions, severity, hospital and intensive care unit (ICU) stay and outcome were analyzed.

Results: Three hundred thirty-three patients having a mean age (SD) of 20 years (2.5) were studied. 87% were males and 72% were UAE nationals. Majority of injured patients were drivers or front-seat passengers (70%), followed by back seat passengers (16%), motorcyclists (5%) and pedestrians (4%). Rollover was the most common crash mechanism (35%), followed by front crash (34%). Twenty seven patients (8%) were ejected during the crash, 14 during roll-over, 7 from quadribikes and three during front crash. 20% of the patients were admitted to the ICU. Median Glasgow Coma Scale was 15 (range 3–15), median Injury Severity Score was 5 (range 1–41), and median total hospital stay was 3 days (range 1–73). Nine (3%) patients died.

Conclusions: Young UAE-national males are at a higher risk of being injured at traffic. Rollover crash was frequent with high risk of ejection. Promotion of traffic safety and enforcement of safety legislation is necessary.

Keywords: Youth, RTC, Traffic injury, Traffic safety

Background

Traffic-related injuries are the most common cause of premature morbidity and a leading cause of death among the youth in the Middle-East [1, 2]. These injuries have a high impact on the affected victims, their families and societies [1]. According to the World Health Organization Global Status Report on Road Safety 2015 there are over 1.2 million road traffic deaths worldwide every year [3]. The estimated road traffic death rate in 2013 in the United Arab Emirates (UAE) was 10.9 per 100.000 population [3]. UAE is a fast developing country with a large proportion of young population. It has a growing number of vehicles

(2.7 million in 2013) [3] and an expanding network of highways.

Specific risk factors for road traffic injuries in youth include inexperience, developmental changes with increased emotionality, overestimation of driving skills, increased risk taking, and response to peer pressure [4]. Prevention of road traffic collisions (RTCs), including use of safety belts and creating safe road environment, has been well-studied [5]. However risk factors vary in different settings. Despite legislation and increased enforcement in the UAE, the use of restraints among the youth is still very low [6]. Information on traffic-related injuries requiring hospitalization for this specific age group in our region is highly needed. We aimed to study the epidemiology, risk factors and outcomes of hospitalized road traffic injured youth patients in order to give recommendations for prevention.

* Correspondence: fabuzidan@uaeu.ac.ae

This paper has been presented as a poster in the 12th World Conference on Injury Prevention and Safety Promotion, held on 18–21 September, 2016 in Tampere, Finland and published as an abstract in Injury Prevention 09/2016; 22(Suppl 2):A188.

[3]Department of Surgery, College of Medicine and Health Sciences, UAE University, Al-Ain, United Arab Emirates

Full list of author information is available at the end of the article

Methods

We prospectively studied all youth patients (15–24 year old) who were admitted to Al Ain City's two major trauma centers or who died after arrival to these hospitals following RTCs during the period of April 2006 to October 2007. Al Ain City had about 460,000 inhabitants during study period [7]. Trauma patients were exclusively admitted to Al Ain Hospital and Tawam hospital. Al Ain hospital has 412 beds and provides a wide range of general and specialist clinical services [8], whereas Tawam Hospital is a highly specialized tertiary care center with 468 beds [9].

Patients or their caregivers were interviewed by a full time Research Fellow. We collected data on demography (age, gender, nationality), crash mechanism, place of injury, road user type, position in the vehicle, speed of the vehicle, use of safety equipment, time of the crash, anatomical body part(s) injured, severity, Revised Trauma Score (RTS), Glasgow coma scale (GCS), intensive care unit (ICU) admission, length of hospital stay, and outcome (survival or death).

Injury severity of different regions was calculated manually using The Abbreviated Injury Scale (AIS) of the Abbreviated Injury Scale Handbook [10]. This scale assigns each region a severity ranging from 1-6 (minor = 1, moderate = 2, serious = 3, severe = 4, critical = 5, unsurvivable = 6). The Injury Severity of the patients was assessed using the ISS [11]. The revised trauma score (RTS) was calculated using the systolic blood pressure, pulse rate, respiratory rate and GCS at arrival to the Hospital [12].

Statistics

Nationality was divided into two categories (UAE nationals and non-UAE nationals) because the traffic risks differ between these two groups [6, 13, 14]. Comparison of continuous or ordinal data was performed using the Mann-Whitney U-test for two groups or the Kruskal-Wallis for more than two groups. Fisher's exact test or Pearson Chi square test were used to compare categorical data of two or more independent groups as appropriate. A p value of less than 0.05 was needed to refuse the null hypothesis and accepting significant differences between the groups. Data were analyzed using Statistical Package for the Social Sciences (IBM-SPSS version 21.0, Chicago, Il, USA).

Results

Personal risk factors: gender, age and nationality

There were 333 patients, 290 males (87%). The mean age (SD) was 20 (2.5) years. Majority were UAE nationals (72%). The annual incidence of RTC hospitalizations using census data was estimated to be 279.4 per 100 000 person-years. Higher incidence was among males (411.1) than females (88.4). Although male to female population ratio was 1.5:1, the traffic-related injury ratio in our study was 6.7:1.

Injuries by type of road user and vehicle type

Majority of injured patients were drivers or front-seat passengers (70%), followed by rear seat passengers (16%), motorcyclists (5%), and pedestrians (4%) (Table 1). The percentage of drivers were significantly higher among UAE nationals comapred with non-UAE nationals ($p < 0001$, Fisher's Exact test). In contrast the percentage of rear seat passengers, pedestrians, and bicycle riders were significantly higher among non-UAE nationals comapred with UAE nationals ($p = 0.04$, $p < 0.001$, and $p = 0.006$ consequetivly, Fisher's Exact test) (Table 1).

There was no significant difference in age, GCS, RTS and ISS between vehicle occupants and vulnerable road users (pedestrians, bicyclists, motorcyclists, and quadri-bike users). Mortality among vehicle occupants was 2% compared with 4% in vulnerable road users.

Motorcyclists and cyclists were all males (100%). Table 2 compares those patients who were less than 18 years old

Table 1 Traffic-related youth injury hospitalisations by road user type and nationality, Al Ain, 2006–2007 ($n = 333^*$)

Road user	UAE ($n = 238$)		Non-UAE ($n = 94$)		p-value	Total ($n = 332$)	
	Number	%	N	%		N	%
Vehicle Occupant							
Driver	129	54.2	26	27.7	$P < 0.0001$	155	46.7
Front seat	52	21.8	25	26.6	0.39	77	23.2
Rear seat	31	13	21	22.3	0.044	52	15.7
Vulnerable road user							
Pedestrian	2	0.8	13	13.8	$P < 0.0001$	15	4.5
Cyclist	0	0	4	4.3	0.006	4	1.2
Motorcyclist	13	5.5	4	4.3	0.79	17	5.1
Quadrubike	11	4.6	1	1.1	0.19	12	3.6

p Fisher's Exact test
*Information on road user type was missing in 1 patient
Numbers may not add to 100 due to rounding

Table 2 Demographic and severity variables by age category (<18 and ≥18), Al Ain, 2006–2007, n = 333

	Age <18 years (n = 62)	Age ≥18 years (n = 271)	p-value
Gender (male)	53 (85.5%)	237 (87.5%)	0.68
UAE nationals	49 (79%)	189 (69.7%)	0.16
Type of patient			p < 0.0001
Driver	12 (19.4%)	143 (53%)	
Front seat	18 (29%)	59 (21.8%)	
Back seat passenger	18 (29%)	34 (12.6%)	
Motorcyclist	6 (9.7%)	11 (4.6%)	
Quadrubike user	6 (9.7%)	6 (2.2%)	
Cyclist	0	4 (1.5%)	
Pedestrian	2 (3.2%)	13 (4.8%)	
ICU admission	12 (19.4%)	52 (19.2%)	0.99
Hospital stay (days)	15 (2–69)	3 (1–58)	0.25
Mortality	1 (1.6%)	8 (2.95%)	0.7
GCS	9 (5–15)	15 (3–15)	0.42
RTS	10 (8–12)	12 (7–12)	0.44
ISS	5 (1–41)	5 (1–41)	0.31

Data are presented as number (%) or median (range) as appropriate
p Fisher's Exact test or Mann Whitney test as appropriate, ICU Intensive Care Unit, GCS Glasgow Coma Scale, RTS Revised Trauma Score, ISS Injury Severity Score

and those who were ≥18 years old. Back seat passengers and motorcyclists were significantly higher in those less than 18 years old (p < 0.001, Fisher's Exact test). Twelve drivers (8%) and 6 motorcyclists (35%) were under the licensing age in the UAE (18 years old). There were also 6 (50%) quadrubike users less than 18 years old. Underaged motorcyclists were injured off-road and in the parking or housing areas. Two underaged quadrubike users were injured on highway or street while four were injured off-road.

Fifty three percent (150/285) vehicle occupants were injured in sedan cars, 44% (124/285) in sport utility vehicles (SUVs) and 4% (11/285) in other vehicles. Male drivers were significantly more injured driving SUVs compared with females (70/148 (39%) comapred with 0/6 (0%), p = 0.032, Fisher's Exact test). Females were driving only sedan cars. Sixty six percent (103/155) of drivers were driving alone; 64% (7/11) of drivers who were less then 18 years old were driving alone.

Crash mechanism

Rollover of the vehicle was the most common crash mechanism of injury (35%), followed by front impact collision (34%) (Table 3). Secondary roll-over of the car was in 50% of rear-end, 37% of side and of 18% of front-impact crashes. Twenty seven patients (8%) were ejected during the crash. More UAE nationals were injured in

rollover crashes compared with front or side angle (p = 0.002) (Table 3). Patients in rollover crashes had a longer stay in the hospital compared with front and side angle crashes (p = 0.03) (Table 3).

Speed of the car

The mean (SD) of car speed was 97.2 (35.8) km/hr, 42% were higher than the legal speed limit of 100 km/hr (Fig. 1).

Place and time of injury

Majority of traffic-related injuries occurred on highways and streets (276/333;83%), 7% (24/333) off road, 6% (20/333) around homes in residential areas, and 4% (13/333) in other locations. Thirty three percent (5/15) of pedestrians and 29% (5/17) of motorcyclists were injured in housing areas. Seventy five percent of quadrubike users (9/12) and 24% of motorcyclists (4/17) were injured off road.

Evening (6–12 pm) was the most common time of crashes (34%) and Friday the most common day of crashes (20%) (Fig. 2). Most of injuries occured in the period of May to October.

Safety equipment, distraction, sleep and alcohol

Only 12% (n = 18) of the drivers, and 4% (3) of front seat passengers were restrained. No back seat passenger used a setabelt. Five motorcyclists used a helmet (17%) and two wore protective clothing (7%). No byclist or quadrubike user used a helmet. Eight drivers (5%) were using mobile phones. Seven drivers were sleepy when they crashed (4%). Alcohol use was found only in one patient.

Severity and anatomical location of injuries

There were 66 patients (20%) admitted to the ICU. Median GCS was 15 (range 3–15), median ISS was 5 (range 1–41), median RTS was 12 (range 7–12) and median total hospital stay was 3 days (range 1–73). Nine patients (2.7%) died.

The head was the most common injured region (67%) followed by extremities and chest (Table 4). The highest AIS score was in the chest (mean AIS 2.5) followed by the spine (mean AIS 2.3) (Table 4). Eighty percent of ejected patients sustained a head injury.

Discussion

Youth is the active period of life with major developments affecting adult health [2]. Traffic-related injuries are the most common cause of morbidity and mortality in the youth. In our study, young UAE-national males were at higher risk of being injured in traffic. Rollover crash was common with a high risk of ejection. Restraint use was extremly low in our study population.

The youth male preponderance has been described in many studies [2, 3, 15, 16]. Young male drivers have a

Table 3 Demographic and severity variables by car crash mechanism, Al Ain, 2006–2007 ($n = 333$)

	Car crash mechanism				p-value
	Front	Side angle	Rollover	Other	
	$n = 96$	$n = 57$	$n = 98$	$n = 29$	
Age (years)	20.2 (2.2)	20.7 (2.6)	19.8 (2.3)	18.9 (2.3)	0.006
Gender (male)	84 (87.5%)	45 (78.9%)	87 (88.8%)	27 (93.1%)	0.26
UAE national	69 (71.9%)	35 (61.4%)	85 (86.7%)	19 (65.5%)	0.002
ICU admission	19 (19.8%)	11 (19.3%)	21 (21.4%)	5 (17.2%)	0.28
Hospital stay (days)	2 (1–68)	3 (1–73)	5 (1–58)	2 (1–44)	0.03
Mortality	2 (2.1%)	2 (3.5%)	1 (1%)	1 (3.4%)	0.72
GCS	15 (5–15)	15 (4–15)	15 (3–15)	15 (7–15)	0.1
RTS	12 (9–12)	12 (9–12)	12 (7–12)	12 (10–12)	0.87
ISS	5 (1–45)	5 (1–34)	5 (1–36)	5 (1–41)	0.29

Data are presented as number (%), mean (SD) or median (range) as appropriate

Other mechanisms include back crash or crash with motorcycle or bicycle

p Fisher's Exact test, Pearson chi square, or Kruskall Wallis test as appropriate, *ICU* Intensive Care Unit, *GCS* Glasgow Coma Scale, *RTS* Revised Trauma Score, *ISS* Injury Severity Score

higher collision rate than women [5] and their death rate is double compared with women [17]. In the UAE, young women drive less and usually drive small cars, which are less prone to rollover. During the cognitive development the ability of youth to make safe decisions on the road is not mature [16, 18]. Adolescents are known to seek out risks when driving [4]. They have lower compliance with restraint use in our region [6, 16].

Despite legislation and increased law enforcement, seat belt use remains low in our setting, especially among young UAE nationals [6]. Only 12% of drivers and 4% of front seat passengers were restrained in our study. This poses a serious risk to all vehicle occupants. There is a high risk of severe injury and fatality for unrestrained passengers, especially in front collisions and rollovers [13].

Rollover crash was the most common crash mechanism in our study with 8% of the passengers being ejected. SUV is a very popular vehicle in the UAE, especially among UAE national families, who like to drive in the desert and off-road. These cars tend to roll-over during collision, because they have a higher center of gravity. Ejection rate is high because of the low use of restraints in our community. Quadrubike use by teenagers in our study caused 4% of all crashes, 75% of them sustained a head injury. Head injury was also common among other vulnerable road

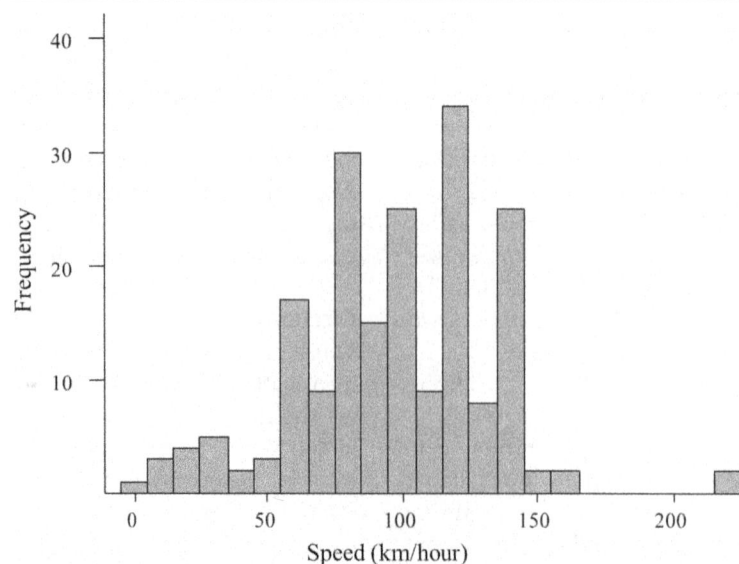

Fig. 1 Distribution of speed of the cars involved in road traffic collision ($n = 196$)

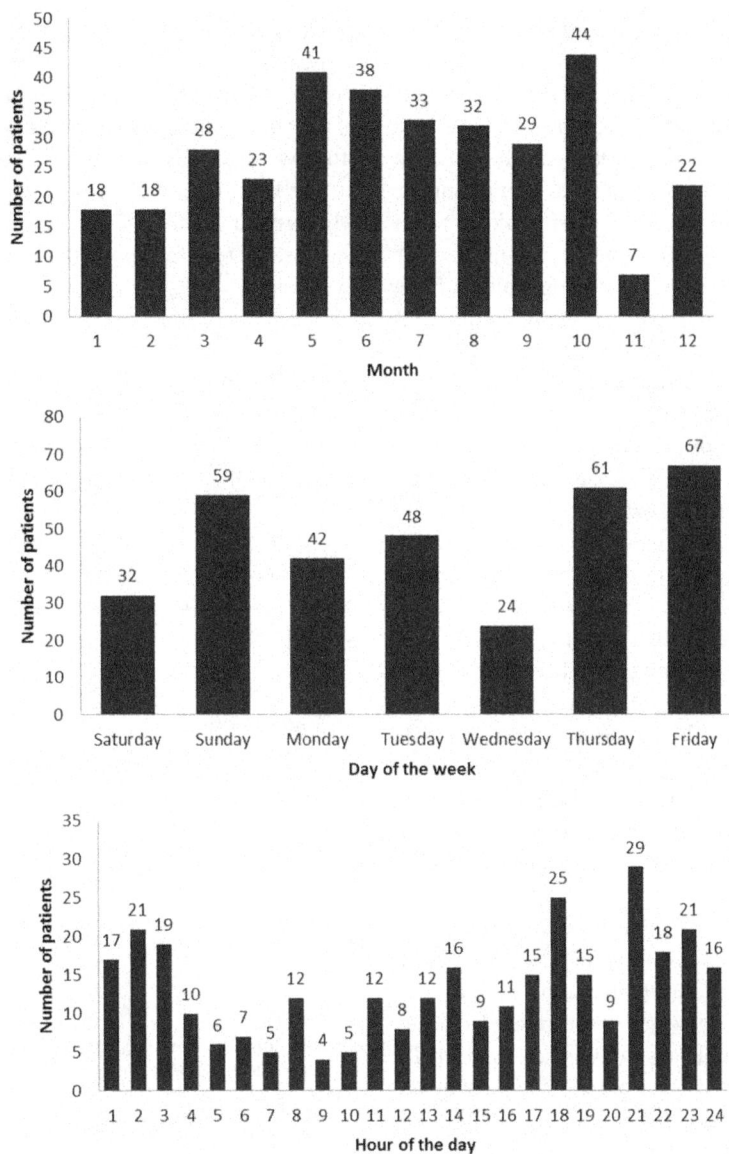

Fig. 2 Distribution of patients by month, day and hour (*n* = 333)

Table 4 Traffic-related youth injury hospitalisations by anatomical region and AIS severity, Al Ain, 2006–2007 (*n* = 333)

Anatomical Region	Number (%)		Injury severity by Maximum AIS*			
			Mean	Median	Min	Max
Head	223	67.0	1.91	2	1	5
Chest	107	32.1	2.50	3	1	5
Abdomen	47	14.1	1.77	1.5	1	4
Spine	43	12.9	2.30	2	2	5
Upper extremity	114	34.2	1.64	2	1	3
Lower extremity	135	40.5	1.79	2	1	3
Superficial	44	13.2	1.02	1	1	2

*Maximum Abbreviated Injury Scale – only the most severe injury per body region was counted for each patient; Some patients have injury in more than one region

users (bicyclists and motorcyclists) who did not use helmets. Bicyclists in our study were only non-UAE nationals. They are usually poor workers using bicycles for their transport. The percentage of pedestrian injuries were also higher among non-UAE nationals comapred with UAE nationals. UAE nationals tend to use the car even for very short distances compared with non-UAE nationals who generally walk to perform their duties.

Distractive driving is a major contributing factor for traffic collisions. US Transportation Department reported that nearly 20% of all crashes involve some distractive driving [19]. Distractive driving causes impairement in driving performance and prolongs reaction time [20]. In our study, 5% of drivers were using mobile phones when they crashed. Despite legislation, use of mobile and smart phones while driving is common in the UAE. Alcohol use in the youth was less than 0.5% in the present study. Overall alcohol use in road traffic injuried patients in our city was 2.1% [21]. This is attributed to legislation, religious believes, and limited accessibility to alcohol.

The age for obtaining driving license in the UAE is 18 years. 8% of injured drivers in our study were younger than this age and 64% of them were driving alone when they crashed. Families ignore the need for a license for short trips and use adolescents for bringing siblings from school and for shopping. A study in Oman found that 33% of students had driven without a license and 34% liked to speed [22]. 35% of motorcycle riders and 50% of quadrubike riders were under 18 years old in our study. Unlicensed driving is a major problem for traffic safety as it often correlates with high-risk behaviors such as speeding, failure to wear a seat belt or motorcycle helmets. Unlicensed drivers were three times more likely to be involved in a collision than licensed drivers [23].

Most of our patients were injured at night (64%). This is possibly contributed to impaired visibility during night and a possibility to drive with high speed because of presence of fewer vehicles. Violation of speed limits is another important contributing factor to RTCs [5]. The traffic design in Al Ain with long roads having 3 lanes between roundabouts allows the youth to speed. Drivers who drive faster or slower than the mean speed of traffic have a higher risk of crash [5].

There was a sharp increase of injuries during the weekend (Thursday and Friday) and in October which was the fasting month of Ramadan during the study period. The Canadian study [24] which assessed the increased crashes during the weekends and holidays, found three main risky behaviors: unsafe speeding, non-use of restraints, and driver intoxication. There is increased risk for traffic collisions during the fasting month of Ramadan, especially in the evenings when tired drivers after a day without food or drinks are rushing home for breaking fast [25, 26]. Sleepeness occured in 4% of drivers involved in road traffic collisions in our city. This risk increased during the fasting month of Ramadan [26].

The police, transportation and the health sectors in the UAE have made active efforts to reduce the burden of RTCs over last decades. This included introduction of new laws and regulations, enforcement of speed limits, improved road design, and educational campaigns [27]. Plans are underway to introduce mandatory seat belts for rear seat passengers and child safety restraints [27].

Limitations of the study

We have to acknowledge that there are certain limitations in our study. We studied only patients who were admitted to the hospital or those who died in the Emergency Department following road traffic collisions. More seriously injured patients may have died before arriving to our hospitals. Furthermore, our study population was from Al Ain City, limiting the generalizability of our results for other parts of the UAE. Finally, our study was a specific time limited research project supported by the UAE University before 2007. It may be questioned whether our results reflect the present situation. We think that risk factors for youth traffic injuries are still the same in our city.

Conclusions

Young UAE-national males are at a higher risk of being injured at traffic. Rollover crashes have high risk of ejection. There is a need for implementation of cultural relevant evidence-based educational programs for all new and existing youth drivers. Promotion of traffic safety and enforcement of safety legislation is neccesary. Distractive and underage driving should be controlled.

Acknowledgments

We would like to thank Faisal Aziz from the Institute of Public Health, College of Medicine and Health Sciences, UAU University for assistance in data analysis and design of tables.

Funding

This study was supported by an Interdisciplinary UAE University grant (No. 02-07-8-1/4).

Authors' contributions

Conceived and designed the experiments: MG HOE FAZ. Retrieved and coded the data: HOE. Analyzed the data: MG HOE FAZ. Wrote the paper: MG FAZ. Critically read the paper: MG HOE FAZ. Approved final version: MG HOE FAZ.

Authors' information

Not applicable.

Competing interests

The authors declare that they have no competing interests.

Author details

[1]Institute of Public Health, College of Medicine and Health Sciences, UAE University, Al-Ain, United Arab Emirates. [2]Department of Surgery, Trauma Group, College of Medicine and Health Sciences, UAE University, Al-Ain, United Arab Emirates. [3]Department of Surgery, College of Medicine and Health Sciences, UAE University, Al-Ain, United Arab Emirates.

References

1. Al-Kharusi W. Update on road traffic crashes: Progress in the Middle East. Clin Orthop Relat Res. 2008;466:2457–64.

2. Makhlouf Obermeyer C. Adolescents in Arab countries: Health statistics and social context. DIFI Family Research and Proceedings 2015:1. http://www.qscience.com/doi/pdf/10.5339/difi.2015.1. Accessed 4 Sep 2016.

3. WHO. Global status report on road safety 2015. Geneva, World Health Organization; 2015. http://www.who.int/violence_injury_prevention/road_safety_status/2015/en/. Accessed 4 Sep 2016.

4. Arnett J. Developmental sources of crash risk in young drivers. Inj Prev. 2002;8(Suppl II):ii17–23.

5. Elvik R, Hoye A, Vaa T, Sorensen M. The handbook of road safety measures. 2nd ed. Bingley, UK: Emerald Group Publishing Limited 64. 2009. p.172-173.

6. Barss P, Al-Obthani M, Al-Hammadi A, Al-Shamsi H, El-Sadig M, Grivna M. Prevalence and issues in non-use of safety belts and child restraints in a high-income developing country: Lessons for the future. Traffic Inj Prev. 2008;9:256–63.

7. Ministry of Health UAE. Annual Report 2008; 2008:4.

8. Al Ain Hospital. 2016. https://www.seha.ae/alain/English/Pages/default.aspx. Accessed 4 Sep 2016.

9. Tawam Hospital. 2016. https://www.seha.ae/tawam/English/Pages/default.aspx. Accessed 4 Sep 2016.

10. Association of the Advancement of Automotive Medicine. Abbreviated Injury Scale. Association for the Advancement of Automotive Medicine, Barrington, IL. 1998

11. Bergeron E, Lavoie A, Moore L, Bamvita JM, Ratte S, Clas D. Paying the price of excluding patients from a trauma registry. J Trauma. 2006;60:300–4.

12. Maurer A, Morris JA Jr. Injury Severity Scoring. In: Moore E, Feliciano D, Mattox K (eds) Trauma (5th ed.), McGraw-Hill Companies, Inc, New York. 2004. p. 87-91.

13. Abu-Zidan FM, Abbas AK, Hefny AF, Eid HO, Grivna M. Effects of seat belt usage on injury pattern and outcome of vehicle occupants after road traffic collisions: prospective study. World J Surg. 2012;36:255–9.

14. Hefny AF, Barss P, Eid HO, Abu-Zidan FM. Motorcycle-related injuries in the United Arab Emirates. Accid Anal Prev. 2012;49:245–8.

15. Mansouri FA, Al-Zalabani AH, Zalat MM. Road safety and road traffic accidents in Saudi Arabia – A systematic review of existing evidence. Saudi Med J. 2015;36:418–24.

16. Sarhan NA. Non-intentional injuries in adolescents and youth: Facts and figures. Bahrain Med Bull. 2012;34:1–7.

17. NHTSA (National Highway Traffic Safety Administration). Traffic Safety Facts 1997. Overview, U.S. Department of Transportation, Washington DC. 1997. Accessed on April 18, 2016 from www-nrd.nhtsa.dot.gov/Pubs/TSF1997.PDF. Accessed 4 Sep 2016.

18. Dunbar G, Hill R, Lewis V. Children's attentional skills and road behaviour. Exp Psychol Appl. 2001;7:227–34.

19. NHTSA (National Highway Traffic Safety Administration). Distracted driving 2009. In Traffic Safety Facts – Research Note. 2010. http://www-nrd.nhtsa.dot.gov/Pubs/811379.pdf. Accessed 4 Sep 2016.

20. WHO. Mobile phone use: a growing problem of driver distraction. Geneva, Switzerland, World Health Organization. 2011. file:///C:/Users/m.grivna/Documents/1UAEU/2Publications/Journals/Youth%20injuries/References/2011%20WHO%20-%20NHTSA%20-%20Mobile%20phone%20use%20-%20A%20growing%20problem%20of%20driver%20distraction.pdf. Accessed 4 Sep 2016.

21. Osman OT, Abbas AK, Eid HO, Salem MO, Abu-Zidan FM. Alcohol-related road traffic injuries in Al-Ain City, United Arab Emirates. Traffic Inj Prev. 2015;16:1–4.

22. Jaffer YA, Afifi M, Al Ajmi F, Alouhaishi K. Knowledge, attitudes and practices of secondary-school pupils in Oman: I. health-compromising behaviours. East Mediterr Health J. 2006;12:35–49.

23. Watson B, Steinhardt D. A comparison of the crash involvement of unlicensed motorcycle riders and unlicensed drivers in Queensland. In Proceedings 2006 Australasian Road Safety Research, Policing, Education Conference, Gold Coast, Quensland. 2006. http://eprints.qut.edu.au/5457/1/5457.pdf Accessed 14 Dec 2016.

24. Anowar S, Yasmin S, Tay R. Comparison of crashes during public holidays and regular weekends. Accid Anal Prev. 2013;51:93–7.

25. Mehmood A, Khan IQ, Mir MU, Moin A, Jooma R. Vulnerable road users are at greater risk during Ramadan – results from road traffic surveillance data. J Pak Med Assoc. 2015;65:287–91.

26. Al-Houqani M, Eid HO, Abu-Zidan FM. Sleep-related collisions in United Arab Emirates. Accid Anal Prev. 2013;50:1052–5.

27. Grivna M, Aw TC, El-Sadeg M, Loney T, Sharif A, Thomsen J, Mauzi M, Abu-Zidan FM. The legal framework and initiatives for promoting safety in the United Arab Emirates. Int J Inj Control Saf Promot. 2012;19:278–89.

Permissions

All chapters in this book were first published in WJES, by BioMed Central; hereby published with permission under the Creative Commons Attribution License or equivalent. Every chapter published in this book has been scrutinized by our experts. Their significance has been extensively debated. The topics covered herein carry significant findings which will fuel the growth of the discipline. They may even be implemented as practical applications or may be referred to as a beginning point for another development.

The contributors of this book come from diverse backgrounds, making this book a truly international effort. This book will bring forth new frontiers with its revolutionizing research information and detailed analysis of the nascent developments around the world.

We would like to thank all the contributing authors for lending their expertise to make the book truly unique. They have played a crucial role in the development of this book. Without their invaluable contributions this book wouldn't have been possible. They have made vital efforts to compile up to date information on the varied aspects of this subject to make this book a valuable addition to the collection of many professionals and students.

This book was conceptualized with the vision of imparting up-to-date information and advanced data in this field. To ensure the same, a matchless editorial board was set up. Every individual on the board went through rigorous rounds of assessment to prove their worth. After which they invested a large part of their time researching and compiling the most relevant data for our readers.

The editorial board has been involved in producing this book since its inception. They have spent rigorous hours researching and exploring the diverse topics which have resulted in the successful publishing of this book. They have passed on their knowledge of decades through this book. To expedite this challenging task, the publisher supported the team at every step. A small team of assistant editors was also appointed to further simplify the editing procedure and attain best results for the readers.

Apart from the editorial board, the designing team has also invested a significant amount of their time in understanding the subject and creating the most relevant covers. They scrutinized every image to scout for the most suitable representation of the subject and create an appropriate cover for the book.

The publishing team has been an ardent support to the editorial, designing and production team. Their endless efforts to recruit the best for this project, has resulted in the accomplishment of this book. They are a veteran in the field of academics and their pool of knowledge is as vast as their experience in printing. Their expertise and guidance has proved useful at every step. Their uncompromising quality standards have made this book an exceptional effort. Their encouragement from time to time has been an inspiration for everyone.

The publisher and the editorial board hope that this book will prove to be a valuable piece of knowledge for researchers, students, practitioners and scholars across the globe.

List of Contributors

Shaoyun Liu, Yuzhi Gao and Mao Zhang
Department of Emergency Medicine, Second Affiliated Hospital, Zhejiang University School of Medicine, No. 88 Jiefang road, Hangzhou 310009, China
Institute of Emergency Medicine, Zhejiang University, No. 88 Jiefang road, Hangzhou 310009, China

Jiefeng Xu
Department of Emergency Medicine, Second Affiliated Hospital, Zhejiang University School of Medicine, No. 88 Jiefang road, Hangzhou 310009, China
Institute of Emergency Medicine, Zhejiang University, No. 88 Jiefang road, Hangzhou 310009, China
Department of Emergency Medicine, Yuyao People's Hospital, Medical School of Ningbo University, Yuyao 315400, China

Peng Shen
Department of Emergency Medicine, Second Affiliated Hospital, Zhejiang University School of Medicine, No. 88 Jiefang road, Hangzhou 310009, China
Institute of Emergency Medicine, Zhejiang University, No. 88 Jiefang road, Hangzhou 310009, China
Department of Emergency Medicine, The First Hospital of Jiaxing/The First Affiliated Hospital of Jiaxing University, Jiaxing 314000, China

Senlin Xia
Department of Emergency Medicine, Second Affiliated Hospital, Zhejiang University School of Medicine, No. 88 Jiefang road, Hangzhou 310009, China
Institute of Emergency Medicine, Zhejiang University, No. 88 Jiefang road, Hangzhou 310009, China
Department of Emergency Medicine, Huzhou Central Hospital, Huzhou 313000, China

Zilong Li
Department of Emergency Medicine, Yuyao People's Hospital, Medical School of Ningbo University, Yuyao 315400, China

Murat Cikot, Kivanc Derya Peker, Mehmet Abdussamet Bozkurt, Ali Kocatas, Osman Kones, Sinan Binboga and Halil Alis
Department of General Surgery, Istanbul Bakirkoy Dr. Sadi Konuk Training and Research Hospital, Zuhuratbaba Mh, Tevfik Saglam Cad. No: 11, 34147 Bakirkoy/Istanbul, Turkey

Asuman Gedikbasi
Department of Biochemistry, Istanbul Bakirkoy Dr. Sadi Konuk Training and Research Hospital, Bakirkoy/Istanbul, Turkey

Belinda De Simone and Fausto Catena
Department of Emergency and Trauma Surgery, University Hospital of Parma, Via Gramsci 11, 43100 Parma, Italy

Federico Coccolini and Luca Ansaloni
Department of General and Emergency Surgery, Papa Giovanni XIII Hospital, Bergamo, Italy

Massimo Sartelli
Department of Surgery, Macerata Hospital, Macerata, Italy

Salomone Di Saverio
Department of Surgery, Maggiore Hospital of Bologna, Bologna, Italy

Rodolfo Catena
Oxford University, Oxford, Great Britain

Antonio Tarasconi
Ospedali Civili di Brescia, Brescia, Italy

Ruben Peralta, Adarsh Vijay, Rafael Consunji, Husham Abdelrahman, Ashok Parchani, Ibrahim Afifi and Hassan Al-Thani
Trauma Surgery Section, Hamad Trauma Center, Hamad General Hospital, Doha, Qatar

Ahmad Zarour
Trauma Surgery Section, Hamad Trauma Center, Hamad General Hospital, Doha, Qatar
Clinical Medicine, Weill Cornell Medical College, Doha, Qatar. 4Department of Surgery, University of Arizona, Tucson, AZ, USA

Rifat Latifi
Trauma Surgery Section, Hamad Trauma Center, Hamad General Hospital, Doha, Qatar
Department of Surgery, University of Arizona, Tucson, AZ, USA

Ayman El-Menyar
Clinical Research, Trauma Surgery Section, Hamad General Hospital, HMC, Doha, Qatar
Clinical Medicine, Weill Cornell Medical College, Doha, Qatar

Kai-Biao Lin
School of Computer and Information Engineering, Xiamen University of Technology, Xiamen 361024, China
Department of Computer Science and Engineering, Yuan Ze University, Taoyuan 32003, Taiwan

K. Robert Lai
Department of Computer Science and Engineering, Yuan Ze University, Taoyuan 32003, Taiwan
Innovation Center for Big Data and Digital Convergence, Yuan Ze University, Taoyuan 32003, Taiwan

Yuan-Hung Liu
Department of Computer Science and Engineering, Yuan Ze University, Taoyuan 32003, Taiwan
Innovation Center for Big Data and Digital Convergence, Yuan Ze University, Taoyuan 32003, Taiwan
Section of Cardiology, Cardiovascular Center, Far Eastern Memorial Hospital, New Taipei City, Taiwan

Nan-Ping Yang
Management Center, Keelung Hospital, Ministry of Health and Welfare, Keelung 20147, Taiwan
Institute of Public Health, National Yang-Ming University, Taipei 11221, Taiwan

Chien-Lung Chan
Department of Information Management, Yuan Ze University, Taoyuan 32003, Taiwan
Innovation Center for Big Data and Digital Convergence, Yuan Ze University, Taoyuan 32003, Taiwan

Ren-Hao Pan
Innovation Center for Big Data and Digital Convergence, Yuan Ze University, Taoyuan 32003, Taiwan

Chien-Hsun Huang
Department of Obstetrics and Gynecology, Taoyuan General Hospital, Ministry of Health and Welfare, Taoyuan, Taiwan

Kyoung Hoon Lim
Department of Surgery, Kyungpook National University Hospital, School of Medicine, Kyungpook National University, 50, Samduk-dong 2ga, Jung-gu, Daegu, South Korea
Andong General Hospital, Department of Surgery, Andong, South Korea

Bong Soo Chung, Jong Yeol Kim and Sung Soo Kim
Andong General Hospital, Department of Surgery, Andong, South Korea

Fu-Yuan Shih, Hsin-Huan Chang, Hung-Chen Wang, Tsung-Han Lee, Yu-Jun Lin, Wu-Fu Chen and Jih-Tsun Ho
Departments of Neurosurgery, Chang Gung University College of Medicine, Kaohsiung, Taiwan

Cheng-Hsien Lu
Departments of Neurology, Chang Gung University College of Medicine, Kaohsiung, Taiwan

Wei-Che Lin
Departments of Radiology, Kaohsiung Chang Gung Memorial Hospital and Chang Gung University College of Medicine, Kaohsiung, Taiwan

Krstina Doklestić, Branislav Stefanović, Pavle Gregorić, Nenad Ivančević, Zlatibor Lončar, Vasilije Jeremić and Aleksandar Karamarković
Faculty of Medicine, University of Belgrade and Clinical Center of Serbia, Clinic for Emergency Surgery, University of Belgrade, Serbia, Pasteur Str

Bojan Jovanović, Vesna Bumbaširević and Branislava Stefanović
Belgrade 11000, Serbia. 2Faculty of Medicine, University of Belgrade and Clinical Center of Serbia, Department for Anesthesiology, University of Belgrade, Serbia, Belgrade, Serbia.

Sanja Tomanović Vujadinović
Faculty of Medicine, University of Belgrade and Clinical Center of Serbia, Clinic for Physical and Rehabilitation Medicine, Clinical Center of Serbia, Belgrade, Serbia

Nataša Milić
Faculty of Medicine and Institute for Medical Statistics and Informatics, University of Belgrade, Belgrade, Serbia

Hidefumi Sano, Junya Tsurukiri, Akira Hoshiai, Taishi Oomura and Yosuke Tanaka
Emergency and Critical Care Medicine, Tokyo Medical University Hachioji Medical Center, 1163 Tatemachi, Hachioji, Tokyo 193-0998, Japan

Shoichi Ohta
Emergency and Disaster Medicine, Tokyo Medical University, 6-7-1 Nishi-shinjuku, Shinjuku, Tokyo 160-0023, Japan

Nurettin Ay
Diyarbakır Gazi Yaşargil Education and Research Hospital, Transplantation Center, Diyarbakır, Turkey

Vahhaç Alp
Department of General Surgery, Diyarbakir Gazi Yaşargil Education and Research Hospital, Diyarbakır, Turkey

İbrahim Aliosmanoğlu
Department of General Surgery, Akdeniz University Hospital, Antalya, Turkey

Utkan Sevük
Department of Cardiovascular Surgery, Diyarbakır Gazi Yaşargil Education and Research Hospital, Diyarbakır, Turkey

Şafak Kaya
Department of İnfectious Disease, Diyarbakır Gazi Yaşargil Education and Research Hospital, Diyarbakır, Turkey

Bülent Dinç
Atatürk State Hospital, Antalya, Turkey

Phillipo L Chalya and Joseph B Mabula
Department of Surgery, Catholic University of Health and Allied Science-Bugando, Mwanza, Tanzania

Sander F.L.van Stigt and Edward C.T. H.Tan
Department of Surgery, Traumasurgery Radboud University Medical Center, Geert Grooteplein-Zuid 10, 6525 GA Nijmegen, The Netherlands

Janneke de Vries
Department of Medical Microbiology, Radboud University Medical Center, Geert Grooteplein-Zuid 10, 6525 GA Nijmegen, The Netherlands

Jilles B. Bijker
Department of Anesthesiology, Gelderse Vallei Hospital, Willy Brandtlaan 10, 6716 RP Ede, The Netherlands

Roland M. H. G. Mollen
Department of Surgery, Gelderse Vallei Hospital, Willy Brandtlaan 10, 6716 RP Ede, The Netherlands

Edo J. Hekma
Department of Surgery, Rijnstate Hospital, Wagnerlaan 55, 6815 AD Arnhem, The Netherlands

Susan M. Lemson
Department of Surgery, Slingeland Hospital, Kruisbergseweg 25, 7009 BL Doetinchem, The Netherlands

Timothy E. Sweeney, Arghavan Salles, David A. Spain and Kristan L. Staudenmayer
Department of Surgery, Stanford University Medical Center, 300 Pasteur Drive, Stanford, CA 94305, USA

Odette A.Harris
Department of Neurosurgery, Stanford University Medical Center, 300 Pasteur Drive, Stanford, CA 94305, USA

Ebru Menekse and Mesut Tez
Department of General Surgery, Ankara Numune Training and Research Hospital, Ankara 06100, Turkey

Belma Kocer
Department of General Surgery, Faculty of Medicine, Sakarya University, Sakarya 54000, Turkey

Ramazan Topcu
General Surgery Clinic, Turhal State Hospital, 60300 Tokat, Turkey

Aydemir Olmez
Department of Surgery, Faculty of Medicine, Mersin University, 33343 Mersin, Turkey

Cuneyt Kayaalp
Department of Surgery, Faculty of Medicine, Inonu University, 44280 Malatya, Turkey

Shokei Matsumoto, Tomohiro Funabiki, Tomohiko Orita, Masayuki Shimizu, Kei Hayashida, Taku Kazamaki, Motoyasu Yamazaki and Mitsuhide Kitano
Department of Trauma and Emergency Surgery, Saiseikai Yokohamashi Tobu Hospital, 3-6-1 Shimosueyoshi, Tsurumi-ku, Yokohama-shi, Kanagawa 230-0012, Japan

Kazuhiko Sekine
Department of Emergency Medicine, Saiseikai Central Hospital, 1-4-17 Mita, Minato, Tokyo 108-0073, Japan

Tatsuya Suzuki
Department of Radiological Technology, Saiseikai Yokohamashi Tobu Hospital, 3-6-2 Shimosueyoshi, Tsurumi-ku, , Yokohama-shi 230-0011, Japan

Masanobu Kishikawa
Division of Emergency Medicine, Fukuoka City Hospital, 13-1 Yoshizukahonmachi, Hakata-ku, Fukuoka 812-0046, Japan

Jin-Young Hwang
Department of Anesthesiology and Pain Medicine, Borame Medical Center, Seoul National University, College of Medicine, Boramae-ro 5-gil, Dongjak-gu, Seoul, Kyoneggido 156-707, South Korea

Jiseok Baik
Department of Anesthesiology and Pain Medicine, Pusan National University Hospital, Biomedical Research Institute, Pusan National University, School of Medicine, 179 Gudeok-ro, Seo-Gu, Busan 602-739, South Korea

Sahngun Francis Nahm, Young-Tae Jeon, Jinhee Kim, Seongjoo Park and Sunghee Han
Department of Anesthesiology and Pain Medicine, Seoul National University Bundang Hospital, Seoul National University, College of Medicine, 300 Gumidong Bundanggu, Seongnamsi, Kyoneggido 463-707, South Korea

Dongjin Kim
Department of Thoracic Surgery, Sejong General Hospital, 489-28 Hohyun-Ro, Sosa-Gu, Bucheon-Si, Kyoneggido 422-711, South Korea

Gaby Jabbour
Department of Surgery, Hamad General Hospital (HGH), Doha, Qatar

Ayman El-Menyar
Clinical Research, Trauma Surgery, Hamad General Hospital, Doha, Qatar
Clinical Medicine, Weill Cornell Medical School, Doha, Qatar

Ruben Peralta, Husham Abdelrahman, Mohamed Ellabib and Hassan Al-Thani
Trauma Surgery Section, Hamad General Hospital, Doha, Qatar

Nissar Shaikh and Insolvisagan Natesa Mudali
Surgical Intensive Care Unit, HGH, Doha, Qatar

Cristiane de Alencar Domingues
All Trauma, São Paulo, SP, Brazil

Raul Coimbra
University of California San Diego Medical Center, San Diego, CA, USA

Renato Sérgio Poggetti
Medical School, University of Sao Paulo, São Paulo, SP, Brazil

Lilia de Souza Nogueira and Regina Marcia Cardoso de Sousa
School of Nursing, University of Sao Paulo, São Paulo, SP, Brazil

Aleksejs Kaminskis, Anna Tolstova, Maksims Mukans, Solvita Stabiņa and Raivis Gailums
Department of General and Emergency Surgery, Riga East University Hospital, 2 Hipokrata Str. Riga, Riga LV 1038, Latvia

Aina Kratovska, Sanita Ponomarjova, Andrejs Bernšteins and Patricija Ivanova
Department of Interventional Radiology, Riga East University Hospital, Riga, Latvia

Viesturs Boka
Riga East University Hospital, Riga, Latvia

Guntars Pupelis
Surgical Department, Riga East University Hospital, Riga, Latvia

M. Sugrue
Department of Surgery, Letterkenny University Hospital and Donegal Clinical Research Academy, Donegal, Ireland

E. E. Moore
University of Colorado, Denver, USA

M. Boermeester
Department of Surgery, Academic Medical Center, Amsterdam, Netherlands

F. Catena
Department of Emergency Surgery, Maggiore Hospital, Parma, Italy

G. Velmahos
Department of Trauma, Emergency Surgery and Surgical Critical Care, Massachusetts General Hospital, Boston, MA, USA

L. Ansaloni
General Surgery Department, Papa Giovanni XXIII Hospital, Bergamo, Italy

F. Abu-Zidan
Department of Surgery, College of Medicine and Health Sciences, UAE University, Al-Ain, United Arab Emirates

M. Paduraru
Milton Keynes University Hospital NHS Foundation Trust, Milton Keynes, UK

L. Pearce
Northwest Research Collaborative, Manchester, UK

B. M. Pereira
Division of Trauma Surgery, Department of Surgery, School of Medical Sciences, University of Campinas, Campinas, Brazil

Paula Ferrada
Trauma, Emergency surgery and Critical Care, Virginia Commonwealth University, 417 N 11th St, Richmond, VA 23298, Richmond, VA 23298-0454, USA

Rachael A. Callcut
University of California San Francisco, San Francisco, USA

David J. Skarupa
University of Florida College of Medicine, Gainesville, USA

Desmond Khor
University of Southern California, California, USA

Vincent Anto and Jason Sperry
University of Pittsburg, Pittsburg, USA

David Turay
Loma Linda University, Loma Linda, USA

Toby Enniss
University of Utah School Medicine, Salt Lake City, USA

Michelle McNutt
McGovern Medical School at the University of Texas Health Science Center at Houston, Houston, USA

Herb Phelan
University of Texas-Southwestern Medical Center, Dallas, USA

Falco Hietbrink and Luke P. H. Leenen
Department of surgery, University Medical Center Utrecht, Utrecht, The Netherlands

Lonneke G. Bode
Department of Medical Microbiology, University Medical Center Utrecht, Utrecht, The Netherlands

Louis Riddez
Department of Surgery, Karolinska Institutet, Solna, Sweden

Marijke R. van Dijk
Department of Pathology, University Medical Center Utrecht, Utrecht, The Netherlands

Shintaro Furugori, Takeru Abe and Masayuki Iwashita
Department of Emergency Medicine, Yokohama City University, 4-57 Urafunecho, Minamiku, Yokohama City, Kanagawa Prefecture 232-0024, Japan

Makoto Kato
Department of Surgery, Yokohama City University, 4-57 Urafunecho, Minamiku, Yokohama City, Kanagawa Prefecture 232-0024, Japan

Naoto Morimura
Department of Acute Medicine, Graduate School of Medicine, The University of Tokyo, 7-3-1 Hongo, Bunkyo-ku, Tokyo 113-0033, Japan

Katayoun Jahangiri, Hasan Ghodsi, Ali Khodadadizadeh and Sadegh Yousef Nezhad
Department of Health in Disasters and Emergencies, School of Health, Safety and Environment, Shahid Beheshti University of Medical Sciences, Tehran, Iran

Sung-Mi Ji
Department of Anesthesiology and Pain Medicine, College of Medicine, Dankook University, Cheonan, South Korea

Eun-Jin Moon, Tae-Jun Kim, Jae-Woo Yi, Hyungseok Seo and Bong-Jae Lee
Department of Anesthesiology and Pain Medicine, Kyung Hee University Hospital at Gangdong, College of Medicine, Kyung Hee University, Seoul 05278, South Korea

Andres Isaza-Restrepo
Escuela de Medicina y Ciencias de la Salud, Universidad del Rosario, Carrera 24 No 63C - 69 Barrio Siete de Agosto, Bogotá, DC, Colombia
Méderi Hospital Universitario Mayor, Carrera 24 No 63C - 69 Barrio Siete de Agosto, Bogotá, DC, Colombia

Marcos Tarazona-Lara
Méderi Hospital Universitario Mayor, Carrera 24 No 63C - 69 Barrio Siete de Agosto, Bogotá, DC, Colombia

Dínimo José Bolívar-Sáenz
Hospital Occidente de Kennedy, Bogotá, D.C., Colombia

José Rafael Tovar
Escuela de Estadística, Facultad de Ingenierías, Universidad delValle, Santiago de Cali, Colombia

Antonio Biondi
Department of Surgery, Vittorio Emanuele Hospital, University of Catania, Via Plebiscito, 628, 95124 Catania, Italy

Carla Di Stefano, Francesco Ferrara, Angelo Bellia, and Luigi Piazza
General and Emergency Surgery Department, Garibaldi Hospital, 95100 Catania, Italy

Marco Vacante
Department of Medical and Pediatric Sciences, University of Catania, 95125 Catania, Italy

Hong-xiang Lu, Jian-hui Sun, Da-lin Wen, Juan Du, Ling Zeng, An-qiang Zhang and Jian-xin Jiang
State Key Laboratory of Trauma, Burns and Combined Injury, Institute of Surgery Research, Daping Hospital, Third Military Medical University, Chongqing 400042, China

Roy Spijkerman, Michel Paul Johan Teuben, Taco Johan Blokhuis, and Luke Petrus Hendrikus Leenen
Department of Trauma, University Medical Centre Utrecht, Heidelberglaan 100, 3584CX Utrecht, The Netherlands

Fatima Hoosain, Liezel Phyllis Taylor and Brian Leigh Warren
Department of Trauma, Tygerberg Hospital (University of Stellenbosch), Francie van Zijl Avenue, Cape Town 7505, South Africa

Timothy Craig Hardcastle
Department of Trauma, Inkosi Albert Luthuli Central Hospital (University of Kwazulu-Natal), 800 Bellair Road, Durban 4091, South Africa

Daniel Clerc, Fabian Grass, Markus Schäfer, Nicolas Demartines and Martin Hübner
Department of Visceral Surgery, University Hospital of Lausanne (CHUV), Lausanne, Switzerland

Alban Denys
Department of Interventional Radiology, University Hospital of Lausanne (CHUV), Lausanne, Switzerland

Hailan Zhang, Yuzuo Bai and Weilin Wang
Department of Pediatric Surgery, Shengjing Hospital of China Medical University, No. 36 SanHao St., Heping District, Shenyang 110004, China

Michal Grivna
Institute of Public Health, College of Medicine and Health Sciences, UAE University, Al-Ain, United Arab Emirates

Hani O. Eid
Department of Surgery, Trauma Group, College of Medicine and Health Sciences, UAE University, Al-Ain, United Arab Emirates

Fikri M. Abu-Zidan
Department of Surgery, College of Medicine and Health Sciences, UAE University, Al-Ain, United Arab Emirates

Index